Spermatozoa: Biology, Function and Chromosomal Abnormalities

Spermatozoa: Biology, Function and Chromosomal Abnormalities

Edited by Bill Young

STATES
ACADEMIC PRESS
www.statesacademicpress.com

States Academic Press,
109 South 5th Street,
Brooklyn, NY 11249, USA

Visit us on the World Wide Web at:
www.statesacademicpress.com

ISBN: 978-1-63989-494-9

Cataloging-in-Publication Data

Spermatozoa : biology, function and chromosomal abnormalities / edited by Bill Young.
p. cm.
Includes bibliographical references and index.
ISBN 978-1-63989-494-9
1. Spermatozoa. 2. Spermatozoa--Physiology. 3. Spermatozoa--Motility--Disorders. 4. Semen. I. Young, Bill.
QP255 .S64 2022
612.61--dc23

Table of Contents

Preface

Spermatozoa are the motile haploid cells that are the male gametes. A spermatozoon fuses with a haploid egg cell to form a zygote. Spermatozoa accounts for nearly half of the genetic material of the diploid offspring. There are two types of sperm cells: one bearing an X chromosome and another bearing a Y chromosome. The sex of the offspring is also determined by the sperm cells. The fusion of the sperm cell having an X chromosome will lead to a female (XX) offspring, while the fusion of the sperm cell having a Y chromosome will lead to a male offspring (XY). A sperm cell has four parts: a head, neck, middle piece and a tail. This book attempts to understand the biology, function and chromosomal abnormalities of spermatozoa. It presents researches and studies performed by experts across the globe. This book will serve as a reference to a broad spectrum of readers.

This book has been the outcome of endless efforts put in by authors and researchers on various issues and topics within the field. The book is a comprehensive collection of significant researches that are addressed in a variety of chapters. It will surely enhance the knowledge of the field among readers across the globe.

It gives us an immense pleasure to thank our researchers and authors for their efforts to submit their piece of writing before the deadlines. Finally in the end, I would like to thank my family and colleagues who have been a great source of inspiration and support.

Editor

Preface

1

Assessment of Human Sperm Cells Morphological Parameters

Kristina Lasiene

Abstract

The quality of spermatozoa has a direct influence on the fertilization and developmental competence of embryos. The aim of this work was to review the methods of spermatozoa morphology assessment, features of the normal spermatozoa and the reasons of their several abnormalities. Three methods can be used for the evaluation of spermatozoa morphology in the *in vitro* fertilization (IVF) laboratory: (1) light microscopy of stained spermatozoa, (2) motile sperm organelle morphology examination (MSOME) and (3) polarized light microscopy. The analysis of spermatozoa morphology includes the assessment of head, neck, midpiece and tail. Morphologically abnormal spermatozoa are categorized into subgroups according to the defects of the head, neck, midpiece and/or tail. Before IVF and intracytoplasmic sperm injection (ICSI), the quality of spermatozoa must be estimated exactly, because this has the high influence on embryo development. Therefore the analysis of the morphological parameters of spermatozoa using the light microscopy, MSOME, in combination with precise head birefringence detection using the polarized microscopy, could give the best fertilization rate and embryo quality after IVF and ICSI.

Keywords: abnormalities, human, morphology, normal, spermatozoa

1. Introduction

The development of *in vitro* produced human embryos is directly dependent on the quality of the oocytes and spermatozoa which are used for *in vitro* fertilization (IVF) and intracytoplasmic sperm injection (ICSI). The examination of oocyte and spermatozoa morphology is currently considered to be a tool devoted to the fertility prognosis. Morphology of spermatozoa has been recognized as the best predictor of outcome for natural fertilization, intrauterine insemination and IVF. The spermatozoa morphology also plays a significant role in ICSI outcome [1].

The aim of this work was to review the methods of spermatozoa morphology assessment, features of the normal spermatozoa and the reasons of their various abnormalities.

2. Semen collection and analysis

The sample of semen should be collected after 2–7 days of sexual abstinence. The first ejaculate gives a correct conclusion in at least 85% of cases. It is helpful to examine two or three samples to obtain more precise data [2, 3].

Semen analysis includes:

- Spermatozoa analysis (number, vitality, motility, morphology),
- Immunological analysis (anti-spermatozoa antibodies detection),
- Seminal fluid analysis (biochemical markers of accessory glands secretions) [3].

2.1. Evaluation of the spermatozoa morphology

2.1.1. Light microscopy of stained spermatozoa

The light microscopy of stained spermatozoa is the fundamental and commonly used method for evaluation of spermatozoa morphology. Two techniques can be used for this evaluation: (1) the microscopic analysis of stained samples as visual observations of spermatozoa (manual method) and (2) computerized analysis. Primarily for both methods, the stained smears of semen must be prepared. The droplet of the semen sample are smeared on a glass slide, dried in the air and fixed. The smears must be stained for providing sharp contrast for defining the spermatozoa outline and cell details. There are a lot of methods for the staining of human and animal spermatozoa. World Health Organization recommends three routine staining methods for the evaluation of morphology of human spermatozoa: Papanicolaou, Shorr or Diff-Quik (Rapidiff) [3, 4]. Some laboratories use a new stain SpermBlue® successfully [5, 6].

The stained smears are analyzed by the magnification 1000× with oil immersion. Using a manual method, the laboratory technician examines 200 spermatozoa and categorizes each spermatozoon as normal or abnormal. Subsequently, the anomalies are classified using strictly defined criteria. The measurement of spermatozoa can be performed using the ocular micrometer. By computerized analysis method, various computer analyzing programs, systems and modules categorize and measure automatically different morphological features of each selected spermatozoon [5, 7–11].

A few classifications of human spermatozoa morphology have been originated and used worldwide: MacLeod's [12], David's [13, 14], Dusseldorf [15, 16], Strict (Tygerberg's) criteria [17, 18] and others. The World Health Organization (WHO) confirmed the Strict (Tygerberg's) criteria as conventional standard for spermatozoa morphology [4].

2.1.2. *Motile sperm organelle morphology examination (MSOME)*

This method is used for evaluating the morphology of the live (non-fixed, non-stained) spermatozoa before the ICSI. Using the high magnification (6000× and more) by the inverted computerized microscope, it is possible to observe the morphological abnormalities in spermatozoa, which are not visible with magnification 400× (**Figure 1**). The neck, tail, midpiece, mitochondria, acrosome and post-acrosomal lamina and the nucleus of spermatozoon are morphologically examined in live motile spermatozoa [19–25].

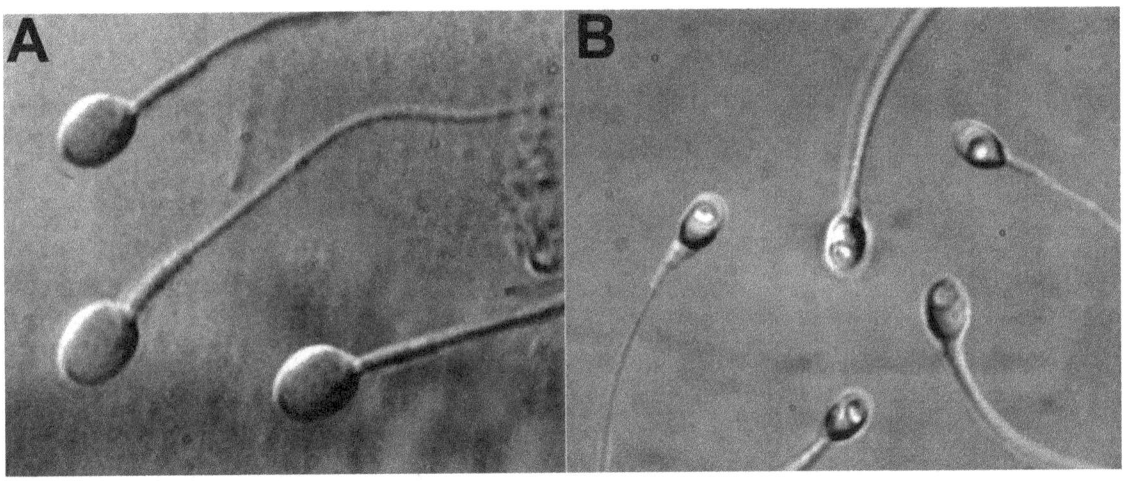

Figure 1. Spermatozoa morphology using MSOME ([19], open access). (A) Normal spermatozoa observed at high magnification (8400×); (B) spermatozoa with large nuclear vacuoles observed at high magnification (8400×).

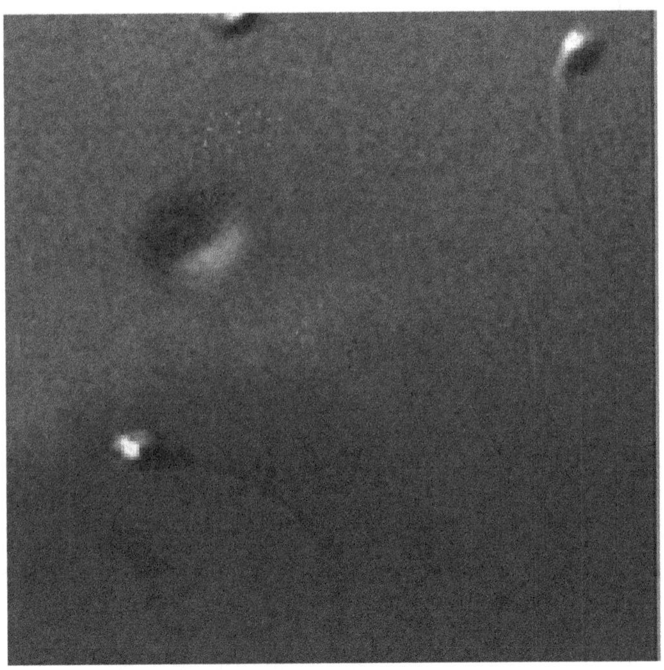

Figure 2. The birefringence of human spermatozoa ([26], with permission).

2.1.3. Polarized light microscopy

An estimation of head birefringence by polarized light using polarized microscope method is used for analysis of live spermatozoa morphological quality. This birefringence is associated with sub-acrosomal protein filaments and nucleoprotein filaments (**Figure 2**). The presence of birefringence in the head indicates the good morphology of a spermatozoon [26–31].

3. Morphology of the normal spermatozoon

The analysis of spermatozoa morphology includes the assessment of head, neck, midpiece and tail. The analysis of the head includes the assessment of head shape and size, nucleus shape and size, acrosomal area (acrosomal index) and acrosomal vacuoles. The shape, size and cytoplasmic droplets are analyzed in the midpiece, principal and terminal pieces of tail (**Table 1**).

The acrosomal vacuoles are concentrated between the inner and outer acrosomal membranes. They present the migration of acrosin to the spermatozoon surface and may be the earliest event characterizing the beginning of the acrosome reaction. The presence of these vacuoles is considered as a significant marker of successful fertilization of oocytes *in vitro* [37, 38].

Normal human spermatozoa carry the X or the Y chromosome. Measuring the spermatozoa sorted by the polymerase chain reaction (PCR) sexing, Cui [39] estimated that the X chromosome-bearing spermatozoa have significantly greater head length, neck and tail length, head perimeter and head area than Y chromosome-bearing spermatozoa. The neck and tail were

	Features		**References**
Head	Shape	Oval	[4]
	Size	Length 4–5 μm, width 2.5–3.5 μm, length-width ratio 1.5–1.75	
	Acrosomal size	40–70% of total head area	
	Nucleus shape	Smooth, symmetric and oval	[1, 32, 33]
	Nucleus size	Length 4.75 ± 0.28 μm, width 3.28 ± 0.20 μm	
	Nuclear inside	No regional nuclear disorders, ≤ 1vacuole that occupies less than 4% of the nuclear area	
Neck		No abaxial implantation	[18]
Midpiece of tail	Shape	Slender	[1, 32–34]
	Size	Length 7–8 μm, width < 1 μm	
	Attachment	Axially attached to the head	
	Cytoplasmic droplets	No cytoplasmic droplets and/or disorders or less than half size of normal head	
	Mitochondria	Not fragmented or damaged	
Principal and terminal pieces of tail	Shape	Straight, uniform, and thinner than the midpiece, uncoiled	[34–36]
	Size	Length 45–50 μm, tail/head length ratio 10.3 ± 0.2	

Table 1. Features of morphologically normal spermatozoon.

	Papanicolaou	Rapidiff®	SpermBlue®	Fresh
Length (μm)	4.28 ± 0.27a	5.17 ± 0.27b	4.73 ± 0.27c	4.79 ± 0.26
Width (μm)	2.65 ± 0.19a	3.12 ± 0.21b	2.75 ± 0.24a	2.82 ± 0.23
Area (μm^2)	9.26 ± 0.99a	12.87 ± 1.19b	10.47 ± 1.21c	—
Perimeter (μm)	11.83 ± 0.69a	14.33 ± 0.75b	12.99 ± 0.80c	—
Ellipticity	1.63 ± 0.11	1.68 ± 0.10	1.75 ± 0.13	1.73 ± 0.12
Width/length ratio	0.62 ± 0.04	0.60 ± 0.04	0.58 ± 0.04	0.59 ± 0.04
Elongation	0.23 ± 0.03	0.25 ± 0.03	0.27 ± 0.03	0.26 ± 0.03
Roughness	0.83 ± 0.02	0.79 ± 0.02	0.78 ± 0.03	—
Regularity	0.96 ± 0.01	0.98 ± 0.01	0.97 ± 0.02	—
Acrosome coverage (%)	32.76 ± 7.43	23.73 ± 7.97	46.29 ± 8.63	—

Table 2. The comparison of sperm head morphometry for the three staining techniques and spermatozoa of fresh semen (mean ± SD) [42].

also significantly longer in X chromosome-bearing spermatozoa. A difference of volume of X- and Y-bearing spermatozoa heads is associated with the difference of DNA content (3.5–4%) [40].

Therefore, the morphometric parameters of normal spermatozoon can differ according to staining method of sperm smear [11, 41]. Maree with co-authors [42] maintained that fixatives and stains can change the size of spermatozoa. They reported that morphometric parameters of SpermBlue® stained spermatozoa head differed least from parameters of fresh non-stained spermatozoa (**Table 2**). Also the results can differ according the technician [17].

The live morphologically normal spermatozoa can be selected by sperm head birefringence for ICSI. Two types of head birefringence are ascertained on the basis of acrosome integrity: (1) partial head birefringence in acrosome-reacted spermatozoa and (2) total head birefringence in acrosome-non-reacted spermatozoa. Using acrosome-reacted spermatozoa shows better ICSI results [28–30]. Spermatozoa with partial head birefringence can present lower ratio of DNA fragmentation and higher ratio of normal nucleus [29]. In other hand, spermatozoa with nuclear vacuoles and DNA fragmentation can show the normal head birefringence. And otherwise, some spermatozoa with normal MSOME morphology and without DNA fragmentation can show no birefringence. Therefore the scientists recommend combining MSOME with evaluation of the head birefringence. It was determined that the lowest amount of DNA fragmentation occurs in sperm selected by MSOME and birefringence, compared to sperm selected *via* just one of the two methods alone [43].

4. Morphological abnormalities of spermatozoa

The abnormalities in morphology of spermatozoa have a negative effect on the outcome of IVF and ICSI. Morphologically abnormal spermatozoa analyzed by light microscopy or MSOME are categorized into subgroups according to the defects of the head, neck, midpiece and/or tail.

4.1. Abnormalities of the head

Spermatozoa, with head size and shape abnormalities (large, small, tapered, pyriform, round and amorphous heads), vacuolated heads, heads with small acrosomal area (<40% of head area), with double or multiple heads and without head are often found in the semen samples (**Figure 3**).

The cause of acephalic spermatozoa can be biallelic *SUN5* mutations or homozygous deletion of *SUN5* or mutation of *BRDT* and other genes [44–46].

Large-headed (macrocephalous) spermatozoa are defined as those with a length > 4.7 μm and a width > 3.2 μm. Large head can indicate insufficient shrinking of the nucleus, abnormally

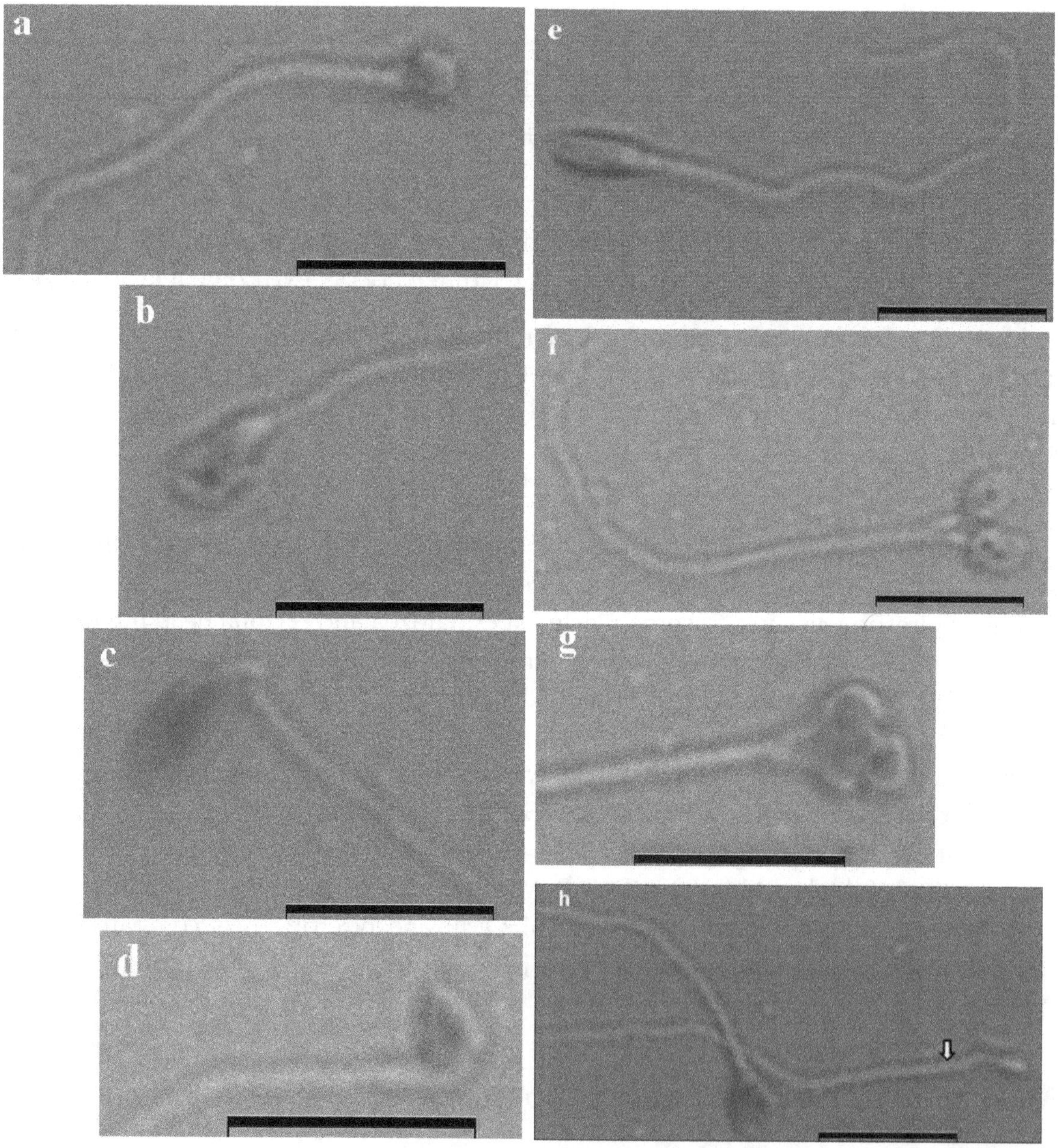

Figure 3. Spermatozoa with abnormal head morphology. (a) Round head; (b) amorphous head; (c) large head and bent neck; (d) small tapered head and bent neck; (e) elongated head; (f) two-headed; (g) multiple-headed and (h) acephalic spermatozoon (arrow). Bar = 10 μm.

condensed chromatin, diploidy and aneuploidy of spermatozoa. Detailed genetic analysis shows that large-headed spermatozoa of some patients can have the homozygous mutation (*c.144delC*) in the *Aurora kinase C* (*AURKC*) gene. These spermatozoa of *AURKC*-deficient patients cannot complete meiosis in the absence of functional *AURKC*. Therefore they can be tetraploid [47–50].

Small-headed (microcephalous) spermatozoa are defined as those with a length < 3.5 μm and a width < 2.5 μm. These spermatozoa can have the excessive shrunk nucleus and abnormally condensed chromatin and fragmented DNA. They may also present with very small, abnormally formed acrosomes [51, 52].

Elongated-headed spermatozoa are described as being a head length > 5 μm with a width < 3 μm or a length of <5 μm and a width of <2 μm. Pyriform heads are also included under elongation of spermatozoa. Elongation of head is generally recognized as a stress-induced sperm morphology aberration, and is prevalent especially in male accessory gland infections and in the presence of a varicocele. An abnormally elongated nucleus shape of these spermatozoa is related with defects in the nuclear membrane, an increased frequency of chromosomal aneuploidies and altered chromatin compaction. Also anomalies of the neck region, persistence of cytoplasmic residues can often exist in these spermatozoa [52, 53].

Globozoospermia (round-headed sperm syndrome) is genetically determined abnormalities of spermatozoa. This disorder is classified into two categories: (1) total and (2) partial *globozoospermia*. In the total *globozoospermia*, the spermatozoa are easily recognizable by their small, round head shape, high DNA fragmentation and the absence of the acrosome. Owing to the absence of acrosomes, the spermatozoa do not contain acrosomal enzymes. Therefore they are unable to bind and penetrate the *zona pellucida* and fuse with the oolemma of the oocyte. In the case of the partial *globozoospermia*, spermatozoa show the oval head shape with less condensed chromatin, a partially present or remnants of acrosome and a disorganized midpiece. Mitochondria are present not only in the midpiece, but in the spermatozoa head too [52, 54–56].

Amorphous-headed spermatozoa indicate the chromosome 18 disomy and sex chromosome aneuploidy. Also, the high incidence of amorphous heads is relative to other abnormal head forms [57].

Multiple-headed spermatozoa have two or more closed or dissociated heads with or without an acrosome or midpiece. Disorders of movement and fragmented DNA are appropriated for these spermatozoa [51].

Human spermatozoa heads often contain vacuoles. They are not visible on standard magnification and can be observed using MSOME method only. According to their size, vacuoles are divided into three types: (1) large (>50% of surface area), (2) medium (50–25% of surface area) and (3) small (<25% of surface area of total sperm head). Based on the location, they are classified as acrosomal, equatorial and post-acrosomal. Also according to the size and the number of vacuoles in the head of one spermatozoon, they can be classified into three categories: (1) one small vacuole, (2) multiple sporadic vacuoles of various sizes and (3) one large vacuole. Head vacuoles are non-acrosomal origin large nuclear indentations of various sizes and positions, packed with membranous material organized in membrane whorls. Vacuoles cannot be considered as degenerative structures but can be regarded as a normal feature of the sperm head and does not affect ICSI outcomes. Therefore, some vacuoles can include vacant or low density DNA or show DNA fragmentation or abnormal chromatin compaction. Large vacuoles in the nucleus can indicate aneuploidy, fragmented DNA and chromatin condensation defects in the cell [24, 55, 58–63].

4.2. Abnormalities of the tail

Spermatozoa without tail or with the neck and midpiece defects (bent neck, asymmetrical insertion of the midpiece into the head, thick or irregular midpiece and abnormally thin midpiece) and principal and terminal pieces of tail defects (short, multiple, hairpin, broken, coiled, bent tail and tails of irregular width) are often found in the semen samples (**Figure 4**).

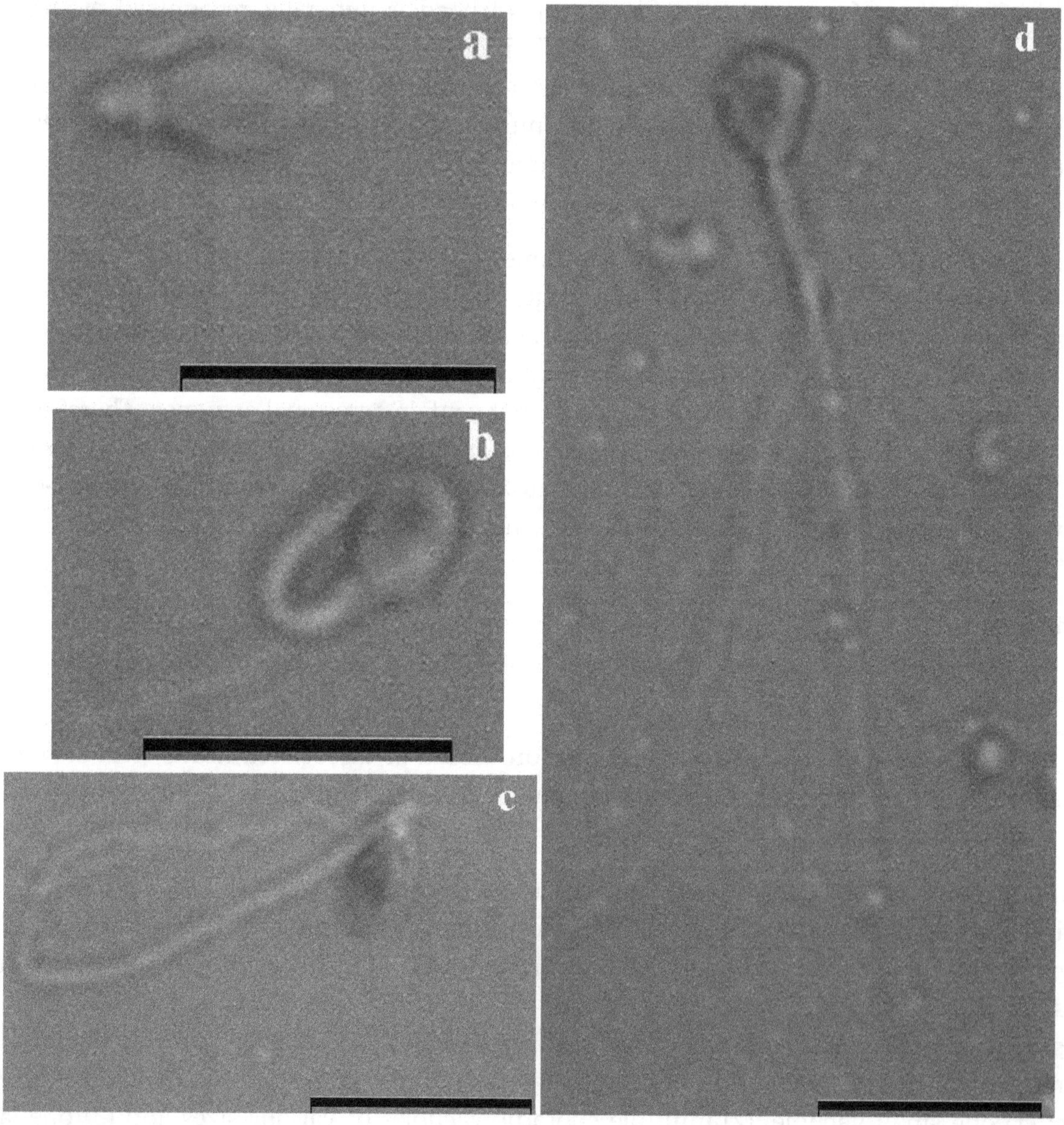

Figure 4. Spermatozoa with abnormal neck and tail morphology. (a) Absent tail; (b) coiled tail; (c) bent neck and (d) two-tailed spermatozoon. Bar = 10 μm.

All abnormalities of spermatozoa neck and tail reduce their motility and therefore have the negative influence on fertilization of oocyte.

Bent necks are associated with DNA fragmentation. Abnormal tails (two-tailed, bent tails, irregular tails) are associated to chromosome 13 disomy, supernumerary chromosomal abnormalities and the cytoskeletal abnormalities (including centriolar defects) [57].

The absence of a tail, the short and broken tail may be related to axonemal abnormalities that are only visible with electron microscopy, and an unknown genetic origin of these abnormalities could be hypothesized [64, 65]. Coiled tails of spermatozoa can be associated with varicocele and epididymal dysfunction [66, 67].

The spermatozoa can often have cytoplasmic droplets and cytoplasmic residues. Cytoplasmic droplets are small, regular osmotically sensitive vesicles which are located at the neck as opposed to the end of the annulus (**Figure 5**). Cytoplasmic droplets of normal human spermatozoa are still present after ejaculation and have no negative influence on cell function.

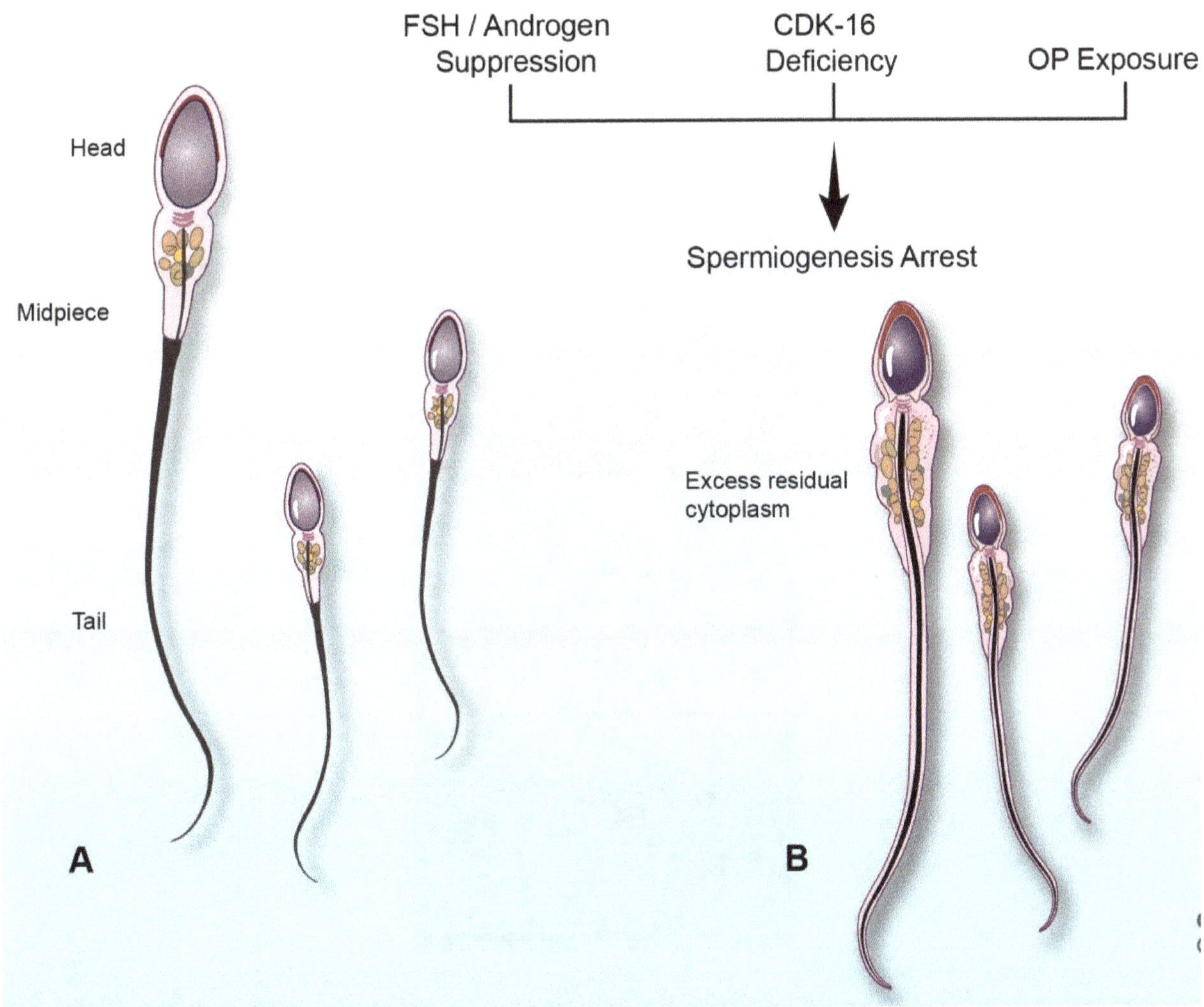

Figure 5. Cytoplasmic droplets and residual cytoplasm structure ([68], open access). (A) Spermatozoa with cytoplasmic droplets and (B) spermatozoa with residual cytoplasm.

Cytoplasmic residues are large, irregular material along the midpiece and can indicate the abnormal spermiogenesis (**Figure 6**). They form as outcome of incomplete cytoplasmic extrusion during spermiogenesis in the causes of suppression of FSH and/or androgens, deficiency of cyclin-dependent kinase 16 (*CDK16*) and organophosphorus pesticide (OP) exposure. In comparison to the cytoplasmic droplet, cytoplasmic residues contain major quantity of cytoplasm enzymes, which produce pathological amounts of reactive oxygen species. These species can negatively affect spermatozoa function including peroxidative damage to the cell membrane, DNA damage, mitochondrial dysfunction, impaired interaction with the female reproductive tract and lead to male infertility [1, 32, 52, 68, 69].

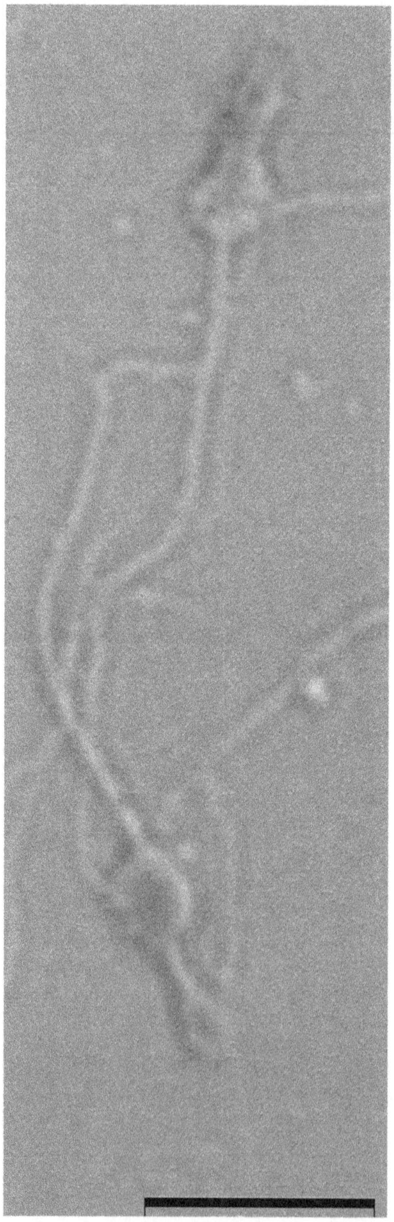

Figure 6. The residual cytoplasm on the spermatozoa tail. Bar = 10 μm.

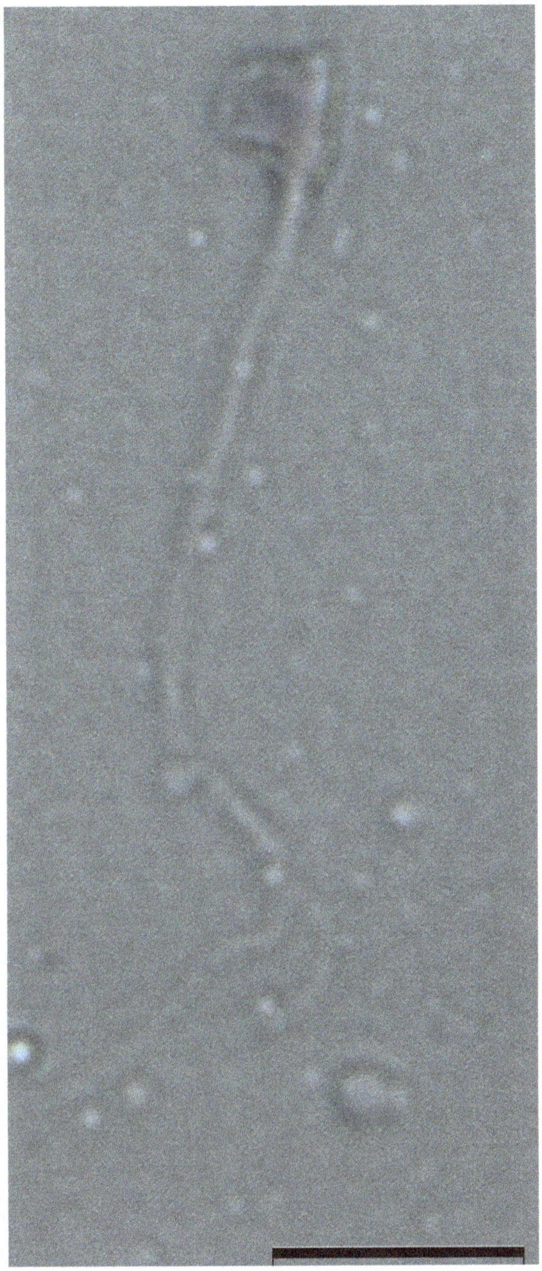

Figure 7. Spermatozoon with multiple abnormalities. Round head, bent neck and duplicate tail. Bar = 10 μm.

Multiple morphological abnormalities in the same patient's spermatozoa tail structure and ultrastructure which impair motility can show the mutation of some genes (*DNAH1*, *DNAJB13*, *CFAP43* and *CFAP44*) [70–73].

The morphologically abnormal spermatozoon can have multiple defects too (**Figure 7**). The most irregularly shaped, multi-tailed spermatozoa is associated with severe male infertility. The multiple gene mutations, high rates of polyploidy and aneuploidy and reduced motility of spermatozoa have been described in these cases [48, 49].

5. Conclusion

The morphology of spermatozoa has a direct influence on the fertilization and developmental competence of embryos. A normal semen sample must have >30% of morphologically normal spermatozoa. Considering on the morphological study of patients spermatozoa, researchers, practicians and WHO have defined the prognosis of IVF treatment. Excellent prognosis is expected when >14% of normal spermatozoa were found in the semen sample. When 4–14% of normal spermatozoa were found, the IVF prognosis is good. When prognosis is poor (<4% of normal spermatozoa were found in the semen), the ICSI should be recommended for these patients [3, 18, 74–76].

Therefore the analysis of the morphological parameters of spermatozoa using the light microscopy, MSOME, in combination with precise head birefringence detection using the polarized microscopy, could give the best fertilization rate and embryo quality after IVF and ICSI.

Author details

Kristina Lasiene

Address all correspondence to: kristina.lasiene@lsmuni.lt

Department of Histology and Embryology, Academy of Medicine, Lithuanian University of Health Sciences, Kaunas, Lithuania

References

[1] Berkovitz A, Eltes F, Yaari S, Katz N, Barr I, Fishman A, Bartoov B. The morphological normalcy of the sperm nucleus and pregnancy rate of intracytoplasmic injection with morphologically selected sperm. Human Reproduction. 2005;**20**:185-190. DOI: 10.1093/humrep/deh545

[2] Rylander L, Wetterstrand B, Haugen TB, Malm G, Malm J, Bjørsvik C, Henrichsen T, Saether T, Giwercman A. Single semen analysis as a predictor of semen quality: Clinical and epidemiological implications. Asian Journal of Andrology. 2009;**11**:723-730. DOI: 10.1038/aja.2009.64

[3] World Health Organization. WHO Laboratory Manual for the Examination and Processing of Human Semen. 5th ed. Cambridge University Press; 2010. 271 p

[4] World Health Organization. WHO Laboratory Manual for the Examination of Human Semen and Semen-Cervical Mucus Interaction. 4th ed. Cambridge University Press; 1999. 138 p

[5] van der Horst G, Maree L. SpermBlue: A new universal stain for human and animal sperm which is also amenable to automated sperm morphology analysis. Biotechnic & Histochemistry 2009;**84**:299-308. DOI: 10.3109/10520290902984274

[6] Rapid SpermBlue® Protocol [Internet]. Available from: http://www.micropticsl.com/products/disposables/morphology/spermblue/

[7] Auger J. Assessing human sperm morphology: Top models, underdogs or biometrics? Asian Journal of Andrology. 2010;**12**:36-46. DOI: 10.1038/aja.2009.8

[8] Bellastella G, Cooper TG, Battaglia M, Ströse A, Torres I, Hellenkemper B, Soler C, Sinisi AA. Dimensions of human ejaculated spermatozoa in Papanicolaou-stained seminal and swim-up smears obtained from the Integrated Semen Analysis System (ISAS(®)). Asian Journal of Andrology. 2010;**12**:871-879. DOI: 10.1038/aja.2010.90

[9] Blanchard M, Haguenoer K, Apert A, Poret H, Barthélémy C, Royère D, Guérif F. Sperm morphology assessment using David's classification: Time to switch to strict criteria? Prospective comparative analysis in a selected IVF population. International Journal of Andrology. 2011;**34**:145-152. DOI: 10.1111/j.1365-2605.2010.01066.x

[10] Butts IA, Ward MA, Litvak MK, Pitcher TE, Alavi SM, Trippel EA, Rideout RM. Automated sperm head morphology analyzer for open-source software. Theriogenology. 2011;**76**:1756-1761. DOI: 10.1016/j.theriogenology.2011.06.019

[11] Soler C, De Monserrat JJ, Gutierrez R, Nunez J, Nunez M, Sancho M, Perez-Sanchez F, Cooper TG. Use of the sperm-class analyser for objective assessment of human sperm morphology. International Journal of Andrology. 2003;**26**:262-270. DOI: 10.1046/j.1365-2605.2003.00422.x

[12] MacLeod J. Human seminal cytology as a sensitive indicator of the germinal epithelium. International Journal of Fertility. 1964;**9**:281-295

[13] Jouannet P, Ducot B, Feneux D, Spira A. Male factors and the likelihood of pregnancy in infertile couples. I. Study of sperm characteristics. International Journal of Andrology. 1988;**11**:379-394. DOI: 10.1111/j.1365-2605.1988.tb01011.x

[14] Auger J, Eustache F, David G. Standardisation de la classification morphologique des spermatozoïdes humains selon la méthode de David modifiée. Andrologie. 2000;**10**:358-373. DOI: 10.1007/BF03034491

[15] Hofmann N, Freundl G, Florack M, Die Formstorungen d. Spermatozoen im sperma und zervikalschleim als spiegel testikularer erkrankungen. Der Gynäkologe. 1985;**18**:189-192

[16] Hofmann N, Hilscher B. Use of aniline blue to assess chromatin condensation in morphologically normal spermatozoa in normal and infertile men. Human Reproduction. 1991;**6**:979-982. DOI: 10.1093/oxfordjournals.humrep.a137472

[17] Kruger TF, Ackerman SB, Simmons KF, Swanson RJ, Brugo SS, Acosta AA. A quick, reliable staining technique for human sperm morphology. Archives of Andrology. 1987;**18**:275-277. DOI: 10.3109/01485018708988493

[18] Menkveld R, Stander FS, Kotze TJ, Kruger TF, Van Zyl JA. The evaluation of morphological characteristics of human spermatozoa according to stricter criteria. Human Reproduction. 1990;**5**:586-592. DOI: 10.1093/oxfordjournals.humrep.a137150

[19] Akl LD, Oliveira JB, Petersen CG, Mauri AL, Silva LF, Massaro FC, Baruffi RL, Cavagna M, Franco JG Jr. Efficacy of the motile sperm organelle morphology examination (MSOME) in predicting pregnancy after intrauterine insemination. Reproductive Biology and Endocrinology. 2011;**9**:120. DOI: 10.1186/1477-7827-9-120

[20] Antinori M, Licata E, Dani G, Cerusico F, Versaci C, d'Angelo D. Intracytoplasmic morphologically selected sperm injection: A prospective randomized trial. Reproductive Biomedicine Online. 2008;**16**:835-841. DOI: 10.1016/S1472-6483(10)60150-2

[21] Nadalini M, Tarozzi N, Distratis V, Scaravelli G, Borini A. Impact of intracytoplasmic morphologically selected sperm injection on assisted reproduction outcome: A review. Reproductive Biomedicine Online. 2009;**19**:S45-S55. DOI: 10.1016/S1472-6483(10)60283-0

[22] Sermondade N, Hafhouf E, Dupont C, Bechoua S, Palacios C, Eustache F, Poncelet C, Benzacken B, Lévy R, Sifer C. Successful childbirth after intracytoplasmic morphologically selected sperm injection without assisted oocyte activation in a patient with globozoospermia. Human Reproduction. 2011;**26**:2944-2949. DOI: 10.1093/humrep/der258

[23] Sermondade N, Sifer C. Motile sperm organelle morphology examination: Toward a consensus? Gynécologie, Obstétrique & Fertilité. 2011;**39**:309-314. DOI: 10.1016/j.gyobfe.2011.03.014

[24] Silva LF, Oliveira JB, Petersen CG, Mauri AL, Massaro FC, Cavagna M, Baruffi RL, Franco JG Jr. The effects of male age on sperm analysis by motile sperm organelle morphology examination (MSOME). Reproductive Biology and Endocrinology. 2012;**10**:19. DOI: 10.1186/1477-7827-10-19

[25] Boitrelle F, Guthauser B, Alter L, Bailly M, Bergere M, Wainer R, Vialard F, Albert M, Selva J. High-magnification selection of spermatozoa prior to oocyte injection: Confirmed and potential indications. Reproductive Biomedicine Online. 2014;**28**:6-13. DOI: 10.1016/j.rbmo.2013.09.019

[26] Ghosh S, Chattopadhyay R, Bose G, Ganesh A, Das S, Chakravarty BN. Selection of birefringent spermatozoa under Polscope: Effect on intracytoplasmic sperm injection outcome. Andrologia. 2012;**44**:734-738. DOI: 10.1111/j.1439-0272.2011.01258.x

[27] Gianaroli L, Magli MC, Collodel G, Moretti E, Ferraretti AP, Baccetti B. Sperm head's birefringence: A new criterion for sperm selection. Fertility and Sterility. 2008;**90**:104-112. DOI: 10.1016/j.fertnstert.2007.05.078

[28] Gianaroli L, Magli MC, Ferraretti AP, Crippa A, Lappi M, Capitani S, Baccetti B. Birefringence characteristics in sperm heads allow for the selection of reacted spermatozoa for intracytoplasmic sperm injection. Fertility and Sterility. 2010;**93**:807-813. DOI: 10.1016/j.fertnstert.2008.10.024

[29] Petersen CG, Vagnini LD, Mauri AL, Massaro FC, Cavagna M, Baruffi RL, Oliveira JB, Franco JG Jr. Relationship between DNA damage and sperm head birefringence. Reproductive Biomedicine Online. 2011;**22**:583-589. DOI: 10.1016/j.rbmo.2011.03.017

[30] Magli MC, Crippa A, Muzii L, Boudjema E, Capoti A, Scaravelli G, Ferraretti AP, Gianaroli L. Head birefringence properties are associated with acrosome reaction, sperm motility and morphology. Reproductive Biomedicine Online. 2012;**24**:352-359. DOI: 10.1016/j.rbmo.2011.12.013

[31] Collodel G, Iacoponi F, Mazzi L, Terzuoli G, Pascarelli NA, Moretti E. Light, polarizing, and transmission electron microscopy: Three methods for the evaluation of sperm quality. Systems Biology in Reproductive Medicine. 2013;**59**:27-33. DOI: 10.3109/19396368.2012.724518

[32] Bartoov B, Berkovitz A, Eltes F, Kogosowski A, Menezo Y, Barak Y. Real-time fine morphology of motile human sperm cells is associated with IVF-ICSI outcome. Journal of Andrology. 2002;**23**:1-8. DOI: 10.1002/j.1939-4640.2002.tb02595.x

[33] Ubaldi F, Rienzi L. Morphological selection of gametes. Placenta. 2008;**29**:S115-S120. DOI: 10.1016/j.placenta.2008.08.009

[34] Oliveira JB, Massaro FC, Mauri AL, Petersen CG, Nicoletti AP, Baruffi RL, Franco JG Jr. Motile sperm organelle morphology examination is stricter than Tygerberg criteria. Reproductive Biomedicine Online. 2009;**18**:320-326. DOI: 10.1016/S1472-6483(10)60088-0

[35] Gergely A, Kovanci E, Senturk L, Cosmi E, Vigue L, Huszar G. Morphometric assessment of mature and diminished-maturity human spermatozoa: Sperm regions that reflect differences in maturity. Human Reproduction. 1999;**14**:2007-2014. DOI: 10.1093/humrep/14.8.2007

[36] Celik-Ozenci C, Catalanotti J, Jakab A, Aksu C, Ward D, Bray-Ward P, Demir R, Huszar G. Human sperm maintain their shape following decondensation and denaturation for fluorescent in situ hybridization: Shape analysis and objective morphometry. Biology of Reproduction. 2003;**69**:1347-1355. DOI: 10.1095/biolreprod.103.019596

[37] Tesarik J, Drahorad J, Peknicova J. Subcellular immunochemical localization of acrosin in human spermatozoa during the acrosome reaction and zona pellucida penetration. Fertility and Sterility. 1988;**50**:133-141. DOI: 10.1016/S0015-0282(16)60021-3

[38] El-Ghobashy AA, West CR. The human sperm head: A key for successful fertilization. Journal of Andrology. 2003;**24**:232-238. DOI: 10.1002/j.1939-4640.2003.tb02667.x

[39] Cui KH. Size differences between human X and Y spermatozoa and prefertilization diagnosis. Molecular Human Reproduction. 1997;**3**:61-67. DOI: 10.1093/molehr/3.1.61

[40] van Munster EB, Stap J, Hoebe RA, te Meerman GJ, Aten JA. Difference in volume of X- and Y-chromosome-bearing bovine sperm heads matches difference in DNA content. Cytometry. 1999;**35**:125-128. DOI: 10.1002/(SICI)1097-0320(19990201)35:23.0.CO;2-H

[41] Henkel R, Schreiber G, Sturmhoefel A, Hipler UC, Zermann DH, Menkveld R. Comparison of three staining methods for the morphological evaluation of human spermatozoa. Fertilily and Sterility. 2008;**89**:449-455. DOI: 10.1016/j.fertnstert.2007.03.027

[42] Maree L, du Plessis SS, Menkveld R, van der Horst G. Morphometric dimensions of the human sperm head depend on the staining method used. Human Reproduction. 2010;**25**:1369-1382. DOI: 10.1093/humrep/deq075

[43] Garolla A, Cosci I, Menegazzo M, De Palo R, Ambrosini G, Sartini B, Pizzol D, Foresta C. Sperm selected by both birefringence and motile sperm organelle morphology examination have reduced deoxyribonucleic acid fragmentation. Fertility and Sterility. 2014;**101**:647-652. DOI: 10.1016/j.fertnstert.2013.11.029

[44] Zhu F, Wang F, Yang X, Zhang J, Wu H, Zhang Z, Zhang Z, He X, Zhou P, Wei Z, Gecz J, Cao Y. Biallelic SUN5 mutations cause autosomal-recessive acephalic spermatozoa syndrome. American Journal of Human Genetics. 2016;**99**:942-949. DOI: 10.1016/j.ajhg.2016.08.004

[45] Elkhatib RA, Paci M, Longepied G, Saias-Magnan J, Courbiere B, Guichaoua MR, Levy N, Metzler-Guillemain C, Mitchell MJ. Homozygous deletion of SUN5 in three men with decapitated spermatozoa. Human Molecular Genetics. 2017. DOI: 10.1093/hmg/ddx200

[46] Li L, Sha Y, Wang X, Li P, Wang J, Kee K, Wang B. Whole-exome sequencing identified a homozygous BRDT mutation in a patient with acephalic spermatozoa. Oncotarget. 2017;**8**:19914-19922. DOI: 10.18632/oncotarget.15251

[47] Benzacken B, Gavelle FM, Martin-Pont B, Dupuy O, Lièvre N. Familial sperm polyploidy induced by genetic spermatogenesis failure: Case report. Human Reproduction. 2001;**16**:2646-2651. DOI: 10.1093/humrep/16.12.2646

[48] Guthauser B, Pollet-Villard X, Boitrelle F, Vialard F. Is intracouple assisted reproductive technology an option for men with large-headed spermatozoa? A literature review and a decision guide proposal. Basic and Clinical Andrology. 2016;**26**:8. DOI: 10.1186/s12610-016-0035-6

[49] Dieterich K, Soto Rifo R, Faure AK, Hennebicq S, Ben Amar B, Zahi M. Homozygous mutation of AURKC yields large-headed polyploid spermatozoa and causes male infertility. Nature Genetics. 2007;**39**:661-665. DOI: 10.1038/ng2027

[50] Dieterich K, Zouari R, Harbuz R, Vialard F, Martinez D, Bellayou H, Prisant N, Zoghmar A, Guichaoua MR, Koscinski I, Kharouf M, Noruzinia M, Nadifi S, Sefiani A, Lornage J, Zahi M, Viville S, Sèle B, Jouk PS, Jacob MC, Escalier D, Nikas Y, Hennebicq S, Lunardi J, Ray PF. The Aurora Kinase C c.144delC mutation causes meiosis I arrest in men and isfrequent in the North African population. Human Molecular Genetics. 2009;**18**:1301-1309. DOI: 10.1093/hmg/ddp029

[51] Gandini L, Lombardo F, Paoli D, Caponecchia L, Familiari G. Study of apoptotic DNA fragmentation in human spermatozoa. Human Reproduction. 2000;**15**:830-839. DOI: 10.1093/humrep/15.4.830

[52] Menkveld R. Clinical significance of the low normal sperm morphology value as proposed in the fifth edition of the WHO Laboratory Manual for the Examination and Processing of Human Semen. Asian Journal of Andrology. 2010;**12**:47-58. DOI: 10.1038/aja.2009.14

[53] Prisant N, Escalier D, Soufr JC, Morillon M, Schoevaert D. Ultrastructural nuclear defects and increased chromosome aneuploidies in spermatozoa with elongated heads. Human Reproduction. 2007;**22**:1052-1059. DOI: 10.1093/humrep/del481

[54] Dam AH, Ramos L, Dijkman HB, Woestenenk R, Robben H, van den Hoven L, Kremer JA. Morphology of partial Globozoospermia. Journal of Andrology. 2011;**32**:199-206. DOI: 10.2164/jandrol.109.009530

[55] Gatimel N, Léandri RD, Foliguet B, Bujan L, Parinaud J. Sperm cephalic vacuoles: New arguments for their non acrosomal origin in two cases of total globozoospermia. Andrology. 2013;**1**:52-56. DOI: 10.1111/j.2047-2927.2012.00011.x

[56] Perrin A, Coat C, Nguyen MH, Talagas M, Morel F, Amice J, De Braekeleer M. Molecular cytogenetic and genetic aspects of globozoospermia: A review. Andrologia. 2013;**45**:1-9. DOI: 10.1111/j.1439-0272.2012.01308.x

[57] Tang SS, Gao H, Zhao Y, Ma S. Aneuploidy and DNA fragmentation in morphologically abnormal sperm. International Journal of Andrology. 2010;**33**:e163-e179. DOI: 10.1111/j.1365-2605.2009.00982.x

[58] Kaneko S, Yoshida J, Takamatsu K. Low density regions of DNA in human sperm appear as vacuoles after translucent staining with reactive blue 2. Journal of Medical Diagnostic Methods. 2013;**2**:145. DOI: 10.4172/2168-9784.1000145

[59] Berkovitz A, Eltes F, Ellenbogen A, Peer S, Feldberg D, Bartoov B. Does the presence of nuclear vacuoles in human sperm selected for ICSI affect pregnancy outcome? Human Reproduction. 2006;**21**:1787-1790. DOI: 10.1093/humrep/del049

[60] Kacem O, Sifer C, Barraud-Lange V, Ducot B, De Ziegler D, Poirot C, Wolf JP. Sperm nuclear vacuoles, as assessed by motile sperm organellar morphological examination,are mostly of acrosomal origin. Reproductive BioMedicine Online. 2010;**20**:132-137. DOI: 10.1016/j.rbmo.2009.10.014

[61] Perdrix A, Travers A, Clatot F, Sibert L, Mitchell V, Jumeau F, Macé B, Rives N. Modification of chromosomal architecture in human spermatozoa with large vacuoles. Andrology. 2013;**1**:57-66. DOI: 10.1111/j.2047-2927.2012.00016.x

[62] Franco JG Jr, Mauri AL, Petersen CG, Massaro FC, Silva LF, Felipe V, Cavagna M, Pontes A, Baruffi RL, Oliveira JB, Vagnini LD. Large nuclear vacuoles are indicative of abnormal chromatin packaging in human spermatozoa. International Journal of Andrology. 2012;**35**:46-51. DOI: 10.1111/j.1365-2605.2011.01154.x

[63] Tanaka A, Nagayoshi M, Tanaka I, Kusunoki H. Human sperm head vacuoles are physiological structures formed during the sperm development and maturation process. Fertility and Sterility. 2012;**98**:315-320. DOI: 10.1016/j.fertnstert.2012.04.034

[64] Moretti E, Pascarelli NA, Federico MG, Renieri T, Collodel G. Abnormal elongation of midpiece, absence of axoneme and outer dense fibers at principal piece level, supernumerary microtubules: A sperm defect of possible genetic origin? Fertility and Sterility. 2008;**90**:1201.e3-e8. DOI: 10.1016/j.fertnstert.2007. 11.050

[65] Mitchell V, Sigala J, Ballot C, Jumeau F, Barbotin AL, Duhamel A, Rives N, Rigot JM, Escalier D, Peers MC. Light microscopy morphological characteristics of the sperm flagellum may be related to axonemal abnormalities. Andrologia. 2015;**47**:214-220. DOI: 10.1111/and.12249

[66] Pelfrey RJ, Overstreet JW, Lewis EL. Abnormalities of sperm morphology in cases of persistent infertility after vasectomy reversal. Fertility and Sterility. 1982;**38**:112-114. DOI: 10.1016/S0015-0282(16)46407-1

[67] Yeung CH, Tüttelmann F, Bergmann M, Nordhoff V, Vorona E, Cooper TG. Coiled sperm from infertile patients: Characteristics, associated factors and biological implication. Human Reproduction. 2009;**24**:1288-1295. DOI: 10.1093/humrep/dep017

[68] Rengan AK, Agarwal A, van der Linde M, du Plessis SS. An investigation of excess residual cytoplasm in human spermatozoa and its distinction from the cytoplasmic droplet. Reproductive Biology and Endocrinology. 2012;**10**:92. DOI: 10.1186/1477-7827-10-92

[69] Cooper TG, Yeung CH, Fetic S, Sobhani A, Nieschlag E. Cytoplasmic droplets are normal structures of human sperm but are not well preserved by routine procedures for assessing sperm morphology. Human Reproduction. 2004;**19**:2283-2288. DOI: 10.1093/humrep/deh410

[70] Amiri-Yekta A, Coutton C, Kherraf ZE, Karaouzène T, Le Tanno P, Sanati MH, Sabbaghian M, Almadani N, Sadighi Gilani MA, Hosseini SH, Bahrami S, Daneshipour A, Bini M, Arnoult C, Colombo R, Gourabi H, Ray PF. Whole-exome sequencing of familial cases of multiple morphological abnormalities of the sperm flagella (MMAF) reveals new DNAH1 mutations. Human Reproduction. 2016;**31**:2872-2880. DOI: 10.1093/humrep/dew262

[71] El Khouri E, Thomas L, Jeanson L, Bequignon E, Vallette B, Duquesnoy P, Montantin G, Copin B, Dastot-Le Moal F, Blanchon S, Papon JF, Lorès P, Yuan L, Collot N, Tissier S, Faucon C, Gacon G, Patrat C, Wolf JP, Dulioust E, Crestani B, Escudier E, Coste A, Legendre M, Touré A, Amselem S. Mutations in DNAJB13, encoding an HSP40 family member, cause primary Ciliary dyskinesia and male infertility. American Journal of Human Genetics. 2016;**99**:489-500. DOI: 10.1016/j.ajhg.2016.06.022

[72] Tang S, Wang X, Li W, Yang X, Li Z, Liu W, Li C, Zhu Z, Wang L, Wang J, Zhang L, Sun X, Zhi E, Wang H, Li H, Jin L, Luo Y, Wang J, Yang S, Zhang F. Biallelic Mutations in CFAP43 and CFAP44 Cause Male Infertility with Multiple Morphological Abnormalities of the Sperm Flagella. American Journal of Human Genetics. 2017;**100**:854-864. DOI: 10.1016/j.ajhg.2017.04.012

[73] Wang X, Jin H, Han F, Cui Y, Chen J, Yang C, Zhu P, Wang W, Jiao G, Wang W, Hao C, Gao Z. Homozygous DNAH1 frameshift mutation causes multiple morphological anomalies of the sperm flagella in Chinese. Clinical Genetics. 2017;**91**:313-321. DOI: 10.1111/cge.12857

[74] Kruger TF, Menkveld R, Stander FS, Lombard CJ, Van der Merwe JP, van Zyl JA, Smith K. Sperm morphologic features as a prognostic factor in *in vitro* fertilization. Fertility and Sterility. 1986;**46**:1118-1123. DOI: 10.1016/S0015-0282(16)49891-2

[75] Kruger TF, Acosta AA, Simmons KF, Swanson RJ, Matta JF, Oehninger S. Predictive value of abnormal sperm morphology in *in vitro* fertilization. Fertility and Sterility. 1988;**49**:112-117. DOI: 10.1016/S0015-0282(16)59660-5

[76] Grow DR, Oehninger S, Seltman HJ, Toner JP, Swanson RJ, Kruger TF, Muasher SJ. Sperm morphology as diagnosed by strict criteria: Probing the impact of teratozoospermia on fertilization rate and pregnancy outcome in a large *in vitro* fertilization population. Fertility and Sterility. 1994;**62**:559-567. DOI: 10.1016/S0015-0282(16)56946-5

2

Male Accessory Glands and Sperm Function

Lozano Hernández Jesús Ricardo

Abstract

With the advent of the techniques of reproduction, the functions of this fluid on the sperm function became a topic of lesser interest to the embryologist, urologist and andrologist. The interaction of spermatozoa with seminal plasma often goes unnoticed, but it is very likely that many substances produced by male accessory glands have impact on the sperm physiology. Seminal fluid contains several components besides spermatozoa; many of them are produced by a specific tissue and can be useful markers of secretion of the glands. The information in the 5th Manual of World Health Organization is very limited with respect to the interpretation in several characteristics abnormally high in semen. Male accessory glands secrete several factors such as alpha-glucosidase, fructose, prostaglandins, bicarbonate and citric acid among others, which are crucial for sperm physiology. This chapter deals with the interpretation of markers of accessory glands and their relation to some pathologies such as varicocele, infections, obstructions of the seminiferous pathways and some hormonal alterations.

Keywords: male accessory glands, seminal plasma, semen hyperviscosity, male infertility, citric acid

1. Introduction

The study of seminal fluid had great importance some decades ago, but with the advent of fertilization *in vitro*, intracytoplasmatic sperm injection and other techniques of reproduction, the functions of this fluid on the sperm function became a topic of lesser interest to the embryologist, urologist and andrologist. The interaction of spermatozoa with seminal plasma often goes unnoticed, but it is very likely that these substances have impact in DNA integrity, in the membranes and organelles on sperm and embryo.

2. Components of the seminal plasma

Seminal plasma has a wide variety of elements, which are formed by the testicle, the seminiferous ducts and the glands. Some proteins of seminal plasma produced by type of tissues are considered markers. The increase or decrease in the levels of these markers may be indicative of a pathological process in a specific tissue [1].

Spermiogram is the most important test in the study of infertile man. In the semen sample, the spermatozoa and the products of secretion of the seminiferous ways and accessory glands are evaluated. The fifth version of the seminal analysis of the Manual of the World Health Organization showed some lower reference index (LRI) established to the seminal characteristics in 95% of a fertile population [2]. However, the information in this manual is very limited in interpretation if some characteristics are abnormally high such as density sperm (polyzoospermia), pH (alkalinity), seminal volume (hyperspermia) and markers of male accessory glands fructose, zinc and neutral alpha glucosidase.

The ejaculated contains sperm, immature germ cells, cell debris, other cells and secretions that come mostly from the accessory glands. After centrifugation of semen, a pellet composed of spermatozoa, cells and cell debris is obtained in approximately 5% of the volume. Seminal plasma is the supernatant remaining after centrifugation and removal of cells and cell debris from seminal liquid forms almost the whole 95%. The accessory glands are prostate and seminal vesicle, whereas the epididymis is an organ located on the posterior border of the testes where the sperm mature and are stored. The epididymis has secretory capacity and is often referred to as an accessory gland. Therefore, seminal vesicles, prostate and epididymis secrete most of the semen around 70, 20 and 10%, respectively [3, 4], **Figure 1**.

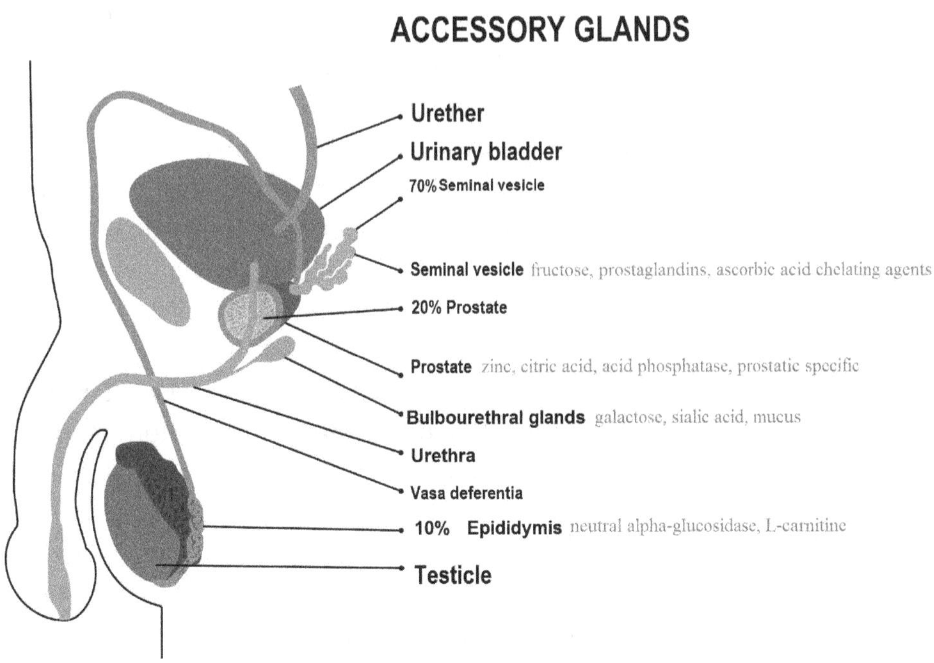

Figure 1. Male accessory glands and their main products of secretions.

The production of the seminal fluid begins in the tubule recti, the rete testis and the epididymis inside the testicle. The testicle and the epididymis are found inside the scrotum. At the time of ejaculation, the sperm exit the scrotum and reach the vasa efferentia [1]. A part from providing the suitable environment for sperm nurturing, transport and maturation, during the transit in male reproductive tract functional and dynamic exchanges of molecules among spermatozoa and reproductive fluids occur. In the epididymis, the first organ in which post-testicular maturation takes place, a gradient of molecules, such as endocannabinoids provide the suitable environment for the acquisition of sperm motility [5] and defective spermatozoa are eliminated through the activity of molecular chaperones/cochaperone and de/ubiquitinating systems [6]. Prior to ejaculation, sexual arousal stimulates Cowper's glands located in the urethra, which produce a mucous and alkaline fluid that helps protect sperm from the remains of acid urine present in the urethra and in the urethral orifice. The secretion of Cowper's glands is known as pre-ejaculatory fluid. Occasionally, during long exciting phase, the secretion can reach up to 1 mL of the fluid, usually contained in one to three drops which appear at the opening of the glans of the penis [7]. The bulbourethral glands secrete galactose, sialic acid and mucus that lubricate semen, allowing more efficient sperm transfer. Despite being rich in components with potential diagnostic value, seminal plasma has been evaluated in the clinic rarely [1]. For these reasons to determine the causes of male infertility, tract genital fluid remains a field still unknown to many specialists in human reproduction.

2.1. Biomarkers of male accessory glands

2.1.1. Fructose

Fructose is the main sugar related to metabolism and sperm motility, it is an important marker of the performance of seminal vesicles. Al-Daghistani et al. proposed a reference range of fructose in fertile men: 367.5 ± 21.8 mg/l [8]; so that in a seemingly normal volume of 1.5 ml as outlined in the fifth WHO manual for seminal analysis concentration, the value of seminal fructose should be 20 μmol/ejaculate, over lower reference limit: 13 μmol/ejaculate [2]. The value of fructose expressed in "lower reference limit" discards if an extremely high value of fructose can be associated to an alteration in the metabolic pathway of sugars. Abnormally high values of fructose had been cited in individuals with diabetes, oligozoospermia and azoospermia [9–11]. The use of testosterone including in men with male accessory glands infection (MAGI) increases the seminal fructose [12]. Besides, lower values of fructose are detected in ejaculates with high sperm density with motile spermatozoa, so that the spermatic fructolysis decreases the concentration of fructose [13]. This controversy makes necessary to correct the fructose levels with the sperm concentration; hence, the value of corrected fructose (mg/ml) may be calculated by the logarithm (log10) of the concentration of spermatozoa/ml. It is necessary to remain in mind that the sperm motile activity and the fructose (mg/ml) must be multiplied by the log10 of the concentration/ml of "motile spermatozoa," to obtain an even more reliable parameter: true corrected fructose (FCV) [14]. Interestingly, the value of FCV has been related to condensation of sperm chromatin, zinc chelation and fertilization. The ejaculate of any fertile man may contain spermatozoa with different degrees of chromatin stability. After the introduction of sperm into the oocyte, an appropriate decondensation of the nuclear chromatin and the subsequent formation of the male pronucleus are essential for fertilization and normal embryonic development. Higher incidence of intact spermatozoa in unfertilized oocytes suggests that sperm has high chromatin stability. In infertile men, the condensation of the sperm chromatin may be elevated. The prostatic zinc condenses the spermatic chromatin, this metal binds to the metallothionein coming from the seminal vesicle and gives greater stability of the chromatin; however, this step is regulated by secretions of seminal vesicles that have a chelating action on zinc to allow decondensation of sperm chromatin during fertilization. For these reasons, insufficiency of seminal vesicles or excessive production of zinc by a prostatic inflammatory process may be associated with infertility due to failure in chromatin stability. The reference value found for FCV is ≥2.5 mg/million sperm/ml [11, 14].

2.1.2. Citric acid and zinc

The prostate produces a variety of substances such as zinc (Zn), citric acid (citrate), acid phosphatase and gamma-glutamyltransferase into others. These four have been considered reliable markers of the prostate gland [15, 16]. Zinc has a tendency to bind with other elements of semen; it can sometimes be bound to the surface of the sperm cells [17]. Zn is an essential trace element for the maintenance of germ cells, the progression of spermatogenesis, and the regulation of sperm motility. In addition, zinc exerts antioxidant functions; it competes with iron and copper for binding to cell membranes and some proteins; it displaces the redox-active metals making it more available to bind to ferritin and metallothionein, respectively; and finally, it binds to the sulfhydryl groups of proteins, protecting them from oxidation. On the other hand, heat-induced oxidative stress causes apoptosis of germ cells [18]. Animals undergoing scrotal heating exhibit a significant reduction in sperm motility and concentration, but the adverse effects of hyperthermia on the seminal parameters of patients with varicocele can be prevented if these are treated with Zn, although this proposal must be supported by larger experimental studies [19]. The LRI established for zinc is ≥2.4 μmol/ejaculate [2].

Citrate is probably the major ligand of zinc. Citric acid levels are regulated by testosterone, and like fructose can be observed elevated in oligozoospermic and azoospermic subjects without a convincing clinical explanation [20]. Citrate is one of the most important anions, although it has an affinity for calcium, magnesium and zinc, and much of the seminal citrate is strongly charged anion [21]. A relationship between seminal citric acid and acrosomal integrity has been found in semen after cryopreservation. This is due to during cryopreservation, the spermatozoa become more permeable to ionic calcium, which is the main inducer of the reaction acrosome; if the sample has high levels of citric acid, it increases the capture of the ionic calcium and reduces the induction of the acrosomal reaction [22]. Conversely, citric acid is lower in semen hyperviscosity and suggests that the hyperviscous samples are inadequate for intrauterine insemination or fertilization in vitro. Citric acid is an important anion with high affinity for ionic calcium, magnesium and zinc; hence, lower concentrations of citrate may to induce premature acrosomal reaction [23]. Citric acid may be found in low concentrations in semen of men with abnormal prostate growth, in hyperviscous samples and with high adiposity. Seminal volume and spermatozoa/ejaculate are reduced in men with morbid obesity, so the hypospermia is more associated with decreased secretion of the prostate than seminal vesicles; an inverse relationship between citric acid and chronic oxidative stress has been observed. Citric acid has antioxidant and anti-inflammatory functions in tissues damaged by environmental factors; also it favors the synthesis of glycosaminoglycans in various tissues. In obese men, abnormal growth of the prostate is associated with low production of prostatic citric acid in addition to other hormonal disorders that compromise testosterone, estrogen, insulin, insulin growth factor (IGF-1) and leptin. In semen of morbid obese men, there is an increase of fructose and lower levels of citric acid [24].

2.1.3. α-1,4 Neutral alpha glucosidase

With respect to the epididymis secretion, an important marker has been mentioned in the last few years, the α-1,4 neutral alpha glucosidase (NAG), there are two forms, an acid of prostatic origin another neutral of epididymal origin. The neutral isoform is secreted primarily in the body of the epididymis and plays a role in the maturation of spermatozoa [25]. L-carnitine and glycerophosphorylcholine had been used as biomarkers of epididymal function, but in the last few years, NAG has been considered the most sensitive and specific epididymal marker [26]. In this face, an infectious/inflammatory process in the epididymis can cause total or partial obstruction of the spermatic transport, causing azoospermia or oligozoospermia respectively. The obstruction generates pressure in the epithelial duct or the efferent ducts, the hemato-testicular barrier is overcome and the production of antisperm antibodies can be triggered [27, 28]. The decrease of NAG in semen is associated with obstruction between epididymis and ejaculatory duct, hypoandrogenism, infection or inflammation of the epididymis [2]. But the importance of NAG as an indicator of obstructive azoospermia is partial; nonetheless, the presence of cysteine-rich secretory protein 1 (CRISP1) in seminal plasma may be considered better marker to distinguish obstructive azoospermia and nonobstructive azoospermia. Seminal plasma samples from nonobstructive azoospermic men have the presence of CRISP1, whereas CRISP1 has been observed absent or very low in samples from patients with obstructive azoospermia [29].

The recommended reference for NAG value is ≥20 mU/ejaculate [2]. In the presence of *Chlamydia trachomatis, Mycoplasma hominis* and *Ureaplasma urealyticum* fructose and NAG are lower than samples of men without infection, suggesting low glandular function in epididymis and seminal vesicles associated lesions in the glandular tissue and at the presence of bacteria [30]. In men with varicocele, there are not alterations in levels of fructose, citric acid, pH nor acid phosphatase activity, but there is an important decrease of NAG associated to epididymal dysfunction in varicoceles grade II-III, possibly associated with a detrimental in sperm quality. The epididymis is located inside the scrotum and posterior to the testis and its function is possibly affected by the scrotal temperature [31]. The epididymis has a reduced function during varicocele, which is associated with decreased NAG activity and lower-quality sperm membrane and nucleus. The epididymis is an important organ involved in sperm maturation. The production of antioxidants by the epididymis is essential to counteract the damaging events resulting from excessive reactive oxygen species (ROS) production originated locally and along the transit through the epididymis from the testis. Reduced NAG activity in human semen of men with varicocele has been shown related to increase in DNA fragmentation, low integrity of sperm membrane and reduction of binding to hyaluronic acid.

Therefore, varicocele may compromise not only the testis but also the epididymis, causing a reduction of seminal quality and impaired quality of the sperm membrane and nucleus [32].

2.1.4. Seminal pH

The seminal pH is close to neutral, in the vaginal acid medium provides the spermatozoa the conditions to reach and penetrate the cervical mucus. The ideal pH of human semen has been a matter of debate [33], there is a considerable variation in pH measurements reported by different researchers. The LRI of seminal pH established by WHO is ≥7.2 [2], unlike most references that had been expressed in ranges 7.2–8.0. The value ≥LRI does not give a clear idea to what extent the semen alkalinity is favorable for sperm physiology. Lower values are associated with low seminal vesicle function and the absence of ejaculatory ducts that affect sperm quality and fertility [2, 32]. In this way, it is important to note that the pH > 7.2 interpreted literally as normal, subtracts the previous information when the pH value was ≥7.8 for infections or seminal inflammations [2, 10, 34]. The alkaline environment of semen is maintained by basic polyamines, such as spermine, spermidine and putrescine [35]. The pH value may depend on the time elapsed since ejaculation and tends to increase immediately after ejaculation as a result of CO_2 loss. High values of pH would not be physiologically favorable for sperm physiology, elevated values are also associated with prolonged collection time associated with fructolysis and lactic acid production alter their value [36, 37].

2.2. Other chemical components of semen

2.2.1. Calcium, magnesium and selenium

Zinc and magnesium concentrations in seminal plasma have been correlated with sperm quality [38]. The administration of selenium, magnesium, and calcium reduces the oxidative stress caused by intoxication. Calcium and magnesium have favorable effects on hematological and other biochemical parameters, but selenium is the most effective, it achieves the best protective effects against arsenic poisoning in humans [39]. Seminal calcium has been related to metabolism and sperm motility, acrosome reaction and fertilization [40]. Magnesium is bound to other molecules, which can sometimes bind to the surface of spermatozoa [41]. Selenium in semen has been correlated positively with concentration, motility and sperm morphology. Selenium has been related to the development of spermatogenesis, in the development of Sertoli cells; furthermore, it is a component of glutathione-peroxidase. Spermatozoa from selenium deficient mice have incomplete chromosome decondensation with increased incidence of DNA breaks. The increase of lipid peroxidation is observed in selenium deficiency but also observed when its intake is excessive. The concentration of selenium in seminal plasma of men with varicocele is lower than in normozoospermic men. Elevation of the scrotal temperature is considered to be one of the main factors that endanger spermatogenesis and steroidogenesis in the varicose testis. Selenium concentration is reduced in varicocele and has been associated with decreased sperm concentration, morphology and motility [19]. Oral selenium treatment may help restore seminal quality in many infertile men with varicocele.

2.2.2. Copper

This ion acts as a cofactor of different important enzymes and is associated with the sperm quality in rodents and humans [42]. Low doses of copper (Cu) may have favorable effects on sperm function [43], and elevated levels of Cu have been observed in the seminal plasma of men with varicocele compared with fertile men [15]. In older men, copper levels in seminal plasma have been positively associated with sperm DNA fragmentation [41]. In semen of infertile men with low seminal quality, copper levels were inversely related to sperm concentration. This relationship is not observed in normal samples of infertile men or in fertile men samples [44].

2.2.3. Proteins

In the human semen thousands of proteins have been reported, of which 7346 of them originate in the testicle. The prostate is the second source of proteins, which has aroused interest in their study because they produce high concentrations of proteomes in cases of prostate cancer. Seminal plasma proteins arise from secretions from seminal vesicles (~65% of semen volume), prostate (~25%), testis and epididymis (~10%) and bulbourethral and periurethral glands (~1%) [1]. Most seminal proteins are derived from the seminal vesicles, although the source of albumin is primarily of prostatic origin [45]. Albumin makes up about one-third of the semen protein content. The amino acid content of semen is much higher than that of plasma, and it increases rapidly (especially glutamic acid) within the first few hours after ejaculation [46].

Some of the proteins or their isoforms detected in the seminal plasma were zinc alpha-2-glycoprotein 1, clusterin, lactotransferrin, prostate specific antigen. Prostate is a very rich source of protein (35–55 g/l). The large variation in the number of proteins identified by any given technique depends mainly on the sample preparation and mass spectrometry technology available. Two proteins responsible for semen coagulation have been detected: the prolactin-induced protein (PIP) and Semenogelin (Sg), which are observed different between fertile and infertile men and could have an impact on sperm physiology. PIP is higher in semen samples of fertile men that in fertile men, while increased Sg concentrations are found in asthenozoospermic samples. Other proteins as epididymal secretory protein EI precursor, albumin preprotein, lactotransferrin, extracellular matrix protein E1 precursor, prosaposin isoform a preprotein and cathepsin D preprotein not play a significant role in sperm physiology [47]. Transferrin is one of the serum proteins, which has been characterized in the seminal plasma, but its role in male infertility is unclear [48]. However, a study found correlation of transferrin with sperm morphology. It demonstrated that seminal plasma transferrin concentration is correlated with sperm count and percent motile sperms. Thus, Sertoli cell-dependent secretion of transferrin has a positive influence over spermatogenesis and can be used as a marker of testicular function [49]. Many proteins have been differentially expressed in the seminal plasma of men with poor sperm quality. The overexpression or underexpression of some proteins suggests their role in male infertility.

3. Volume and seminal viscosity

Low reference index of seminal volume in fertile men is 1.5 ml. The term hyperpermia is not included in the last manual of seminal analysis. In a previous study of healthy men, the 95th percentile of the skewed data distribution was 6.3 ml and nearly 50% of them had low sperm concentrations. Seminal volume increase (hyperspermia) has been associated to male accessory gland in patients with bilateral prostate-vesiculo-epididymitis (PVE) more than those with monolateral PVE or prostatitis [50, 51].

The prevalence of hyperviscosity in subfertile men is around 26.2%, and it may be mild, moderate or severe. Treatment may be completely successful only in subjects with mild hyperviscosity with a positive semen culture. In these subjects, progressive motility percentage, straight line velocity and linearity of sperm increase. Pathogenesis was strictly related to infective/inflammatory factors in only 48.0% of cases; therefore, it is possible that biochemical, enzymatic or genetic factors have a role in this condition [52].

Human papillomavirus (HPV) has been detected in semen samples of infertile men, 10.5% of them showed only single type of virus, 5.7% corresponded to the high risk type and 6.1% were type low risk, in 6.1 were more than one type of HPV. Increase of semen viscosity was observed in the samples infected with the virus in single and multiple forms. Hypospermia, leukocytospermia and increased pH are found in infected samples with multiple types of HPV, probably the seminal changes are related to the negative effects of different forms of HPV in the prostate secretion and the fertility [53].

4. Male accessory glands and hormonal control

Male accessory sex glands display a consistent pattern of differential sensitivity to androgens and estrogens and that these hormones may exert their action on different cell types within the organ [25]. The development and differentiation of the male reproductive system in the fetus are directed by the fetal testis through the production of testosterone and anti-Müllerian hormone. In the fetal testes, Leydig cells produce testosterone, a steroidal hormone that promotes the growth and differentiation of Wolff's ducts such as epididymis and prostate. At the same time, the Sertoli testicular cells produce the Anti-müllerian hormone (HAM) that causes the regression of the Müllerian ducts. The development of the external sexual organs is generated from the differentiation of the genital tubercle, eminence (protuberance) located in front of the cloaca of the embryo. The secretion of the enzyme 5-α-reductase allows the transformation of testosterone to dihydrotestosterone (DHT), a hormone that differentiates the genital tubercle to the male external sex organs [54]. However, the possible impact of other glucocorticoid hormones has been proposed in experimental animals. Betamethasone has been used for inducing fetal lung maturation. Some studies reported that prenatal treatment with this drug reduced testosterone levels in the male fetus. In adulthood stage of these animals, lower values of FSH and sperm quality were observed; seminal vesicle weight was decreased while testicular and ventral prostate weights were increased. The betamethasone exposure leads to long-term reproductive impairment in male rats. It is important to considerate the implications for humans, considering the use of this glucocorticoid in pregnant women [55].

Other drug that has negative impact on secretion of male accessory glands is atorvastatin because reduce acid phosphatases, NAG and L-carnitine in semen during the therapy, indicating an alteration of prostatic and epididymal functions with reduction of seminal parameters. The mechanism of the effect of atorvastatin on the function of accessory glands is not clear; possibly, the reduction in LDL-cholesterol levels affects the synthesis of testosterone by Leydig cells [56]. Dihydrotestosterone (DHT), estradiol, progesterone and prolactin receptors have been found in prostates of rats. It has been shown in these species that testosterone induces hyperplasia and also has an anti-inflammatory effect on that gland [57].

The effect of prolactin on the prostate was studied in hypophysectomized animals treated with LH and FSH without any supply of exogenous prolactin, the animals showed low weight in prostate and seminal vesicles [58]. Prolactin potentiates the effect of androgens on the prostate and seminal vesicles in rodents, possibly favoring the conversion of testosterone to dihydrotestosterone. Hyperprolactinemia in mice produces structural changes in the cells with the highest amount of androgen receptor in the epididymis and prostate [59]. Studies in castrated rats showed that prolactin stimulates the expression of epididymal and sialic acid alpha glucosidases, independent of androgens [60]. The reduction of glandular markers in the absence of infection could be related to unknown hormonal changes.

5. Markers of male accessory glands and infection

Infection of male accessory glands (MAGI) can occur as prostatitis, prostatic-vesiculitis and prostate-vesiculo-epididymitis. MAGI can have a negative impact on the secretory function of the glands and on fertility. MAGI is often acquired as a urethral infection, it has a chronic course and it spreads to one or more accessory glands, being able to cover one or both sides, rarely causing obstruction of the seminal routes. The seminal alterations are more evident when the infection reaches two or more glands. The inflammatory response has been associated with the alteration of the seminal parameters when affecting function of the epididymis, seminal vesicles and prostate, especially by diminishing the antioxidant properties of the seminal plasma [61].

Several protein components of seminal plasma are produced by certain types of tissues of the male urogenital tract; therefore, the difference in the concentration of these semen proteins could be indicators of a specific organ disease. This concept is best illustrated by the value of prostate-specific antigen (PSA) as a marker of prostate diseases. The PSA was originally discovered in semen and was isolated from it and is the most used marker to identify prostate cancer, being higher in semen than in blood serum [62]. PSA is a serine protease that cleaves semenogelin by hydrolysis and thus liquefies the semen coagulum and facilitates sperm motility and capacitation [63].

Soufir evaluated the markers fructose, acid phosphatase and citric acid as tools in the differential diagnosis of infectious processes and hypogonadism. The decrease of markers suggested that it is necessary to evaluate hormonal status and to rule out infection of accessory glands, which can affect sperm function and inability to achieve pregnancy naturally [64]. Glandular markers tend to be low in the presence of leukocytes and most likely in infection; nevertheless, these are significantly lower in hypogonadism. An infection could cause permanent damage of the secretory epithelium, so even after treatment may remain low [65]. This implies that in cases of seminal vesicle, infection levels of seminal fructose may be increased or decreased.

Male accessory glands infection may alter the elasticity in semen. Changes in levels of oxidative products in semen are related to seminal viscosity. Hyperviscosity has been associated with reactive oxygen species (ROS) generation, levels of cytokines TNF-α, IL-6 and IL-10 and seminal leucocyte concentration, and whether ROS production was related to the extent of infections/inflammations at one PR (prostatitis) or two PV (prostato-vesiculitis) male accessory glands. ROS production in PV was higher than in prostatitis. Seminal IL-10 levels in PV and PR patients were lower than those found in the controls. In PR men, the levels of hyperviscosity are positively related to TNF-α; the seminal hyperviscosity is associated with increased oxidative stress in infertile men and increased pro-inflammatory interleukins in patients with male accessory gland infection, more when the infection was extended to the seminal vesicles [66]. Seminal hyperviscosity is often associated with prostate infection, reduce citric acid and asthenozoospermia [52, 66]. These alterations have been reversed when properly treated with antibiotics, decreasing the concentration of leukocytes and proinflammatory cytokines. Around one-third of cases of seminal hyperviscosity does not respond to treatment with antibiotics because viscosity depends on other glandular factors that have not yet been clarified [52].

Many compounds secreted by the male reproductive tract may be important in the study of infertile man. It is advisable that before choosing any technique of assisted reproduction, the causes of infertility in man are more accurately evaluated, especially in cases of idiopathic infertility. Disorders of the male accessory glands are often associated with bacterial infections. These alterations must be carefully treated with the antibiotic therapy to which these bacteria show susceptibility [67]. The diagnosis and antibiogram would allow controlling resistance to antibiotics, but taking into account that when there is infection of the glands, antimicrobials have limited efficacy because they are anatomical compartments with barriers that can limit their reach, such as blood-prostatic barrier. Tissue lesions are greater as time progresses, for example prostatitis responds faster to treatment than prostate-vesiculitis and prostate-vesicle-epididymitis, that is, more glands are involved as time progresses [68]. In addition, it is possible to find the compartment of some microorganisms that tend to encapsulate or attach more strongly to the glycocalyx of the extracellular matrix of the gland or probably because of changes in local pH of seminal vesicles (alkaline) or prostate (acid), between others that limit antimicrobial efficacy [64]. Treatment of subclinical infections and secretory failure of male accessory glands can improve sperm physiology to achieve spontaneous pregnancies. It should be noted that the cost of assisted reproduction reflects a much lower percentage of live births than other less costly techniques for many infertile couples. Assisted reproduction already accounts for as many as 5% of live births in some European countries [69] so it is not negligible to investigate the factors that modulate the function of gametes.

6. Conclusions

The study of secretory products of male accessory glands in conjunction with correct seminal evaluation may help to exclude the high percentage of idiopathic infertility. Infectious or post-infectious processes in the epididymis, prostate and seminal vesicles can alter the seminal plasma quality and the physiology of spermatozoa.

The evaluation of compounds of the seminal plasma is useful to understand the process of natural fertilization and to achieve pregnancy naturally when the causes of infertility in man have been clearly established. These evidences suggest that the components of the seminal plasma participate in key events related to sperm function, fertilization and embryonic development in the female reproductive tract. However, the subject of sperm interaction and seminal plasma should continue to be studied to help explain the failure rates in assisted reproduction techniques.

Author details

Lozano Hernández Jesús Ricardo

Address all correspondence to: ricardolozanoh@hotmail.com

Cátedra de Fisiopatología, Facultad de Farmacia y Bioanálisis, Universidad de Los Andes, Mérida, Venezuela

References

[1] Drabovich AP, Saraon P, Jarvi K, Diamandis EP. Seminal plasma as a diagnostic fluid for male reproductive system disorders. Nature Reviews. Urology. 2014;**11**(5):278-288

[2] WHO Laboratory Manual for the Examination of Human Semen and Semen-cervical Mucus Interaction. Vol. 74, N° 3, September 2014. 5ª edition. Cambridge: Cambridge University Press; 2010

[3] Jones R, Lopez Kristin. Human Reproductive Biology. Colorado: Elsevier Inc.; 2014. pp. 78-81

[4] Lozano-Hernández R, Vivas-Acevedo G. Análisis Bioquímico del Plasma Seminal. En: Manual Básico del Semen. México: Ed Prado; 2013. pp. 81-98

[5] Cobellis G, Ricci G, Cacciola G, Orlando P, Petrosino S, Cascio MG, Bisogno T, De Petrocellis L, Chioccarelli T, Altucci L, Fasano S, Meccariello R, Pierantoni R, Ledent C, Di Marzo V. A gradient of 2-arachidonoylglycerol regulates mouse epididymal sperm cell start-up. Biology of Reproduction. 2010;**82**(2):451-458

[6] Meccariello R, Chianese R, Ciaramella V, Fasano S, Pierantoni R. Molecular chaperones, cochaperones, and ubiquitination/deubiquitination system: Involvement in the production of high quality spermatozoa. BioMed Research International. 2014;**2014**:561426. DOI: 10.1155/2014/561426. Epub 2014 Jun 19. Review

[7] Zukerman Z, Weiss DB, Orvieto R. Short communication: Does preejaculatory penile secretion originating from cowper's gland contain sperm? Journal of Assisted Reproduction and Genetics. 2003;**20**(4):157-159

[8] Al-Daghistani HI, Hamad AW, Abdel-Dayem M, Al-Swaifi M, Abu Zaid M. Evaluation of serum testosterone, progesterone, seminal antisperm antibody, and fructose levels among jordanian males with a history of infertility. Biochemistry Research International. 2010;**2010**:409640

[9] Vaishwanar PS, Fructose AHN. Citric acid in human semen. The Indian Journal of Medical Research. 1968;**56**(11):1728-1731

[10] Padrón RS, Alemán G, Mas J. Resultados del tratamiento de la azoospermia secretoria. Rev Cub Obstet Ginecol (Spanish). 1982;**8**:192-196

[11] Gonzales GF. Corrected seminal fructose test. Archives of Andrology. 1994;**33**:17-22

[12] La Vignera S, Condorelli RA, Mongioi LM, Vitale SG, Russo GI, Laganà AS, Calogero AE. Hormonal treatment with transdermal testosterone in patients with male accessory gland inflammation (MAGI): Effects on sperm parameters. Andrologia. 2017;**49**(8). DOI: 10.1111/and.12745

[13] Mauss J, Borsch G, Torok L. Differential diagnosis of low or absent seminal fructose in man. Fertility and Sterility. 1974;**25**:411-415

[14] Gonzales GF, Sanchez A. High sperm chromatin stability in semen with high viscosity. Archives of Andrology. 1994;**32**:31-35

[15] Comhaire FH, Vermeulen L, Pieters O. Study of the accuracy of physical and biochemical markers in semen to detect infectious dysfunction of the accessory sex glands. Journal of Andrology. 1989;**10**:50-53

[16] Kawakami K, Fujita Y, Matsuda Y, Arai T, Horie K, Kameyama K, Kato T, Masunaga K, et al. Gamma-glutamyltransferase activity in exosomes as a potential marker for prostate cancer. BMC Cancer. 2017;**17**(1):316

[17] Mandal A, Bhattacharyya AK. Physical properties and non-enzymatic components of human ejaculates. Relationship to spontaneous liquefaction. International Journal of Andrology. 1985;**8**:224-231

[18] Agarwal A, Sekhon LH. Oxidative stress and antioxidants for idiopathic oligoasthenoteratospermia: Is it justified? Indian Journal of Urology. 2011;**27**(1):74-85

[19] Camejo MI, Abdala L, Vivas-Acevedo G, Lozano-Hernández R, Angeli-Greaves M, Greaves ED. Selenium, copper and zinc in seminal plasma of men with varicocele, relationship with seminal parameters. Biological Trace Element Research. 2011;**143**:1247-1254

[20] Jathar VS, Hirwe R, Desai S. Seminal fructose, citric acid and phosphatase levels and their relation to the sperm count in man. Indian Journal of Physiology and Pharmacology. 1977;**21**:186-190

[21] Banjoko SO, Adeseolu FO. Seminal plasma pH, inorganic phosphate, total and ionized calcium concentrations in the assessment of human spermatozoa function. Journal of Clinical and Diagnostic Research: JCDR. 2013;**7**(11):2483-2486. http://doi.org/10.7860/JCDR/2013/6194.3585

[22] Liu DY, Baker HWJ. Inducing the human acrosome reaction with a calcium ionophore A23187 decreases sperm-zona pellucida binding with oocytes that failed to fertilize in *vitro*. Journal of Reproduction and Fertility. 1990;**89**(1):127-134

[23] Ricardo L-H, Javier G, Daniel N, Alejandra RLM. Efecto de la hiperviscosidad seminal sobre la integridad acrosómica y la movilidad espermática antes y después de la criopreservación. Investigacion Clinica [Internet]. 2016 Sep [citado 2017 Sep 30];**57**(3): 267-279. Disponible en: http://www.scielo.org.ve/scielo.php?script=sci_arttext&pid=S0535-51332016000300005&lng=es

[24] Lozano-Hernández R, Gualdrón J, Camejo MI, Velasco J, Villavicencio A. Markers of accessory glands and seminal parameters in infertile men with overweight and obesity. Journal of Metabolic Syndrome. 2017;**6**(3):1000229

[25] Orgebin-Crist MC, Eller BC, Danzo BJ. The effects of estradiol, tamoxifen, and testosterone on the weights and histology of the epididymis and accessory sex organs of sexually immature rabbits. Endocrinology. 1983;**113**(5):1703-1715

[26] Loko F, Alihonou E, Goufodji B, Fagla B, Hounton M. Neutral alpha-glucosidase, a specific marker for epididymal secretion in seminal pathology. Contraception, Fertilité, Sexualité (1992). 1997;**25**(12):939-941

[27] Fourie MH, Bornman MS, Viljoen E. A comparative study of the EpiScreen kit and a conventional method for the determination of seminal alpha-glucosidase activity. Andrologia. 1998;**30**:133-139

[28] Munoz MG, Witkin SS. Autoimmunity to spermatozoa, asymptomatic chlamydia trachomatis genital tract infection and gamma delta T lymphocytes in seminal fluid from the male partners of couples with unexplained infertility. Human Reproduction. 1995;**10**: 1070-1074

[29] Légaré C, Cloutier F, Makosso-Kallyth S, Laflamme N, Jarvi K, Tremblay RR, et al. Cysteine-rich secretory protein 1 in seminal plasma: Potential biomarker for the distinction between obstructive and nonobstructive azoospermia. Fertility and Sterility. 2013;**100**(5):1253-1260

[30] Ricardo L-H, Giovanny V-A, de Vera María Gladys M. Mycoplasmas y anticuerpos anti-Chlamydia en semen de hombres infértiles y su relación con la calidad seminal y los marcadores de glándulas sexuales accesorias masculinas. Investigación Clínica [Internet]. 2012 Jun [citado 2017 Sep 30];**53**(2):138-147. Disponible en: http://www.scielo.org.ve/scielo.php?script=sci_arttext&pid=S0535-51332012000200003&lng=es.http://www.scielo.org.ve/scielo.php?script=sci_arttext&pid=S0535-51332012000200003&lng=es

[31] Vivas-Acevedo G, Lozano-Hernandez R, Camejo MI. Markers of accessory sex glands function in men with varicocele, relationship with seminal parameters. The Canadian Journal of Urology. 2011;**18**(5):5884-5889

[32] Vivas-Acevedo G, Lozano-Hernández R, Camejo MI. Varicocele decreases epididymal neutral α-glucosidase and is associated with alteration of nuclear DNA and plasma membrane in spermatozoa. BJU International. 2014;**113**:642-649

[33] Meacham OR. Perspectives and editorials: From androlog. Journal of Andrology 2002; **23**:330-331. http://onlinelibrary.wiley.com/doi/10.1002/j.1939-4640.2002.tb02238.x/pdf

[34] Aziz N. The importance of semen analysis in the context of azoospermia. Clinics. 2013; **68**(Suppl 1):35-38. DOI: 10.6061/clinics/2013(Sup01)05

[35] Mann T. Secretory function of the prostate, seminal vesicle and other male accessory organs of reproduction. Journal of Reproduction and Fertility. 1974;**37**:179-188

[36] Makler A, David R, Blumenfeld Z, Better OS. Factors affecting sperm motility. VII. Sperm viability as affected by change of pH and osmolarity of semen and urine specimens. Fertility and Sterility. 1981;**36**:507-511

[37] Wolters-Everhardt E, Dony JM, Peters WH, De Pont JJ. Buffering substances of human semen. Fertility and Sterility. 1987;**48**:159-161

[38] Homonnai ZT, Matzkin H, Fainman N, Paz G, Kraicer PF. The cation composition of the seminal plasma and prostatic fluid and its correlation to semen quality. Fertility and Sterility. 1978;**29**:539-542

[39] Srivastava D, Subramanian RB, Madamwar D, Flora SJ. Protective effects of selenium, calcium, and magnesium against arsenic-induced oxidative stress in male rats. Archives of Industrial Hygiene and Toxicology. 2010;**61**(2):153-159

[40] Sorensen MB, Bergdahl IA, Hjøllund NH, Bonde JP, Stoltenberg M, Zinc EE. Magnesium and calcium in human seminal fluid: Relations to other semen parameters and fertility. Molecular Human Reproduction. 1999;**5**:331-337

[41] Hirsch IH, Jeyendran RS, Sedor J, et al. Biochemical analysis of electroejaculates in spinal cord injured men: Comparison to normal ejaculates. The Journal of Urology. 1991; **145**:73-76

[42] Zhang RS, Sun HJ, Zheng LW. Correlation of the contents of trace elements in male body fluids with sperm quality. Zhonghua Nan Ke Xue. 2010;**16**:1019-1022

[43] Olson GE, Winfrey VP, Nagdas SK, Hill KE, Burk RF. Selenoprotein P is required for mouse sperm development. Biology of Reproduction. 2005;**73**:201-211

[44] Schmid TE, Grant PG, Marchetti F, Weldon RH, Eskenazi B, Wyrobek AJ. Elemental composition of human semen is associated with motility and genomic sperm defects among older men. Human Reproduction. 2013;**28**(1):274-282

[45] Lilja H, Oldbring J, Rannevik G, Laurell CB. Seminal vesicle-secreted proteins and their reactions during gelation and liquefaction of human semen. Journal of Clinical Investigation. 1987;**80**(2):281-285

[46] Verma PK, Singh JN, Quadros M. Modifications in the seminal protein pattern and concentration among infertile men. Ind. Journal of Medical Sciences. 1993;**47**:61-67

[47] Bharshankar RN, Bharshankar JR. Relationship of seminal plasma transferrin with seminal parameters in male infertility. Indian Journal of Physiology and Pharmacology. 2000;**44**(4):456-460

[48] Sharma R, Agarwal A, Mohanty G, Jesudasan R,Gopalan B, Willard B,Yadav S, Sabanegh E. Functional proteomic analysis of seminal plasma proteins in men with various semen parameters. Reproductive Biology and Endocrinology: RB&E. 2013;**11**:38

[49] Arunakaran J, Balasubramanian K, Srinivasan N, Aruldhas MM, Govindarajulu P. Interaction of androgens and prolactin on prostatic enzymes of the pyruvate-malate cycle involved in lipogenesis in castrated mature monkey, *Macaca radiata*. Cytobios. 1992;**70**:33-40

[50] Cooke S, Tyler JP, Driscoll GL. Hyperspermia: The forgotten condition? Human Reproduction. 1995;**10**(2):367-368

[51] La Vignera S, Calogero AE, Cannizzaro MA, Vicari E. Mono or bilateral inflammatory postmicrobial prostato-vesciculo-epididymitis: Differences in semen parameters and reactive oxygen species production. Minerva Endocrinologica. 2006;**31**(4):263-272

[52] Elia J, Delfino M, Imbrogno N, Capogreco F, Lucarelli M, Rossi T, Mazzilli1 F. Human semen hyperviscosity: Prevalence, pathogenesis and therapeutic aspects. Asian Journal of Andrology. 2009;**11**(5):609-615

[53] Damke E, Kurscheidt FA, Balani VA, Takeda KI, Irie MMT, Gimenes F, et al. Male partners of infertile couples with seminal infections of human papillomavirus have impaired fertility parameters. BioMed Research International. 2017;**2017**:4684629

[54] Desjardins C. Endocrine regulation of reproductive development and function in the male. Journal of Animal Science. 1978;**47**(Suppl 2):56-79

[55] Borges CD, Dias AF, Silva PV, Rosa JL, Guerra MT, Silva RF, Kiguti LR, Pupo AS, et al. Long-term adverse effects on reproductive function in male rats exposed prenatally to the glucocorticoid betamethasone. Toxicology. 2017;**376**:15-22

[56] Pons-Rejraji H, Brugnon F, Sion B, Maqdasy S, Gouby G, Pereira B, et al. Evaluation of atorvastatin efficacy and toxicity on spermatozoa, accessory glands and gonadal hormones of healthy men: A pilot prospective clinical trial. Reproductive Biology and Endocrinology. 2014;**12**:65

[57] Yatkin E, Bernoulli J, Talvitie EM, Santti R. Inflammation and epithelial alterations in rat prostate: Impact of the androgen to oestrogen ratio. International Journal of Andrology. 2009;**32**:399-310

[58] Słuczanowska G. The effect of hyperprolactinemia on morphology and function of androgen receptor expressing cells in rat testis, epididymis and prostate. Annales Academiae Medicae Stetinensis. 2004;**50**:123-134

[59] Thomas JA, Keenan EJ. Prolactin influences upon androgen action in male accessory sex organs. Advances in Sex Hormone Research. 1976;**2**:425-470

[60] Gautam R, Pereira BM. Modulation in activity of some epididymal glycosidases by prolactin. Indian Journal of Experimental Biology. 1993;**31**:410-413

[61] La Vignera S, Vicari E, Condorelli RA, D'Agata R, Calogero AE. Male accessory gland infection and sperm parameters (review). International Journal of Andrology. 2011;**34**(5 Pt 2): e330-e347

[62] Robert M, Gibbs BF, Jacobson E, Gagnon C. Characterization of prostate-specific antigen proteolytic activity on its major physiological substrate, the sperm motility inhibitor precursor/semenogelin I. Biochemistry. 1997;**36**:3811-3819

[63] de Lamirande E. Semenogelin, the main protein of the human semen coagulum, regulates sperm function. Seminars in Thrombosis and Hemostasis. 2007;**33**(1):60-68

[64] Soufir JC. Biochemical exploration of human sperm. La Revue du Praticien. 1983;**33**: 3141-3147

[65] Zdrodowska-Stefanow B, Ostaszewska-Puchalska I, Badyda J, Galewska. The evaluation of markers of prostatic inflammation and function of the prostate gland in patients with chronic prostatitis. Archivum Immunologiae et Therapiae Experimentalis (Warsz). 2008;**56**(4):277-282

[66] Castiglione R, Salemi M, Vicari LO, Vicari E. Relationship of semen hyperviscosity with IL-6, TNF-α, IL-10 and ROS production in seminal plasma of infertile patients with prostatitis and prostato-vesiculitis. Andrologia. 2014;**46**(10):1148-1155. DOI: 10.1111/and.12207 Epub 2013 Dec 16

[67] Vicari E, La Vignera S, Castiglione R, Calogero AE. Sperm parameter abnormalities, low seminal fructose and reactive oxygen species overproduction do not discriminate patients with unilateral or bilateral post-infectious inflammatory prostato-vesiculo-epididymitis. Journal of Endocrinological Investigation. 2006;**29**(1):18-25

[68] Lozano-Hernández R, Vivas-Acevedo G. Impacto del tratamiento con antibiótico sobre la calidad seminal y los marcadores glandulares en presencia de Mycoplasma hominis and Ureaplasma urealyticum. Revista de la Facultad de Farmacia. 2011;**53**(2):13-21

[69] de Mouzon J et al. Assisted reproductive technology in Europe, 2007: Results generated from European registers by ESHRE. Human Reproduction. 2012;**27**:954-966

3

Environmental Factors and Male Infertility

Qiuqin Tang, Wei Wu, Jing Zhang, Rong Fan and
Mu Liu

Abstract

A significant decrease in human fertility has been observed in the last 50 years. Approximately 15% of couples of reproductive age have fertility problems and about half of these cases are because of male factors. A growing body of evidence suggests that environmental factors play an important role in the causes of male infertility. Our environment is contaminated by natural and synthetic chemicals, which could interact with the endocrine system, resulting in the reduction of human fertility. Studies carried out in recent years have proven that endocrine-disrupting chemicals may disturb fertility of men. Improper lifestyle factors such as smoking, alcohol consumption, high temperature, radiation also have negative impact on male fertility. This chapter is an overview of recent developments about the importance of endocrine-disrupting chemicals and lifestyle factors' effects on sperm counts and male fertility in human.

Keywords: male infertility, endocrine-disrupting chemicals, EDCs, lifestyle factors, spermatogenic failure

1. Introduction

Approximately, 10–15% of human couples of reproductive age have impaired fertility and male factor is responsible in 50% of these cases. As is well-known, human reproduction is precisely regulated and extremely fragile to the environmental changes. Let alone harmful chemicals, even body temperature could affect sperm quality. In this chapter, we discuss two well-known major aspects that contribute to male infertility such as endocrine-disrupting chemicals (EDCs) and lifestyle factors.

2. EDCs and male infertility

The focus of male infertility is that our environment is contaminated by natural and synthetic chemicals. These chemicals could interact with the endocrine system [1]. People's exposure to chemicals is thought to be extensive, especially to EDCs, which supposed to alter the male reproductive tract. Mass industrial production and widespread use of EDCs have resulted in worldwide contamination.

EDCs are exogenous agents with the ability to mimic endogenous hormones, interfering with their biosynthesis, metabolism, and normal functions. These natural hormones are responsible for self-balance, reproduction, development and behavior of natural hormone synthesis, secretion, and transport. They mimic and inhibit the action of natural endogenous hormones or alter the normal regulatory function of the endocrine system and have potential hazardous effects on male reproductive axis causing infertility [2]. EDCs are estrogen-like and antiandrogenic chemicals in the environment. Bisphenol A (BPA), phthalates, polychlorinated biphenyls (PCBs), dichlorodiphenyltrichloroethane (DDT), dioxin, and some pesticides are the representatives of EDCs [2]. The first estrogenic and antiandrogenic endocrine disruptors that were reported to have transgenerational effects of spermatogenic failure were methoxychlor and vinclozolin [3].

2.1. Bisphenol A (BPA)

BPA is used in industries to synthesize polycarbonate and epoxy resins. Since the 1960s, it has been used in the manufacturing of plastic bottles, suction cup, inner coating of food and beverage cans, and so on. BPA is ubiquitous, from mineral water bottles, medical devices to food packaging, and has its shadow. This widespread chemical can do great harm to male fertility, having the potential of causing cryptorchidism, hypospadias, low sperm counts, or even testicular cancer [4–6]. It was also one of the important causes of occupational infertility [7]. Acting as an endocrine and metabolic disruptor, BPA can mimic the effect of endogenic estrogen. Even a very low dose of BPA can make the animals develop precocious puberty, low sperm count, prostatic hyperplasia, and so on [8]. It was reported that BPA could have greater impact on the development of human fetal testis [9]. Due to its potential harm to not only the reproductive ability but also the functions of other organs, BPA was banned from being used in baby care in many countries.

2.2. DDT

As an effective pesticide, DDT was widely used in agriculture and forestry. Its metabolites (p,p′-DDT, and p,p′-DDE) have estrogenic effects in males by blocking the androgen receptors [10]. DDT exposure was estimated by the level of p,p′-dichlorodiphenyl dichloroethylene in blood plasma, the major metabolite of DDT. Crude regression analysis showed that several sperm motion parameters, including the percentage of motile sperm and sperm with morphological tail defects, decreased and increased respectively with higher plasma p,p′-DDE concentration. Insufficient sperm chromatin condensation was observed in 46.6% of participants and the most severe category of incomplete DNA condensation was also positively correlated with p,p′-DDE concentration [11]. Therefore, nonoccupational exposure to DDT, as assessed by plasma p,p′-DDE concentrations, is associated with poorer semen parameters in men, indicating adverse effects on testicular function and/or the regulation of reproductive hormones.

2.3. Dioxins and dioxin-like compounds

Dioxins had been shown to exhibit antiestrogenic activity [12]. The association between dioxins/dioxin-like compounds exposure and impaired reproductive function had been strengthened by both epidemiological evidence and experimental studies [13–15]. Sexually mature laboratory animals exposed to relatively high doses of dioxin displayed decreased spermatogenesis, decreased testicular weight, and abnormal testes with reduced fertility [11]. By using gas chromatography/high-resolution mass spectrometry (GC/HRMS), Galimova et al. examined the concentration of dioxin-like compounds in semen of infertile males and fertile controls [14]. They found the dioxin/furan level in seminal fluid of infertile males was higher than that of fertile controls. The toxicity of dioxins is mediated by the AhR/ARNT receptor complex. The effects of high exposure to 2,3,7,8-tetrachlorodibenzo-p-dioxin (TCDD) and "TCDD-like" compounds on important sites for the development and reproduction have been recognized for years. The reproductive system has even been thought as the most sensitive "end point" for dioxin.

2.4. Heavy metal

It is beyond argument that cadmium and lead can induce male reproductive toxicity. World Health Organization (WHO) indicated that even low-level exposure to lead and cadmium (400 μg/l and 10 μg/l, respectively) can enable the semen has a significant quality descend, although it did not show conclusive evidence of male hormonal changes in reproduction.

Typically, testicular toxins and various derivatives in the animal model do harm to the testis by causing a severe damage to the seminiferous epithelium. However, cadmium prefers the way of damaging the Sertoli cells, causing testicular damage directly. The morphological changes under the scanning electron microscopy can account for this mechanism. It also works in a way by interfering with the normal functioning of mitochondrial enzymes [16].

Results from testicular biopsies, such as vacuolation, peritubular fibrosis, and oligospermia, prove that lead has direct testicular toxicity, and some researchers found that lead exposure can also have an effect on hormonal feedback mechanism at the hypothalamic pituitary level. But further investigation should be done as these studies are insufficient to make detailed evaluations in humans.

2.5. Phthalates

Phthalates are substances used in the manufacturing of automobiles, medical supplies, plastics, beverage containers, coating of metal cans, and so on. Data have demonstrated that perinatal exposure to a variety of phthalate esters alters the development of the male reproductive tract in an antiandrogenic way, causing underdevelopment and agenesis of the epididymis at relatively low doses [16]. Environmental exposure to di-n-butyl phthalate (DBP) and di-2-ethylhexyl phthalate (DEHP) may contribute to a decline in semen quality [17]. Additionally, our recent study demonstrated that prenatal exposure to DBP has transgenerational effects of impaired spermatogenesis. We also revealed that metabolic and epigenetic changes induced by the aberrant expression of betaine homocysteine S-methyltransferase (BHMT) represent a novel mechanism linking in utero DBP exposure to transgenerational spermatogenesis failure [18].

2.6. Mechanism(s) of action of endocrine disruptions on hypothalamic-pituitary-gonadal (HPG) axis

A large amount of substances has the ability to inhibit the biosynthesis of a variety of hormones. Some substances can inhibit the specific enzymes in steroidogenesis such as aminoglutethimide, cyanoketone, and ketoconazole. Some fungicides inhibit estrogen synthesis by inhibiting aromatase activity in the testis, which has an effect on testosterone to estrogen. Through a set of signals at transcriptional and translational levels, EDCs make further efforts to transform the biosynthesis of protein mediated by gonadal steroids [19].

Hormones react with their target tissues directly by interacting with membrane-bound receptors or intracellular receptors. The vital procedure in the function of hormones is the specific binding of natural ligand to its receptors. Intracellular or nuclear receptors interact with specific DNA sequences regulating gene transcription in a ligand-dependent pattern. This procedure might be changed by many environmental factors through mimicking the natural ligand and serving as an agonist or inhibiting the binding and serving as an antagonist. The most notable examples are methoxychlor, chlordecone, DDT, some polychlorinated biphenyls, and alkylphenols, which can disturb the function of estrogen receptors [20].

Epigenetic modifications characterized by DNA methylation, histone modifications, and chromatin remodeling are important regulators in spermatogenesis. Studies have shown that aberrant epigenetic modifications are associated with disturbed spermatogenesis and male infertility [21–23]. Exposure of gametes to environmental factors may cause alterations in sperm. In addition, more and more studies have demonstrated that many EDCs have transgenerational effect of spermatogenic failure through epigenetic mechanism [3, 24].

Clearly, there should be more studies to explore the data gaps. In addition to a few exceptions (e.g., diethylstilbestrol [DES]), the causal relationship between exposure to specific agents and endocrine disruptor-mediated adverse health effects has not been determined. The development and validation of short-term screening studies should be used to clarify the mechanism.

It is possible that these environmental agents such as alkyl phenol ethylate and their degradation products, chlorinated dibenzodioxins, and PCBs can induce irreversible decline in male fertility [2].

3. Lifestyle factors and male infertility

In general, lifestyle factors affect male reproductive system in various ways. In today's society, male infertility has become a more and more important problem. People’s unhealthy lifestyle may be one of the great reasons. Sperm needs a suitable internal and external environment to complete several physiological links such as occurrence, development, maturity, and transportation. Some physical and chemical factors can lead to the damage of the testis and accessory glands, the disorders of the internal environment, and spermatogenesis dysfunction to some extent. Several studies have found that occupation, behavioral habit, dietary habit, and other factors can play a role in the decreased fertility. The following discussion focuses on the association between male infertility and lifestyle factors such as smoking, alcohol consumption, and diet.

3.1. Smoking

As we know, smoking is associated with variable diseases, including respiratory diseases, cardiovascular diseases and cancer of the lung, kidney, urinary bladder, pancreas, and so on [25, 26]. The relationship between smoking and infertilities has been studied for several years.

A vast amount of studies showed the negative effects of smoking on various parameters of semen analysis. In an experiment conducted in Denmark from 1987 to 2004, 2562 men participated; researchers found that heavy smokers had a 19% lower sperm concentration than nonsmokers [27]. Moreover, in another cohort study which involves 1786 men, researchers proved that smoking was associated with a significant decrease in sperm density, total sperm count, total number of motile sperm, and citrate concentration. In addition, sperm vitality, ejaculate volume, and fructose concentration were slightly but nonsignificantly affected [28]. In other aspects, smokers had a significantly decreased semen volumes, sperm motility, and viability compared with nonsmokers. All sperm motion parameters were lower in the smokers except for beat-cross frequency (Hz). Further, the percentage of normal morphology sperm was decreased significantly in smokers, and the sperm morphology was worse with increasing degree of smoking [29]. The experiments have already shown that smoking in daily life damages the semen quality.

Existing data indicate that varicocele plays an important role in male infertility. There are also experiments trying to figure out the relationship between varicocele and smoking. In a study conducted in Iran, percentage of varicocele was significantly higher in smokers compared with nonsmokers [30].

The mechanism behind the negative effect of smoking on semen quality remains vague until today. There are evidences showing that people who smoke possess a higher proportion of spermatozoa with an alteration of the histone to protamine ratio than those who do not smoke, which may lead to male infertility [31]. Also there was a research that revealed the relationship between smoking and seminal plasma zinc level. Semen parameters were also significantly decreased among smokers with abnormal zinc levels, while there was no significant difference between nonsmokers with normal zinc and nonsmokers with abnormal zinc levels [32]. In addition, DNA methylation pattern in sperm DNA can be influenced by cigarette smoking [33]. Aberrant DNA methylation had been shown to be associated with male infertility [34].

3.2. Alcohol consumption

Excessive alcohol intake is always thought of as a cause of liver diseases, kidney diseases, and so on. In addition, alcohol consumption is considered to have an adverse impact on reproductive function. We discuss about its negative influence on the sperm parameters and the endocrine.

There was an interesting case report showing that an azoospermic patient regained normal sperm parameters 3 months after the discontinuation of alcohol consumption, which strongly supported the negative impact of alcohol consumption on male infertility [35]. Firstly, available literatures stated that alcohol consumption may give rise to spermatozoon morphological changes and the changes including breakage of the sperm head, distention of the midsection, and curling of its tail [36]. Moreover, in an experiment conducted by researchers in Argentina, which involved 537 men, it was found that alcohol consumption evoked a tendency toward diminished sperm concentration, motility, viability, and normal morphology [37].

As for its effect on the endocrine, there are masses of such studies reminding people of the impact of alcohol consumption that might cause structural testicular changes, decreased level of testosterone, which might be involved in the phenotype of hypogonadism and feminization. Alcohol and its metabolite acetaldehyde can cause a reduction in luteinizing hormone (LH) binding to Leydig cells, which may inhibit the enzymes involved in the formation of sex hormones [38]. With regard to the mechanism of its negative effects, alcohol seems to exert a dual effect on the HPG axis by directly inhibiting testicular steroidogenesis and by blocking the release of LH-releasing hormone/LH from the hypothalamic-pituitary axis [39].

3.3. Diet

3.3.1. Dietary bias

Scientists found that our daily consumption of cereals, fruits, and each meal a day had a strong bearing on semen quality. Taking proper amounts of minerals, antioxidant vitamins, and essential amino acids can maintain and improve it effectively [40]. There was also a case report conducted in Spain which showed that frequent intake of lipophilic foods like meat products or milk may negatively affect the semen quality in humans, whereas some fruits or vegetables may maintain or improve semen quality [41].

3.3.2. High-energy diets

High-energy diets, especially poor nutritional food intake with lots of unhealthy fat negatively affect semen parameters and fertility. It was described that the intake of processed meat, a source of saturated fats, is associated with poor semen quality [42]. In a cohort study conducted in the America, researchers found high intake of saturated fats was negatively related to sperm concentration whereas higher intake of omega-3 fats was positively related to sperm morphology [43]. However, studies with larger sample size are required to confirm these findings.

High-energy diets may alter testicular metabolism. Testis provides an environment that nurtures the germs cells, ultimately ensuring spermatogenesis and fertility. However, the overconsumption of high-energy diets enables the increase of fatty acid supply within testicular milieu and consequently compromises the key testicular metabolic mechanisms that ultimately compromise germ cells fate [44, 45]. High-energy diets intake disturbs whole-body metabolism and the normal function of the male reproductive axis. Existing data showed that metabolism and reproduction are closely connected [46]. Obesity toxicant from the high-energy foods can promote the development of obesity and the storage of lipid-soluble toxicants in the body. Thereafter, the molecular mechanisms that regulate appetite and energy intake will gradually be disrupted. The abovementioned process cannot be separated from the mediation of gut and adipose hormones. While the major function of gut and adipose tissues is to perceive the energy status of the body, recently, some gut and fat derived hormones are thought to be a regulatory factor in reproductive events. Hence, disruption of the endocrine activity of these tissues may affect the reproductive function [45].

3.4. Other factors

3.4.1. High temperature

Some people who work under an environment with a high temperature such as blacksmith and kettleman or who had to wear clothes which are too tight for them, both factors bring about heat stress to men's testis. The process of spermatogenesis is closely related to the appropriate temperature and occurs optimally at temperature slightly lower than that of the body. Adequate adjustment of the temperature is imperative to maintain a proper testicular temperature. Raised testicular temperature has a harmful effect on spermatogenesis and the resultant spermatozoa. Therefore, thermoregulatory failure leading to heat stress can compromise the sperm quality and increase the risk of infertility [47]. Both the epididymal sperm and testicular germ cells are sensitive to damage by heat stress, which leads to the apoptosis and the damage of DNA [48, 49].

3.4.2. Radiation

Cell phone usage is an indispensable part in people's daily life. As a result of which, several researchers have conducted a lot of experiments. There is a study investigating an association between characteristics of cell phone usage and semen quality [50]. It showed that talking for ≥1 h/day and during device charging was associated with higher rate of abnormal semen concentration. Among men who reported holding their phones ≤50 cm from the groin, a non-significantly higher rate of abnormal sperm concentration was found. Multivariate analysis revealed that talking while charging the device and smoking were risk factors for abnormal sperm concentration. It suggests that certain aspects of cell phone usage may bear adverse effects on sperm concentration.

Concerning the usage of wireless internet, researchers have demonstrated that continuous Wi-Fi exposure with 2.45 GHz affected the testes of growing rats. Avendano et al. divided the motile spermatozoa, from 29 healthy donors, into two aliquots and one of them was exposed to a Wi-Fi computer but not the other. 4 h later, research findings showed that the sperm motility and the sperm DNA fragmentation in Wi-Fi group were significantly decreased and increased, respectively [51]. However, current studies are not able to reveal the relationship well enough, and, therefore, larger scales of studies concerned about this aspect are needed.

4. Conclusion

Accumulating evidence suggests that environmental factors are posing major threats to human reproductive health (**Figure 1**). Impaired spermatogenesis can be incurred by exposures in

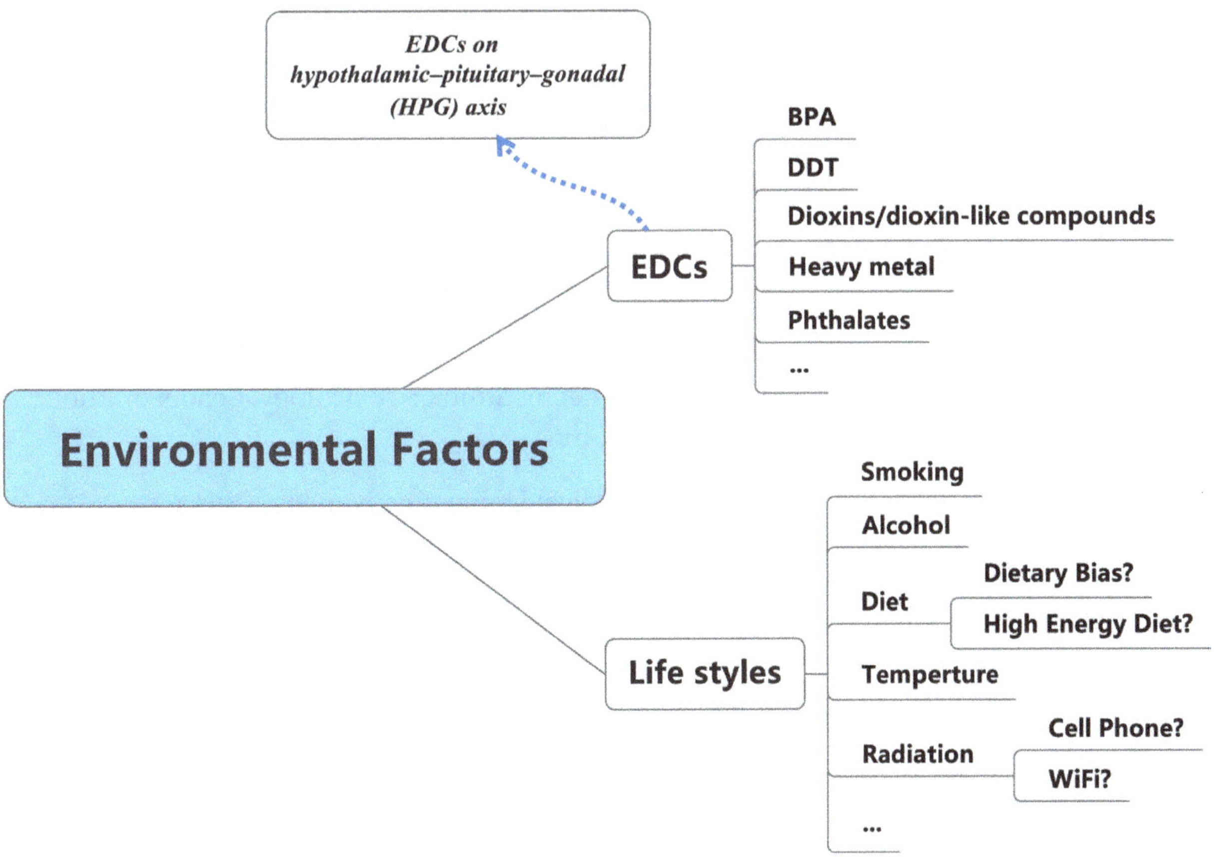

Figure 1. Schematic representation of environmental risk factors of male infertility.

utero, in the neonatal or adolescent periods, or in adulthood, and can have transgenerational effects. Despite promising discoveries, a causal relationship between male infertility and exposure to specific EDC or mixtures of EDCs is yet to be established, due to the degree of EDCs exposure, the sample size of the subjects examined, the complexity of the clinical protocols used, and the determination of the variables measured. Future studies are needed to focus on a uniform system of examining human populations with regard to the exposure to specific EDCs and its direct effect on male infertility. Considering all the lifestyle factors which result in the male infertility, to improve the severe situation of the male infertility, we should try to discontinue smoking and alcohol drinking, avoid high temperature and radiation, and maintain a balanced diet. From now on, if a good and healthy lifestyle is maintained, we will have offspring, bringing endless happiness.

Acknowledgements

This work was supported by National Natural Science Foundation of China (no. 81401213, 81673217), Jiangsu Overseas Visiting Scholar Program for University Prominent Young & Middle-aged Teachers and Presidents, National Key Research and Development Program (2016YFC1000207), and the Priority Academic Program for the Development of Jiangsu Higher Education Institutions (Public Health and Preventive Medicine).

Author details

Qiuqin Tang[1], Wei Wu[2*], Jing Zhang[2], Rong Fan[2] and Mu Liu[3]

*Address all correspondence to: wwu@njmu.edu.cn

1 State Key Laboratory of Reproductive Medicine, Department of Obstetrics, Nanjing Maternity and Child Health Care Hospital Affiliated to Nanjing Medical University, Nanjing, China

2 State Key Laboratory of Reproductive Medicine, Institute of Toxicology, School of Public Health, Nanjing Medical University, Nanjing, China

3 School of Basic Medical Sciences, Nanjing Medical University, Nanjing, China

References

[1] Pasqualotto FF, et al. Effects of medical therapy, alcohol, smoking, and endocrine disruptors on male infertility. Revista do Hospital das Clinicas; Faculdade de Medicina da Universidade de Sao Paulo. 2004;**59**(6):375-382

[2] Sikka SC, Wang R. Endocrine disruptors and estrogenic effects on male reproductive axis. Asian Journal of Andrology. 2008;**10**(1):134-145

[3] Anway MD, et al. Epigenetic transgenerational actions of endocrine disruptors and male fertility. Science. 2005;**308**(5727):1466-1469

[4] Komarowska MD, et al. Serum Bisphenol a level in boys with cryptorchidism: A step to male infertility? International Journal of Endocrinology. 2015;**2015**:973154

[5] Bonde JP, et al. The epidemiologic evidence linking prenatal and postnatal exposure to endocrine disrupting chemicals with male reproductive disorders: A systematic review and meta-analysis. Human Reproduction Update. 2016;**23**(1):104-125

[6] Sifakis S, et al. Human exposure to endocrine disrupting chemicals: Effects on the male and female reproductive systems. Environmental Toxicology and Pharmacology. 2017; **51**:56-70

[7] Bonde JP. Occupational causes of male infertility. Current Opinion in Endocrinology, Diabetes, and Obesity. 2013;**20**(3):234-239

[8] Fenichel P, Chevalier N, Brucker-Davis F. Bisphenol A: An endocrine and metabolic disruptor. Annales d'endocrinologie. 2013;**74**(3):211-220

[9] Rouiller-Fabre V, Habert R, Livera G. Effects of endocrine disruptors on the human fetal testis. Annales d'endocrinologie. 2014;**75**(2):54-57

[10] Mattison DR. The mechanisms of action of reproductive toxins. American Journal of Industrial Medicine. 1983;**4**(1-2):65-79

[11] Brouwer A, et al. Characterization of potential endocrine-related health effects at low-dose levels of exposure to PCBs. Environmental Health Perspectives. 1999;**107**(Suppl 4): 639-649

[12] Bonefeld-Jorgensen EC, Ghisari M, Wielsoe M, Bjerregaard-Olesen C, Kjeldsen LS, Long M. Biomonitoring and hormone-disrupting effect biomarkers of persistent organic pollutants in vitro and ex vivo. Basic Clin Pharmacol Toxicol. Jul 2014;**115**(1):118-28

[13] Bruner-Tran KL, et al. Developmental exposure of mice to dioxin promotes transgenerational testicular inflammation and an increased risk of preterm birth in unexposed mating partners. PLoS One. 2014;**9**(8):e105084

[14] Galimova EF, Amirova ZK, Galimov Sh N. Dioxins in the semen of men with infertility. Environmental Science and Pollution Research International. 2015;**22**(19):14566-14569

[15] Oguz F, et al. Aminoguanidine prevents testicular damage-induced-2,3,7,8-tetrachlorodibenzo-p-dioxin (TCDD) in male rats. Andrologia. 2013;**45**(4):225-231

[16] Queiroz EK, Waissmann W. Occupational exposure and effects on the male reproductive system. Cadernos de Saúde Pública. 2006;**22**(3):485-493

[17] Wang Q, et al. Developmental exposure to the organophosphorus flame retardant tris(1,3-dichloro-2-propyl) phosphate: Estrogenic activity, endocrine disruption and reproductive effects on zebrafish. Aquatic Toxicology. 2015;**160**:163-171

[18] Yuan B, et al. From the cover: Metabolomics reveals a role of betaine in prenatal DBP exposure-induced epigenetic transgenerational failure of spermatogenesis in rats. Toxicological Sciences. 2017;**158**(2):356-366

[19] Manavathi B, Kumar R. Steering estrogen signals from the plasma membrane to the nucleus: Two sides of the coin. Journal of Cellular Physiology. 2006;**207**(3):594-604

[20] White R, et al. Environmentally persistent alkylphenolic compounds are estrogenic. Endocrinology. 1994;**135**(1):175-182

[21] Wu W, et al. Idiopathic male infertility is strongly associated with aberrant promoter methylation of methylenetetrahydrofolate reductase (MTHFR). PLoS One. 2010;**5**(11): e13884

[22] Rotondo JC, et al. Methylation loss at H19 imprinted gene correlates with methylenetetrahydrofolate reductase gene promoter hypermethylation in semen samples from infertile males. Epigenetics. 2013;**8**(9):990-997

[23] Urdinguio RG, et al. Aberrant DNA methylation patterns of spermatozoa in men with unexplained infertility. Human Reproduction. 2015;**30**(5):1014-1028

[24] Guerrero-Bosagna C, Skinner MK. Environmentally induced epigenetic transgenerational inheritance of male infertility. Current Opinion in Genetics & Development. 2014; **26**:79-88

[25] Sasco AJ, Secretan MB, Straif K. Tobacco smoking and cancer: A brief review of recent epidemiological evidence. Lung Cancer. 2004;**45**(Suppl 2):S3-S9

[26] Jung KJ, Jeon C, Jee SH. The effect of smoking on lung cancer: Ethnic differences and the smoking paradox. Epidemiology and Health. 2016;**38**:e2016060

[27] Ramlau-Hansen CH, et al. Is smoking a risk factor for decreased semen quality? A cross-sectional analysis. Human Reproduction. 2007;**22**(1):188-196

[28] Jarow JP. Semen quality of male smokers and nonsmokers in infertile couples. The Journal of Urology. 2003;**170**(2 Pt 1):675-676

[29] Zhang ZH, et al. Decline of semen quality and increase of leukocytes with cigarette smoking in infertile men. Iranian Journal of Reproductive Medicine. 2013;**11**(7):589-596

[30] Shafi H, et al. Prevalence of Varicocele among primary and secondary infertile men: Association with occupation, smoking and drinking alcohol. North American Journal of Medical Sciences. 2014;**6**(10):532-535

[31] Hamad MF, et al. Impact of cigarette smoking on histone (H2B) to protamine ratio in human spermatozoa and its relation to sperm parameters. Andrology. 2014;**2**(5):666-677

[32] Liu RZ, et al. Seminal plasma zinc level may be associated with the effect of cigarette smoking on sperm parameters. The Journal of International Medical Research. 2010;**38**(3):923-928

[33] Laqqan M, et al. Aberrant DNA methylation patterns of human spermatozoa in current smoker males. Reproductive Toxicology. 2017;**71**:126-133

[34] Rajender S, Avery K, Agarwal A. Epigenetics, spermatogenesis and male infertility. Mutation Research. 2011;**727**(3):62-71

[35] Sermondade N, et al. Progressive alcohol-induced sperm alterations leading to spermatogenic arrest, which was reversed after alcohol withdrawal. Reproductive Biomedicine Online. 2010;**20**(3):324-327

[36] Hadi HA, Hill JA, Castillo RA. Alcohol and reproductive function: A review. Obstetrical & Gynecological Survey. 1987;**42**(2):69-74

[37] von Kanel R, et al. Effects of dark chocolate consumption on the prothrombotic response to acute psychosocial stress in healthy men. Thrombosis and Haemostasis. 2014;**112**(6): 1151-1158

[38] Muthusami KR, Chinnaswamy P. Effect of chronic alcoholism on male fertility hormones and semen quality. Fertility and Sterility. 2005;**84**(4):919-924

[39] Kuller LH, May SJ, Perper JA. The relationship between alcohol, liver disease, and testicular pathology. American Journal of Epidemiology. 1978;**108**(3):192-199

[40] Eskenazi B, et al. Antioxidant intake is associated with semen quality in healthy men. Human Reproduction. 2005;**20**(4):1006-1012

[41] Mendiola J, et al. Food intake and its relationship with semen quality: A case-control study. Fertility and Sterility. 2009;**91**(3):812-818

[42] Jensen TK, et al. High dietary intake of saturated fat is associated with reduced semen quality among 701 young Danish men from the general population. The American Journal of Clinical Nutrition. 2013;**97**(2):411-418

[43] Attaman JA, et al. Dietary fat and semen quality among men attending a fertility clinic. Human Reproduction. 2012;**27**(5):1466-1474

[44] Rato L, et al. High-energy diets may induce a pre-diabetic state altering testicular glycolytic metabolic profile and male reproductive parameters. Andrology. 2013;**1**(3):495-504

[45] Rato L, et al. High-energy diets: A threat for male fertility? Obesity Reviews. 2014; **15**(12):996-1007

[46] Crown A, Clifton DK, Steiner RA. Neuropeptide signaling in the integration of metabolism and reproduction. Neuroendocrinology. 2007;**86**(3):175-182

[47] Durairajanayagam D, Agarwal A, Ong C. Causes, effects and molecular mechanisms of testicular heat stress. Reproductive Biomedicine Online. 2015;**30**(1):14-27

[48] Zhu B, et al. Effect of paternal heat stress on the development in vitro of preimplantation embryos in the mouse. Andrologia. 2004;**36**(6):384-394

[49] Yin Y, DeWolf WC, Morgentaler A. p53 is associated with the nuclear envelope in mouse testis. Biochemical and Biophysical Research Communications. 1997;**235**(3):689-694

[50] Zilberlicht A, et al. Habits of cell phone usage and sperm quality—does it warrant attention? Reproductive Biomedicine Online. 2015;**31**(3):421-426

[51] Avendano C, et al. Use of laptop computers connected to internet through Wi-Fi decreases human sperm motility and increases sperm DNA fragmentation. Fertility and Sterility. 2012;**97**(1):39-45 e2

4

Spermatozoa - Facts and Perspectives

Rosanna Chianese and Rosaria Meccariello

1. Spermatozoa morphology and physiology: an introduction

Sperm cells (SPZ) are derived from spermatogenesis, a highly regulated developmental process starting from diploid precursors—spermatogonial stem cells—that undergo strictly orchestrated mitotic and meiotic divisions to form round spermatids. Extensive morphological and biochemical transformations in post-meiotic phase are required to differentiate round spermatids into highly specialized SPZ [1–3]. Thus, during spermiogenesis, the round spermatids transform into specialized and polarized cells that exhibit: at proximal end, the head containing an elongated and transcriptionally inactive nucleus which is apically surrounded by the Golgi-derived acrosome, and at the distal end, a tail surrounded at its proximal mid-pieces by mitochondrial sheet. A part from acrosome biogenesis, the spermiogenesis accounts for a radical chromatin remodeling that causes genome silencing [4] through histone replacement with transition proteins, firstly, and protamines later, to obtain a tightly packaged chromatin [5]. In parallel, a global reorganization of cytoplasmatic/cytoskeleton architecture drives elongation step with the development of a flagellum and the formation of cytoplasmic droplets which contain the excess cytoplasm.

In mammals, two post-testicular maturational events are required so that SPZ may reach their fertilization ability: the former occurring in the epididymis, the latter in female reproductive tract. The epididymis is a long convoluted tubule characterized by three main morphologically and functionally distinct regions (proximal caput, elongated corpus, and distal cauda) [6]. It represents the extracellular microenvironment in which a fine crosstalk between SPZ and epididymis epithelial cells takes place, generally through vesicles known as epididymosomes [7]. During their journey along the epididymis, SPZ remodel the lipid content of plasma membrane, especially cholesterol, receive a rich and complex repertoire of protein and non-coding RNAs (ncRNAs), especially microRNAs (miRNAs), long non-coding RNA

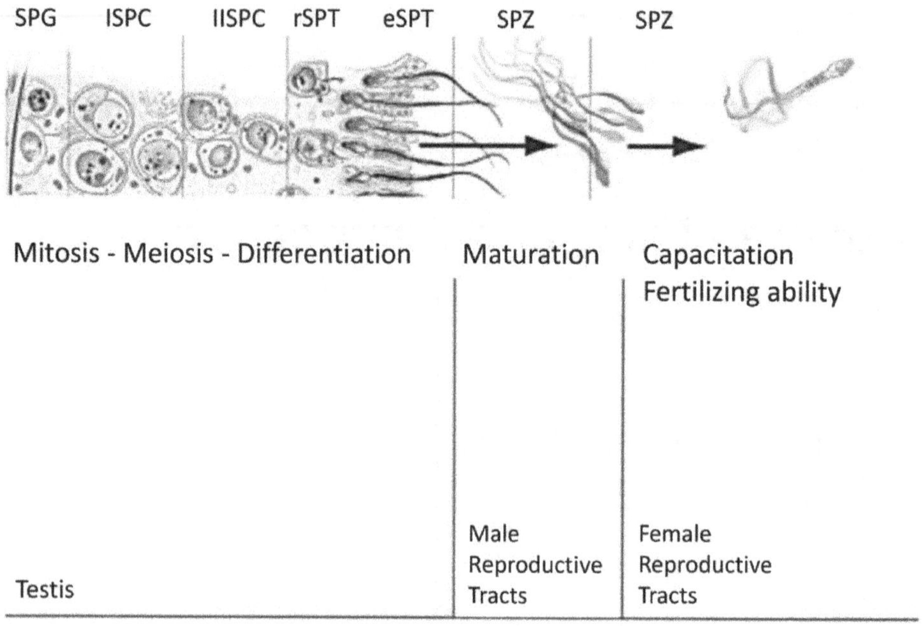

Figure 1. Schematic view of the main events characterizing spermatogenesis in testis, followed by spermatozoa (SPZ) maturation in male reproductive tracts and capacitation/fertilizing ability in female reproductive tracts. SPG: spermatogonia; ISPC: primary spermatocytes; IISPC: secondary spermatocytes; rSPT: round spermatids; eSPT: elongating spermatids; SPZ: spermatozoa.

(lncRNA), and tRNA fragments (tRFs) [8], and lastly they acquire progressive motility. After epididymal maturation, SPZ are still incapable to fertilize eggs; they have to spend some time in the female reproductive tract before they acquire this competence (fertilizing ability) through the capacitation process [9]. During this phase, SPZ undergo other important biochemical modifications in terms of steroid removal or protein modifications [10]; after that, they interact with cumulus-cell oocyte complex to penetrate the matrix of the cumulus oophorus [11]. Capacitated SPZ are subjected to acrosome reaction, a prerequisite event for sperm-egg fusion [12], then they penetrate the zona pellucida, to meet and fuse with the egg plasma membrane [13]. After this fusion, finely controlled by a large body of proteins, SPZ deliver to the oocyte their haploid genome. **Figure 1** summarizes the main features of spermatogenesis and SPZ maturation.

2. The control of spermatogenesis and sperm quality

Intricate neuronal circuitries, mainly governed by hypothalamic kisspeptin and gonadotropin releasing hormone (GnRH) reciprocal communications, centrally orchestrate reproduction [1] and lead to pituitary gonadotropin discharge and sex steroid biosynthesis in order to sustain spermatogenesis and sperm release. In addition to hormonal milieu, a complex network of intratesticular cell-to-cell communications regulates germ cell progression, coordinating mitosis, meiosis, differentiation, and maturation [2, 3]. Thus, SPZ morphological feature is critical to ensure proper physiological activity.

Spermatogenesis is highly sensitive to environmental stressors as energy availability, stress, life style, temperature, pollutants, heavy metals, or endocrine disruptor chemicals that act at several levels along the hypothalamus-pituitary-gonad axis [14–16]. In this respect, the activity of molecular chaperone/cochaperone, ubiquitination, but also DNA repair systems and antioxidants defenses ensures the physiological progression of spermatogenesis, avoids that damaged germ cells differentiate into SPZ, and deeply contributes to produce high-quality mature SPZ [17–19].

Conversely, impaired autocrine/paracrine/endocrine communication along the hypothalamus-pituitary-gonadal axis may impact spermatogenesis and have deleterious effects on male fertility due to: (1) spermatogenesis arrest and lack of SPZ, as in the case of hypogonadotropic hypogonadism; (2) defective production of gonadotropins/sex steroids with outcomes on spermatogenesis onset/progression and SPZ maturation; and (3) low sperm count and/or the production of defective spermatozoa with morphological abnormalities or impaired motility [20]. However, in 30–40% of male infertility cases, the etiology remains unknown and infertility is therefore idiopathic, being a multifactorial disorder in which molecular defects in spermatogenesis and sperm function occur [21].

3. Upcoming issue for paternal epigenetic inheritance

Once considered just a "carrier" for male haploid genome at fertilization, nowadays, the functional role of SPZ has been revised. In fact, a part haploid genome, SPZ, preserve some sperm-specific RNA components, absent in the oocyte, such as fragments of longer transcripts, able to control early embryogenesis [22–24]. Mature SPZ also contain a rich repertoire of ncRNAs, such as miRNAs, tRFs, lncRNAs, and PIWI-interacting RNAs (piRNAs). Their deregulation not only alters SPZ physiology but may affect SPZ contribution to a regular embryo development, through epigenetic dynamics [25], since there is a need to focus more attention on SPZ as carrier of transgenerational epigenetic inheritance.

The specific epigenetic signatures of SPZ include DNA methylation status, chromatin remodeling, and ncRNA pools. Unlike somatic cells, germ cells have hypomethylated DNA [26], and genome-wide hypermethylation of sperm DNA status is associated with pregnancy failure [27]. As reported in the previous paragraph, chromatin remodeling, made possible through histone replacement by protamines, is a key step of spermiogenesis and does not occur in ovogenesis [5, 28]. Interestingly, a deregulated histone-protamine exchange induces DNA damage and male subfertility [29]. A small percentage of paternal genome retains histones and reveals a nucleosome organization, in not random distribution, thus affecting transcription factor accessibility to DNA at specific gene loci [30]. Furthermore, together with a well-known histone code, a protamine code has been suggested in SPZ [31]. Lastly, sperm RNA cargo plays an important role in SPZ epigenetic landscape. Several classes of RNAs have been identified in SPZ [32] and their possible contribution in the regulation of gene expression in embryo is currently under investigation. Surely these small RNAs take part in the sperm epigenetic transgenerational pattern of inheritance because they are vulnerable to paternal exposure to various forms of stress and they are able to regulate developmental trajectories of the offspring. In fact, a high-fat diet (HFD) in male mice alters sperm miRNA content and, thus, glucose tolerance in both male and female offspring [33]. Similarly, sperm tRNA fragments injected from HFD males or from male mice with a protein restriction status to normal zygotes are vehicles of transgenerational transmission of metabolic disorders in the offspring [34, 35].

Therefore, DNA methylation, posttranslational histone modifications, chromatin remodeling, and ncRNA activity are plastic epigenetic mechanisms, modifiable in response to environmental and behavioral events and heritable from father to the offspring as an acquired mark [36]. This also means that paternal lifestyle or experiences, including physical activity, nutrition, and exposure to pollutants, can alter SPZ epigenome, with male infertility, embryo development failure, abnormal embryonic molecular makeup, and disease susceptibility of the offspring as a result [37].

4. Conclusions

The assessment of SPZ quality represents the main bioindicator of male fertility and the analysis of seminal plasma is a valid diagnostic instrument for male fertility, since it is enriched with molecules indicative of SPZ quality status. Furthermore, impressive advances have been made in conferring to SPZ a role in embryo development and in considering SPZ a carrier of "paternal experience" to the offspring. As a consequence, the combined assessments of SPZ quality and (epi)genetic study are necessary for the diagnosis and the development of personalized treatment for male infertility and to preserve embryo development and offspring health.

Acknowledgements

The authors apologize for unintended omission of any relevant references.

Conflict of interest

The authors declare that there is no conflict of interest regarding the publication of this chapter.

Author details

Rosanna Chianese[1] and Rosaria Meccariello[2]*

*Address all correspondence to: rosaria.meccariello@uniparthenope.it

1 Department of Experimental Medicine sec. "F. Bottazzi", University of Campania "L. Vanvitelli", Italy

2 Department of Movement Sciences and Wellbeing, University of Naples "Parthenope", Naples, Italy

References

[1] Pierantoni R, Cobellis G, Meccariello R, Fasano S. Evolutionary aspects of cellular communication in the vertebrate hypothalamo-hypophysio-gonadal axis. International Review of Cytology. 2002;**218**:69-141

[2] Cobellis G, Meccariello R, Pierantoni R, Fasano S. Intratesticular signals for progression of germ cell stages in vertebrates. General and Comparative Endocrinology. 2003; **134**:220-228

[3] Meccariello R, Chianese R, Chioccarelli T, Ciaramella V, Fasano S, Pierantoni R, Cobellis G. Intra-testicular signals regulate germ cell progression and production of qualitatively mature spermatozoa in vertebrates. Frontiers in Endocrinology (Lausanne). 2014;**5**:69

[4] Marcon L, Boissonneault G. Transient DNA strand breaks during mouse and human spermiogenesis: new insights in stage specificity and link to chromatin remodeling. Biology of Reproduction. 2004;**70**:910-918

[5] Miller D, Brinkworth M, Iles D. Paternal DNA packaging in spermatozoa: more than the sum of its parts? DNA, histones, protamines and epigenetics. Reproduction. 2010;**139**:287-301

[6] Cornwall GA. New insights into epididymal biology and function. Human Reproduction. 2009;**15**:213-227

[7] Sullivan R, Saez F. Epididymosomes, prostasomes, and liposomes: Their roles in mammalian male reproductive physiology. Reproduction. 2013;**146**:R21-R35

[8] Belleannée C, Calvo É, Caballero J, Sullivan R. Epididymosomes convey different repertoires of microRNAs throughout the bovine epididymis. Biology of Reproduction. 2013;**89**:30

[9] Chang MC. Fertilizing capacity of spermatozoa deposited into the fallopian tubes. Nature. 1951;**168**:697-698

[10] De Jonge C. Biological basis for human capacitation. Human Reproduction Update. 2005; **11**:205-214

[11] Sun F, Bahat A, Gakamsky A, Girsh E, Katz N, Giojalas LC, Tur-Kaspa I, Eisenbach M. Human sperm chemotaxis: both the oocyte and its surrounding cumulus cells secrete sperm chemoattractants. Human Reproduction. 2005;**20**:761-767

[12] Cross NL, Meizel S. Methods for evaluating the acrosomal status of mammalian sperm. Biology of Reproduction. 1989;**41**:635-641

[13] Ikawa M, Inoue N, Benham AM, Okabe M. Fertilization: a sperm's journey to and interaction with the oocyte. Journal of Clinical Investigation. 2010;**120**:984-994

[14] Chianese R, Cobellis G, Chioccarelli T, Ciaramella V, Migliaccio M, Fasano S, Pierantoni R, Meccariello R. Kisspeptins, Estrogens and male fertility. Current Medicinal Chemistry. 2016;**23**:4070-4091

[15] Chianese R, Troisi J, Richards S, Scafuro M, Fasano S, Guida M, Pierantoni R, Meccariello R. Bisphenol A in reproduction: Epigenetic effects. Current Medicinal Chemistry. 2018;**25**:748-770

[16] Chianese R, Coccurello R, Viggiano A, Scafuro M, Fiore M, Coppola G, Operto FF, Fasano S, Layé S, Pierantoni R, Meccariello R. Impact of dietary fats on brain functions. Current Neuropharmacology. Oct 17, 2017. DOI: 10.2174/1570159X15666171017102547

[17] Meccariello R, Chianese R, Ciaramella V, Fasano S, Pierantoni R. Molecular chaperones, cochaperones, and ubiquitination/deubiquitination system: Involvement in the production of high quality spermatozoa. Biomed Research International. 2014;**2014**:561426

[18] Sutovsky P, Moreno R, Ramalho-Santos J, Dominko T, Thompson WE, Schatten G. A putative, ubiquitin-dependent mechanism for the recognition and elimination of defective spermatozoa in the mammalian epididymis. Journal of Cell Science. 2001;**114**:1665-1675

[19] Hartl FU, Hayer-Hartl M. Molecular chaperones in the cytosol: from nascent chain to folded protein. Science. 2002;**295**:1852-1858

[20] Ray PF, Toure A, Metzler-Guillemain C, Mitchell MJ, Arnoult C, Coutton C. Genetic abnormalities leading to qualitative defects of sperm morphology or function. Clinical Genetics. 2017;**91**:217-232

[21] Bracke A, Peeters K, Punjabi U, Hoogewijs D, Dewilde S. A search for molecular mechanisms underlying male idiopathic infertility. Reproductive Biomedicine Online. 2018;**36**:327-339

[22] Miller D, Ostermeier GC. Towards a better understanding of RNA carriage by ejaculate spermatozoa. Human Reproduction Update. 2006;**12**:757-767

[23] Lalancette C, Miller D, Li Y, Krawetz SA. Paternal contributions: new functional insights for spermatozoal RNA. Journal of Cellular Biochemistry. 2008;**104**:1570-1579

[24] Sendler E, Johnson GD, Mao S, Goodrich RJ, Diamond MP, Hauser R, Krawetz SA. Stability, delivery and functions of human sperm RNAs at fertilization. Nucleic Acids Research. 2013;**41**:4104-4117

[25] Casas E, Vavouri T. Sperm epigenomics: Challenges and opportunities. Frontiers in Genetics. 2014;**5**:330

[26] Oakes CC, La Salle S, Smiraglia DJ, Robaire B, Trasler JM. A unique configuration of genome-wide DNA methylation patterns in the testis. Proceedings of the National Academy of Sciences USA. 2007;**104**:228-233

[27] Benchaib M, Braun V, Ressnikof D, Lornage J, Durand P, Niveleau A, Guérin JF. Influence of global sperm DNA methylation on IVF results. Human Reproduction. 2005;**20**:768-773

[28] Steger K, Klonisch T, Gavenis K, Drabent B, Doenecke D, Bergmann M. Expression of mRNA and protein of nucleoproteins during human spermiogenesis. Molecular of Human Reproduction. 1998;**4**:939-945

[29] Ni K, Spiess AN, Schuppe HC, Steger K. The impact of sperm protamine deficiency and sperm DNA damage on human male fertility: A systematic review and meta-analysis. Andrology. 2016;**4**:789-799

[30] Siklenka K, Erkek S, Godmann M, Lambrot R, McGraw S, Lafleur C, Cohen T, Xia J, Suderman M, Hallett M, Trasler J, Peters AH, Kimmins S. Disruption of histone methylation in developing sperm impairs offspring health transgenerationally. Science. 2015; **350**:aab2006

[31] Brunner AM, Nanni P, Mansuy IM. Epigenetic marking of sperm by post-translational modification of histones and protamines. Epigenetics & Chromatin. 2014;**7**:2

[32] Carrell DT, Aston KI, Oliva R, Emery BR, De Jonge CJ. The "omics" of human male infertility: integrating big data in a systems biology approach. Cell and Tissue Research. 2016;**363**:295-312

[33] Fullston T, Ohlsson Teague EM, Palmer NO, DeBlasio MJ, Mitchell M, Corbett M, Print CG, Owens JA, Lane M. Paternal obesity initiates metabolic disturbances in two generations of mice with incomplete penetrance to the F2 generation and alters the transcriptional profile of testis and sperm microRNA content. FASEB Journal. 2013;**27**:4226-4243

[34] Chen Q, Yan M, Cao Z, Li X, Zhang Y, Shi J, Feng GH, Peng H, Zhang X, Zhang Y, J3 Q, Duan E, Zhai Q, Zhou Q. Sperm tsRNAs contribute to intergenerational inheritance of an acquired metabolic disorder. Science. 2016;**351**:397-400

[35] Sharma U, Conine CC, Shea JM, Boskovic A, Derr AG, Bing XY, Belleannee C, Kucukural A, Serra RW, Sun F, Song L, Carone BR, Ricci EP, Li XZ, Fauquier L, Moore MJ, Sullivan R, Mello CC, Garber M, Rando OJ. Biogenesis and function of tRNA fragments during sperm maturation and fertilization in mammals. Science. 2016;**351**:391-396

[36] van Otterdijk SD, Michels KB. Transgenerational epigenetic inheritance in mammals: How good is the evidence? FASEB Journal. 2016;**30**:2457-2465

[37] Schagdarsurengin U, Steger K. Epigenetics in male reproduction: effect of paternal diet on sperm quality and offspring health. Nature Reviews Urology. 2016;**13**:584-595

5

Interacytoplasmic Morphologically Selected Sperm Injection: A Tool for Selecting the Best Sperm in Real Time

Yona Barak and Adrian Ellenbogen

Abstract

Routine sperm parameters are used to evaluate fertility potential of the male partner. Since the introduction of intracytoplasmic sperm injection (ICSI), it seems that the importance of routine parameters of sperm morphology has decreased in the field of assisted reproduction. ICSI has facilitated to achieve fertilization, embryo development, and pregnancies, from the treatment of males with poor-quality spermatozoa. Morphology is the only criteria for sperm aspiration during ICSI. Routine criteria are based on the raw ejaculate-stained sperm cells. Thus, it is important to score and aspirate a good-quality motile spermatozoon, which will contribute to the quality of the developing embryo after ICSI, in real time of the procedure. In ICSI, assessment of sperm morphology is limited due to the low magnification (200 × 400×) and concomitant low resolution. By using intracytoplasmic morphologically selected sperm injection (IMSI), it was demonstrated that a spermatozoon with normal morphology, and more precisely normal nucleus, might affect the incidence of pregnancy. Although the usage of IMSI is currently wider, it is necessary to standardize which sperm to aspirate, due to criteria based on accumulating data. Correlation to DNA integrity, embryo development in vitro, female age, male age, or the routine use of IMSI for all cases are raised in order to maximize the efficiency of IMSI technology.

Keywords: IMSI, high magnification, sperm morphology, ICSI, embryo quality, sperm quality, real time sperm selection, IVF

1. Introduction

Following dedicated research and treatment of Patrick Steptoe and Robert G Edward in Bourn Hall, Cambridge, the first in vitro fertilization (IVF) baby girl Louise Brown was born in 1978. This revolutionary assisted reproductive technology (ART) attempt brought the fulfillment of a vision to hundreds of thousands of infertile couples to conceive and deliver. The main idea behind the development of the technique was treating women with mechanical factor infertility. Despite the great success of IVF, poor results were obtained in cases of severe male infertility. IVF outcome was satisfactory when oocytes were inseminated with >1.5 million spermatozoa and at least 50% motility could be observed in the specimen. This major limitation of sperm insemination in routine IVF was overcome by intracytoplasmic sperm injection (ICSI), introduced by Palermo in 1992 [1]. The injection of a single sperm into an oocyte, which revealed fertilization and development of viable in vitro embryos, gave a rapid solution to men with severe forms of male factor infertility, allowed application to other forms of infertility. Nowadays, it serves as the main tool for assisting couples to fulfill their wish to conceive [2]. Furthermore, it is also used for various infertility indications as low number and poor morphology of oocytes, thick zona pellucida, pre-implantation genetic diagnosis or screening (PGD, PGS), cases of hepatitis C and human immunodeficiency virus, in vitro maturation, and oocyte cryopreservation. The usage of ICSI enabled to achieve fertilization, embryo development, pregnancies, and deliveries. It has been reported that strict morphologic criteria do not affect ICSI outcomes [3–9]. On the other hand, scientists indicated that the paternal gamete influences the resulting embryo, mainly at the level of blastocyst formation. Several points of negative paternal impact, both genetic and epigenetic, have been identified in embryos following the injection of poor-quality spermatozoa into the oocyte. Using ICSI also clarified some points of the paternal influence on the embryo development, mainly in vitro [10–20]. The specific injected sperm might affect the health of the newborns [21]. Several years ago, a series of reports pointed out that children born as a result of ART were found to have increased frequencies of a number of diseases known to have an epigenetic etiology [22–26], mainly after ICSI [27, 28]. Recently, Santos et al. evaluated the genome-wide DNA methylation together with chromatin organization in human embryos derived by either IVF or ICSI. In this report it was found that infertility per se, rather than ART procedures, may play an important part in predisposition to epimutations that leads to diseases of an epigenetic basis. Interestingly, embryos developing to the blastocyst stage had an apparently normal epigenotype irrespective of the procedure used. These investigators concluded that ICSI per se does not lead to an increased incidence of epigenetic errors [29]. It is accepted that routine morphology characteristics may not necessarily describe the quality of the specific single spermatozoon that was injected into the oocyte. Semen analyses, which describe the general picture of sperm quality of the raw ejaculate, are based on the examination of fixed and stained sperm cells. The latest, obviously, is not suitable for treatment any more. Aspiration of a specific sperm cell, and its injection into the oocyte, during ICSI, regularly takes place under the magnification of 200× or 400×. The sperm cell is randomly chosen when spermatozoa with major morphological abnormalities are generally omitted due to the experienced eyes of the embryologist. It is questionable as to what tool should be used to evaluate morphological criteria in real time during ICSI, which will enable to select a specific spermatozoon, with the highest predictive value for better fertilization, embryo developmental, implantation and pregnancy. De Vos et al. showed a correlation between the gross morphology of the individual injected sperm cell and the formation and development of the resultant embryo. These scientists admitted that the low magnification (e.g. magnification of 400× during ICSI) and concomitant low resolution of the morphology of the motile sperm cell have been the limiting factors of their study [30]. It was demonstrated that using a high-power inverted light microscope with a zoom ≥6000× for the examination of motile spermatozoa in real time might positively affect the outcome of ICSI, in terms of fertilization rate, embryo development, and the occurrence of pregnancies [31–35].

2. Intracytoplasmic morphologically selected sperm injection step by step

2.1. The principle of the IMSI microscope

The term IMSI was defined by Bartoov et al. [32, 33]. The idea was based on the magnification up to 6000× and more of the motile sperm cell in real time [33, 35–38]. The sperm analysis is performed using an interference phase contrast inverted microscope with the optics of Nomarski. The magnified image of the sperm cell is displayed on a screen. The final magnification of the "on-screen image" is actually a combination of the magnification of the objective, the camera adapter, ratio between the diagonal screen size in mm, diagonal of the camera chip size in mm, and internal magnification of the microscope. Depending upon these specific characteristics of an IMSI system, the final value of the magnification might vary from 6000× to 6600× as described earlier. It should be clarified that the final various magnifications achieved in IMSI are actually a result of zoom on the image of the sperm cell, which magnifies the structures of its surface and cannot be observed in magnification of 200–400×, due to objective limitations of the human eyes.

2.2. Preparation of the IMSI dish

The high magnification of the objective (100×) with the optics of Nomarski requires a dish with a glass bottom. Droplets of the medium, approximately droplets from 1 to 4 μl, should be located on the dish as described in the diagram of an IMSI dish (**Figure 1**).

In **Figure 1**, the diagram of the IMSI dish describes the arrangement of the observation droplets with spermatozoa, droplets with PVP, droplets of clean medium for the selected spermatozoa, and clean droplets for the injection of the oocytes. The latest should be replaced with fresh droplets of media, prior to the ICSI procedure.

Observation droplets: three droplets of 2 μl are located in the left side of the dish. In these droplets, 1 μl of the processed sperm cells of the sperm ejaculate will be inserted. These droplets of the sperm culture medium might contain, in correlation with the intensity of the sperm motility, between 0 and 10% polyvinylpyrrolidone (PVP) solution [34].

Clean droplets of a clean sperm culture medium: this is required to host the scored sperm cells after the evaluation. In each droplet, aspirated spermatozoa with a distinct morphological score are located.

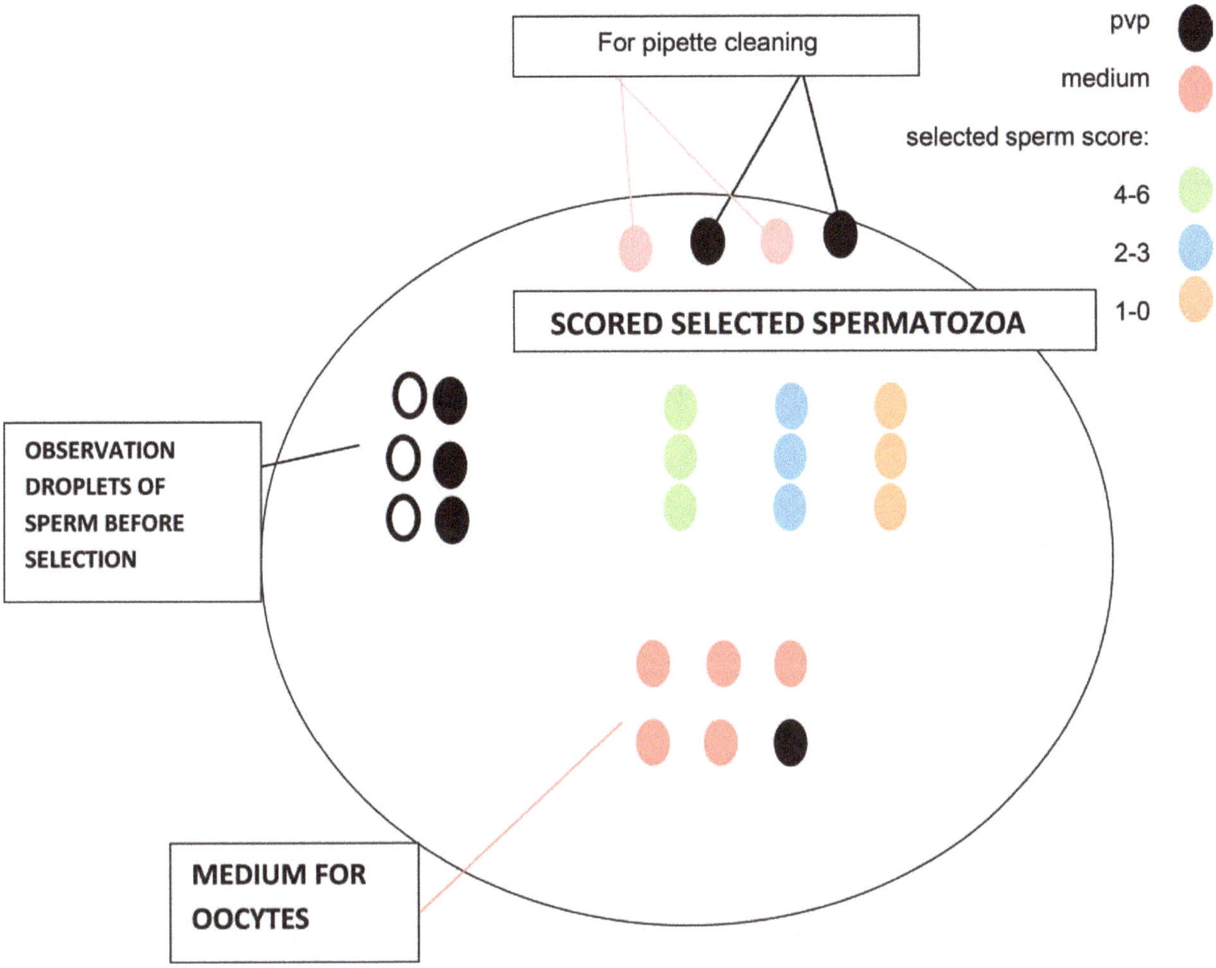

Figure 1. Diagram of an IMSI dish.

Clean droplet of PVP 10%: droplets of 1 μl are located in parallel to the droplets with the spermatozoa. When the intensity of the processed spermatozoa is not high, the authors like to create tiny "bridges" between these two droplets. The tiny bride will allow the passage of spermatozoa to the 10% PVP droplet and it eases the detection on the spermatozoa, as motility of the examined spermatozoa is slowed down. It is recommended to draw tiny extensions from the rim of the PVP droplets to capture the heads of the motile sperm cells. All droplets should be covered by mineral culture oil, which is generally used for the ICSI procedure.

The authors recommend that based on their existing design of the IMSI dish, each laboratory should adapt its special design for the arrangement of the droplets, in accordance with the preference of the laboratory where the ICSI procedure takes place.

3. IMSI in practice

The freshly ejaculated semen is centrifuged at approximately 360 ×*g* for 10 min. In cases when sperm concentration is <5 × 10^6, centrifugation is performed for 1520 min. The pellet is resuspended in 0.5 ml of sperm wash solution (Sperm Preparation Medium, Origio, Denmark). Further assessment is performed by using the bilayer density gradient: 0.5 ml of 50% gradient solution and 0.5 ml of 80% (Supra Sperm Origio, Denmark) for 15 min. In severe oligospermic cases, 0.3 ml of each of the gradient layers is used and centrifugation in 300 × *g* should last up to 1 h [39, 40]. Final sperm pellet is resuspended in 50–100 μl. Approximately a droplet of 1 μl is placed inside the observation droplet of the pre-prepared IMSI dish. During the observation, motile spermatozoa with rough morphological abnormalities are omitted and not aspirated. Other motile sperm cells are aspirated and evaluated inside the ICSI pipette or in the clean PVP droplet and scored as mentioned above. The individual scored sperm cell is then placed into the appropriate droplet, in the IMSI dish [32, 35]. Aspiration of sperm cells is performed by the means of micromanipulations. There is no preference for a certain micromanipulation system. One should work with a system which is the easiest to handle, with his own hands.

3.1. Choosing the sperm

The group of Bartoov classified the selected spermatozoa morphology as "normal" and "second" choice, based on the data collected by scanning and transmission electron microscopy. Some characteristics of the morphology of the head of the sperm cell such as smoothness, symmetry, oval configuration, average length and width (4.75 ± 0.28 and 3.28 ± 0.20 mm, respectively), and nuclear chromatin mass containing no more than one vacuole were defined for normalcy of the sperm nucleus [32, 33]. The "second-choice" motile sperm was not clearly depicted. One might only speculate that during IMSI, when no normal head spermatozoa can be found, the alternative then is to select motile sperm cells that are morphologically the second-best choice.

The Cassuto and Barak Score was developed in order to define more precisely the preferable spermatozoon that should be injected into the oocyte, in real time [35]. This scoring system was established after checking and taking into consideration the sperm defects, which negatively affect the development of the embryo in vitro and had the name of HAVBIC: **H**ead: normalcy and shape, **A**crosome: presence or absence, **V**acuoles: presence or absence, **B**asis of the sperm head, **I**nsertion: the axial position of the sperm, and **C**ytoplasmic droplet: presence or absence. Logistic regression was used for fertilization and embryo development as dependent variables. Coefficients were calculated and tested by comparing receiver operating characteristic (ROC) curves. The best results were achieved with an area under the curve of 0.618, deriving the following formula: Score of spermatozoa = 2 × Head + 3 × Vacuole + 1 × Base. Following these findings, this classification system took into consideration three major parameters of the sperm nucleus: normalcy of shape and size of sperm head, lack of vacuoles and normalcy of the base of the head of the specific spermatozoon. Each of the normal parameter received a value = 1 when normal or = 0 when abnormal. Classification of the individual sperm cell, with a maximum of score 6, is calculated by the embryologist, who performs the IMSI, with this friendly formula, described above, and distinguishes between three classes:

Class 1: spermatozoa of highest quality, score 4–6; class 2: spermatozoa, score 1–3; class 3: low-quality spermatozoa, score 0. In their study a difference was noted between the fertilization rate of oocytes with regard to the classification of the injected spermatozoa ($P < 0.04$; chi square = 6.31). A pair-wise comparison showed a higher fertilization rate in oocytes injected with class 1 spermatozoa in comparison to class 3 ($P < 0.01$; chi square = 6.3). A difference was noted in the development rate into expanded blastocyst ($P < 0.03$; chi square = 6.71), no expanded blastocyst was observed in embryos resulted from injection of class 3 spermatozoa (score of 0) [35].

4. IMSI in patients with a high rate of sperm DNA fragmentation

DNA integrity was assessed by Hazout et al. in 72 patients, referred to IMSI and ICSI. DNA fragmentation rate was evaluated by TUNEL assay. Improvement of clinical outcomes was evident both in patients with an elevated degree of sperm DNA fragmentation and in those with normal sperm DNA status [36]. Similar results were obtained by de Almeida Ferreira Braga et al. and Setti et al., who showed that fertilization and high-quality embryo rates were similar in patients with a high incidence of sperm DNA fragmentation tested in sibling oocytes split into ICSI and IMSI. Their observation suggested that IMSI, but not DNA sperm fragmentation assay per se, could be a beneficial tool in improving IVF-ICSI results [41, 42]. In another independent study no correlation was found between abnormal sperm head morphology as assessed by high magnification (score 0) and DNA fragmentation. However, the rate of chromatin decondensation of their score 0 spermatozoa was twice as high as the spermatozoa that scored 4–6 (19.5% vs. 10.1%; $P < 0.0001$) [43]. This finding might explain the former observation of these researchers that no expanded blastocyst was developed following the injection of spermatozoa with the lowest morphology score [35].

5. IMSI and head-sperm vacuoles

Vanderzwalmen et al., classified the spermatozoa according to the presence and size of vacuoles into four groups: Grade I: normal shape and no vacuoles; Grade II: normal shape and maximum of two small vacuoles; Grade III: normal shape and more than two small vacuoles or one large vacuole; and Grade IV: large vacuoles in conjunction with abnormal head shapes or other abnormalities at the level of the base of the sperm head. The outcome of embryo development in a group of 25 patients after sibling oocyte injection with the four different grades of spermatozoa showed no significant difference in embryo quality up to day 3. However, the occurrence of blastocyst formation was 56.3 and 61.4% with grade I and II spermatozoa, respectively, compared with 5.1% with grade III and 0% with grade IV, respectively ($P < 0.001$) [44]. It is not clear yet why presence of vacuoles in the sperm head is such an important parameter of sperm quality. Some reports showed no correlation between the appearances of vacuoles to male infertility [45–47]. One of these studies was an unpowered investigation [47] and another evaluated the sperm under magnification of 1000× [45]. Many others reported that vacuoles might negatively be associated with male fertility potential [32–37, 44, 48–54]. Moreover, investigation of the relation between sperm vacuoles and acrosome reaction suggested that there might be a negative link between presence of vacuoles and acrosome reaction of the sperm [55, 56]. Consequently, IMSI could be a method for assisting the removal of the acrosome reaction-resistant spermatozoa.

The personal attitude of the authors of the current dissertation is that majority of abnormalities observed under the high magnification of IMSI in real time are probably not visible while using routine conditions with lower magnifications. It is likely, though, that the benefit of scoring scale of the sperm cell is a kind of "fine tuning"; IMSI therefore is more beneficial for motile spermatozoa which have normal morphological appearance under magnification 200–400×.

6. IMSI should not be used for all

It seems that IMSI was a promising revolutionary technique in terms of improving the outcome of ICSI treatments. One might agree that high magnification achieved by the technique contributes with a better evaluation of the aspirated sperm cell for the injection providing encouraging results. On the other hand, prolonged sperm manipulation, special instrumentation, additional number of embryologists who should be trained and expertly perform the technology, and the additional cost for the patients might increase the cost effectiveness of the procedure. Taking all the above into consideration, patients should be given counseling to undergo IMSI, for a better chance to conceive.

It appears that there is no advantage or benefit over standard ICSI in terms of clinical outcome in an unselected infertile population. Although there were trends for higher implantation, clinical pregnancies, and live birth rates in the IMSI group, using the technique did not reveal an improvement in the clinical outcome compared with ICSI [57, 58]. The authors of the current publication, therefore, will try to discuss the benefits of IMSI in cases of patients with repeated implantation failures, severe male factor infertility, and advanced paternal and maternal age.

6.1. Patients with repeated implantation failures

Sixty-two couples with at least two previous consequent pregnancy failures after routine ICSI cycles underwent IMSI in the following cycle. The matched control group comprised 50 couples, who underwent routine ICSI treatment and previously experienced the same number of ICSI failures in the same center. Fertilization and top-quality embryo rates were similar in both groups. A higher pregnancy rate with a lower miscarriage rate were achieved in the IMSI group, in comparison to the control group (66.0% vs. 30.0%; $P < 0.01$; 33.0% vs. 9.0%; $P < 0.01$, respectively) [33]. Following that study, this new concept of sperm selection prior to ICSI was undertaken in additional centers, with encouraging results. Efficacy of IMSI was examined, for instance, in 12 couples with two or more repeated conventional ICSI failures, who underwent an additional conventional ICSI attempt, followed by a high magnification IMSI attempt. Fertilization and cleavage rates and embryo morphology were similar when we compared the two sequential attempts (ICSI attempt vs. the following IMSI cycle). However, improved clinical outcomes such as implantation, pregnancy, delivery, and birth rates were observed in IMSI attempts when compared with ICSI (20.3% vs. 0.8%, 37.6% vs. 2.4%, 33.6% vs. 0.0%, 17.6% vs. 0.0%, respectively; $P < 0.001$) [36]. Another meta-analysis compared the outcomes of conventional ICSI vs. IMSI cycles. It was concluded that IMSI not only improves the percentage of top-quality embryos, implantation, and pregnancy rates but also reduces miscarriage rates as compared with ICSI [59]. Findings of a retrospective study in 42 couples supported the former as well. These scientists examined the efficiency of the IMSI technique in patients with at least three repeated IVF-ICSI failure. The investigators demonstrated superior implantation, clinical pregnancy, and live birth rates in the IMSI group, moreover a lower miscarriage rate [60]. These data, in addition to the abovementioned, pointed toward IMSI as an important tool for the selection of the best spermatozoon for the injection of oocytes in cases of repeated IVF treatment failure.

6.2. IMSI in cases of severe male factor infertility

Usage of IMSI had a significant contribution to the accumulated knowledge of male infertility. At present, few randomized controlled trials are available assessing the advantages of IMSI over the conventional ICSI procedure. Antinori et al. assessed 446 couples, randomly referred to ICSI or IMSI, with at least 2 previous diagnoses of male factors due to severe oligoasthenoteratozoospermia [53]. Despite their initial poor reproductive prognosis, patients with two or more previous failed attempts benefited the most from IMSI not only in terms of increased pregnancy rate (29.8% vs. 12.9%; $P = 0.017$) but also lower miscarriage rates. Patients diagnosed with poor reproductive prognosis with two or more previous failed attempts benefited the most from IMSI. Study of patients with motile sperm less than 0.1×10^6/ml after the swim-up technique showed a positive influence of IMSI on fertilization, implantation, and pregnancy rates [42, 61]. More reports regarding patients with isolated teratozoospermia or severe oligospermia pointed to the benefits following the selection of injected sperm cell using IMSI. Higher clinical pregnancy and higher implantation rates were observed, in comparison to the conventional aspiration of spermatozoa in ICSI [62, 63].

7. IMSI: maternal age and pre-implantation genetic screening

Age-related decline in the quality of the oocytes, which affects the ICSI outcome, is a known phenomenon. Cassuto et al. distinguished between the quality of embryos resulting from oocytes of women younger than 30 years and those from women of 30 years and older, following the injection of spermatozoa selected using IMSI. When class 2 or 3 spermatozoa (moderate and bad morphological score) was injected, a lower rate of best and good embryos developed in the group of the older female patients (>30 years old) in comparison with the rate in the younger group (maternal age ≤ 30). Conversely, when a high-quality spermatozoon (score 4–6) was injected, the age-related quality of the oocyte is negligible; no difference was detected when the ratio of high-quality embryos was compared in young and older women. This is logical because these "top spermatozoa" do not need any repair. According to their findings, these researchers have pointed at the important contribution of a high-quality spermatozoon, scored in a high magnification microscope, for the injection of oocytes aspirated from women of 30 years and older [35]. This outcome is not surprising because younger oocytes are capable of "repairing" the DNA of the injected spermatozoon. In ICSI, the direct sperm deposition probably does not have a delay in the cell cycle, as it might happen due to insemination in vitro of the oocytes. The extra time helps to save maternal ribonucleic acid (mRNA), which partially might overcome epigenetic defects [11, 16, 19, 64].

Embryo chromosomal status was examined in couples who underwent their first IVF-PGS cycle for aneuploidy due to advanced maternal age [65]. Couples were randomly addressed to routine ICSI or IMSI (n = 60). All cases of sperm concentration less than 1×10^6/ml and sperm motility less than 20% were excluded from the study to minimize the influence of male factor infertility.

There was an increased incidence for sex chromosome aneuploidy in ICSI embryos when compared with IMSI (23.5% vs. 15.0%, respectively). IMSI was associated with a lower risk of sex chromosome abnormalities (odds ratio 0.57; confidence interval 0.37–0.90). The incidence of chaotic embryos was also higher with the ICSI procedure in comparison to IMSI (27.5% vs. 18.8%). An unexpected difference in gender incidence rates of euploid embryos was detected. The latest was supported by Setti et al., when a higher incidence of XX embryos derived from IMSI cycles in comparison with ICSI was noticed (66.9% vs. 52.5%, respectively) [42]. It is possible that IMSI-selected "normal" spermatozoa may carry a higher proportion of the X chromosome, which might lead to such findings.

Data also demonstrated a consistent decline in semen quality, as reflected by morphological evaluation by high-power microscope magnification, with increased age, suggesting the use of IMSI as routine in the older group of patients [66, 67].

7.1. IMSI and paternal age

Regarding the question of sperm quality in correlation to male age, it was described that increased male age is associated with a decrease in semen volume of 3–22%, a decrease in sperm motility of 3–37%, and a decrease in percentage of normal sperm of 4–18%, when comparing 30-year-old men with 50-year-old men, with no consistent effect on sperm concentration. Moreover, with control for a female partner, a relative decrease in pregnancy rates of 23 and 38%, increased risks for subfecundity ranging from 11 to 25%, and relative increase in months to achieve pregnancy up to 20% were found, comparing men <30 years old with men >50 years old, respectively [66]. Recently, IMSI provided remarkable information. Considering assessment of semen samples from 975 men who underwent IMSI, two forms of spermatozoa were considered: normal spermatozoa and spermatozoa with large nuclear vacuoles (LNV) [67]. At least 200 spermatozoa per sample were evaluated and the percentages of normal and LNV spermatozoa were determined. The subjects were divided into three groups according to age: Group I ≤ 35 years old; Group II: 3640 years; and Group III ≥ 41 years. Ratio of normal sperm cells in the older group (Group III) was lower than in the younger groups (I and II; $P < 0.05$). Percentage of LNV spermatozoa was higher in the older group (III) than in the younger (I and II) groups ($P < 0.05$). Regression analysis demonstrated a decrease in the incidence of normal sperm with increasing age ($P < 0.05$; $r = -0.10$). There was a positive correlation between the percentage of spermatozoa with LNV and male age ($P < 0.05$, $r = 0.10$).

These results demonstrated a consistent decline in semen quality, as reflected by morphological evaluation following IMSI with increased age, and support the routine use of IMSI for ICSI as a criterion for semen analysis in older group of patients.

8. Conclusions

The introduction to IMSI enabled to morphologically evaluate the individual motile sperm cell prior to its injection into the oocyte. The possibility to correlate each injected spermatozoon to the specific in vitro developing embryo has led to a better understanding of which sperm characteristics should be examined. Selecting a good-quality spermatozoon with normal morphology by using IMSI might be beneficial to embryonic development and to increased implantation and pregnancy rates. Taking into consideration the vast amount of knowledge accumulated, it seems that there is no advantage to recommend IMSI as a routine procedure for the entire populations referred to IVF-ICSI. In regard to the aforementioned studies and the experience accumulated, the authors pointed out that the following populations will have higher chances to conceive, while addressed to IMSI are couples with repeated implantation failures, cases of severe male factor infertility, advanced male age (>41 years old), and advanced maternal age (>30 years old). However, the latest should be considered in combination with deteriorated sperm quality.

It is also suggested to perform an independent observational diagnosis, using high magnification for the motile spermatozoa on a processed specimen prior to the time of the ICSI/IMSI procedure. This gives the laboratory an idea about the percentage of high-quality spermatozoa. In normospermia cases, according to routine sperm analyses, it is recommended to refer the couples to IMSI only when IMSI pre-analysis demonstrated less than 7% of high-scored (score 4–6) motile spermatozoa (Barak and Ellenbogen, personal communication). Moreover, according to the current knowledge no prenatal or postnatal complications in the mothers and offspring were observed following the IMSI procedure. The effectiveness of IMSI is still controversial mainly due to variations in inclusion criteria, stimulation protocols, sperm and oocyte qualities, and many additional confounding variables frequent in the IVF cycles.

However, there is no doubt that usage of the IMSI technique definitely opened a wider door for the hope of couples in their journey to fulfill their wish for a child. Further investigations should take place, to improve our knowledge in using this technique.

A. Appendix

General view of spermatozoa during IMSI.

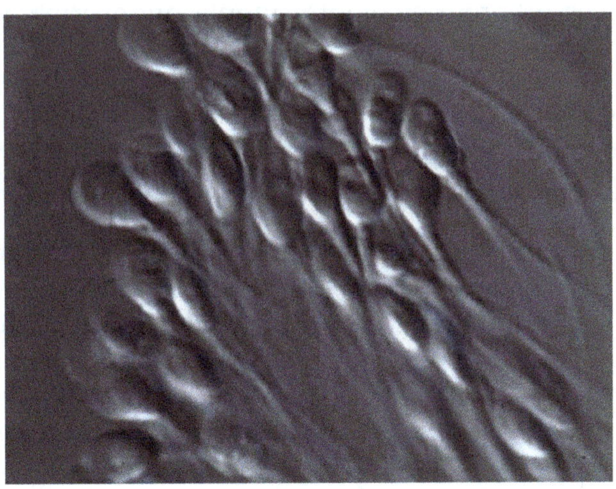

Author details

Yona Barak[1]* and Adrian Ellenbogen[2,3,4,†]

*Address all correspondence to: barak_yp@017.net.il

1 Dr Yona Barak Laboratories Ltd., Rosh Ha'Ayin, Israel

2 Rappaport School of Medicine, Technion-Israel Institute of Technology, Haifa, Israel

3 IVF Unit, Hillel Yaffe Medical Center, Hadera, Israel

4 Meuheded Female Health Center, Bnai-Brack, Israel

† Director (retired)

References

[1] Palermo G, Joris H, Devroy P, Van Steirteghem AC. Pregnancies after intracytoplasmic sperm injection of single spermatozoon into an oocyte. Lancet. 1992;**340**:17-18

[2] Pereira N, Neri QV, Lekovich JP, Spandorfer SD, Palermo GD, Rosenwaks Z. Outcomes of intracytoplasmic sperm injection cycles for complete teratozoospermia: A case-control study using paired sibling oocytes. BioMed Research International. 2015; Article ID: 470819. DOI: 10.1155/2015/470819

[3] Mansour RT, Aboulghar MA, Serour GI, Amin YM, Ramzi AM. The effect of sperm parameters on the outcome of intracytoplasmic sperm injection. Fertility and Sterility. 1995;**64**:982-986

[4] Nagy ZP, Liu J, Joris M, Verheyen G, Tournaye H, Camus M, et al. The result of intracytoplasmic sperm injection is not related to any of the three basic sperm parameters. Human Reproduction. 1995;**10**:1123-1129

[5] Svalender P, Forsberg AS, Jakobsson AH, Wikland M. Factors of importance for the establishment of a successful program of intracytoplasmic sperm injection treatment for male infertility. Fertility and Sterility. 1995;**63**:828-837

[6] Nagy ZP, Verheyen G, Tournaye H, Van Steirteghem AC. Special applications of intracytoplasmic sperm injection: The influence of sperm count, motility, morphology, source and sperm antibody on the outcome of ICSI. Human Reproduction. 1998;**13**:143-154

[7] Oehninger S, Chaturvedi S, Toner J, Morshedi M, Mayer J, Lanzendorf S, et al. Semen quality: Is there a paternal effect on pregnancy outcome in *in-vitro* fertilization/intracytoplasmic sperm injection? Human Reproduction. 1998;**13**:2161-2164

[8] Sukcharoen N, Sithipravej T, Promviengchai S, Chinpilas V, Boonkasemsanti W. Sperm morphology evaluated by computer (IVOS) cannot predict the fertilization rate *in vitro* after intracytoplasmic sperm injection. Fertility and Sterility. 1998;**69**:564-568

[9] Kupker W, Schulze W, Diedrich K. Ultrastructure of gametes and intracytoplasmic sperm injection: The significance of sperm morphology. Human Reproduction. 1998;**13**:99-106

[10] Menezo Y, Dale B. Paternal contribution to successful embryogenesis. Human Reproduction. 1994;**10**:1326-1328

[11] Janny L, Menezo YJ. Maternal age effect on early human embryonic development and blastocyst formation. Molecular Reproduction and Development. 1996;**45**:31-37

[12] Jones GM, Trouson AO, Lolatgis N, Wood C. Factors affecting the success of human blastocyst development and pregnancy following *in vitro* fertilization and embryo transfer. Fertility and Sterility. 1998;**70**:1022-1029

[13] Shoukir Y, Chardonnens D, Campana A, Sakkas D. Blastocyst development from supernumerary embryos after intracytoplasmic sperm injection: A paternal influence? Human Reproduction. 1998;**13**:1632-1637

[14] Hewitson L, Simerly C, Schatten G. Inheritance defects of the sperm centrosome in humans and its possible role in male infertility. International Journal of Andrology. 1997;**3**:35-43

[15] Hewitson L, Dominko T, Takahashi D, Martinovich C, Ramalho-Santos J, Sutovsky P, et al. Unique checkpoints during the first cell cycle of fertilization after intracytoplasmic sperm injection in rhesus monkeys. Nature Medicine. 1999;**5**:431-433

[16] Ménézo Y, Barak Y. Comparison between day-2 embryos obtained either from ICSI or resulting from short insemination IVF: Influence of maternal age. Human Reproduction. 2000;**8**:1776-1780

[17] Miller JE, Smith T. The effect of intracytoplasmic sperm injection and semen parameters on blastocyst development *in vitro*. Human Reproduction. 2001;**16**:918-924

[18] Barak Y, Goldman S. Development of *in vitro* human embryo. In: Allahbadia G, Merchant R, editors. Contemporary Perspectives on Assisted Reproductive Technology. New Delhi: Reed Elsevier; 2006. pp. 80-88

[19] Menezo Y. Paternal and maternal factors in pre-implantation embryogenesis: Interaction with the biochemical environment. Reproductive Biomedicine Online. 2006;**12**:616-621

[20] Loutradi KE, Tarlatzis BC, Goulis DG, Zepiridis L, Pagou T, Chatziioannou E, et al. The effects of sperm quality on embryo development after intracytoplasmic sperm injection. Journal of Assisted Reproduction and Genetics. 2006;**23**:69-74

[21] Ludwig M, Katalinic A. Pregnancy course and health of children born after ICSI depending on parameters of male factor infertility. Human Reproduction. 2003;**18**:351-357

[22] DeBaun MR, Niemitz EL, Feinberg AP. Association of in vitro fertilization with Beckwith-Wiedemann syndrome and epigenetic alterations of LIT1 and H19. American Journal of Human Genetics. 2003;**72**:156-160

[23] Gicquel C, Gaston V, Mandelbaum J, Siffroi JP, Flahault A, Le Bouc Y. In vitro fertilization may increase the risk of Beckwith-Wiedemann syndrome related to the abnormal imprinting of the KCN1OT gene. American Journal of Human Genetics. 2003;**72**:1338-1341

[24] Maher ER, Afnan M, Barratt CL. Epigenetic risks related to assisted reproductive technologies: Epigenetics, imprinting, ART and icebergs? Human Reproduction. 2003;**18**:2508-2511

[25] Moll AC, Imhof SM, Cruysberg JR, Schouten-van Meeteren AY, Boers M, van Leeuwen FE. Incidence of retinoblastoma in children born after *in-vitro* fertilisation. Lancet. 2003; **361**(9354):309-310

[26] Halliday J, Oke K, Breheny S, Algar E, Amor DJ. Beckwith-Wiedemann syndrome and IVF: A case-control study. American Journal of Human Genetics. 2004;**75**:526-528

[27] Cox GF, Bürger J, Lip V, Mau U, Sperling K, Bai-Lin Wu BL, Horsthemke B. Intracytoplasmic sperm injection may increase the risk of imprinting defects. American Journal of Human Genetics. 2002;**71**:162-164. DOI: 10.1086/341096

[28] Ørstavik KH, Eiklid K, van der Hagen CB, Spetalen S, Kierulf K, Skjeldal O, Buiting K. Another case of imprinting defect in a girl with Angelman syndrome who was conceived by intracytoplasmic semen injection. American Journal of Human Genetics. 2003;**72**: 218-219

[29] Santos F, Hyslop L, Stojkovic P, Leary C, Murdoch A, Reik W, et al. Evaluation of epigenetic marks in human embryos derived from IVF and ICSI. Human Reproduction. 2010;**25**:2387-2395. DOI: 10.1093/humrep/deq151

[30] De Vos A, Van De Velde H, Joris H, Verheyen G, Devroey P, Van Steirteghem A. Influence of individual sperm morphology on fertilization, embryo morphology and pregnancy outcome of intracytoplasmic sperm injection. Fertility and Sterility. 2003;**79**:42-48

[31] Bartoov B, Berkovitz A, Eltes F. Selection of spermatozoa with normal nuclei to improve the pregnancy rate with intracytoplasmic sperm injection. The New England Journal of Medicine. 2001;**345**:1067-1068

[32] Bartoov B, Berkovitz A, Eltes F, Kogosowski A, Menezo Y, Barak Y. Breakthroughs in andrology: Real-time fine morphology of motile human sperm cells is associated with IVF–ICSI outcome. Journal of Andrology. 2002;**23**:1-8

[33] Bartoov B, Berkovitz A, Eltes F, Kogosovsky A, Yagoda A, Lederman H, Artzi S, et al. Pregnancy rates are higher with intracytoplasmic morphologically selected sperm injection than with conventional intracytoplasmic injection. Fertility and Sterility. 2003;**80**:1413-1419

[34] Antinori M, Vanderzwalman P, Barak Y. IMSI as a valuable tool for sperm selection during ART. In: Racowsky C, Schlegel PN, Fauser BC, Carrell DT, editors. Evolving Controversies in Reproductive Medicine—Biennial Reviews of Infertility. Springer International Publishing, AG; 2001. pp. 263-276

[35] Cassuto NG, Bouret D, Plouchart JM, Jellad S, Vanderzwalmen P, Balet R, et al. A new real-time morphology classification for human spermatozoa: A link for fertilization and improved embryo quality. Fertility and Sterility. 2009;**92**:1616-1625. DOI: 10.1016/j.fertnstert.2008.08.088

[36] Hazout A, Dumont-Hassan M, Junca AM, Bacrie PC, Tesarik J. High-magnification ICSI overcomes paternal effect resistant to conventional ICSI. Reproductive Biomedicine Online. 2006;**12**:19-25

[37] Franco JG, Baruffi RL, Mauri AL, Petersen CG, Oliveira JB, Vagnini L. Significance of large nuclear vacuoles in human spermatozoa: Implications for ICSI. Reproductive Biomedicine Online. 2008;**17**:42-45

[38] Garolla A, Fortini D, Menegazzo M, De Toni L, Nicoletti V, Moretti A, et al. High power microscopy for selecting spermatozoa for ICSI by physiological status. Reproductive Biomedicine Online. 2008;**17**:610-616

[39] Barak Y. ICSI—A step too soon? In: Allahbadia G, Merchant R, editors. Gynecology Endoscopy and Infertility-Lessons Learnt and Future Challenges Jaypee Brothers Publishers (p) Ltd. 1 ed. 2005. pp. 300-306. DOI: 10.5005/jp Books/10334_36

[40] Barak Y. Preparation of sperm for ICSI. Embryo Talk. 2006;**1**:193-202

[41] de Almeida Ferreira Braga DP, Setti AS, Figueira RC, Nichi M, Martinhago CD, Iaconelli A Jr, et al. Sperm organelle morphologic abnormalities: Contributing factors and effects on intracytoplasmic sperm injection cycles outcomes. Urology. 2011;**78**:786-791. DOI: 10.1016/j.urology.2011.06.018

[42] Setti AS, Figueira RD, Braga DP, Iaconelli A, Borges E. Intracytoplasmic morphologically selected sperm injection benefits for patients with oligoasthenozoospermia according to the 2010 World Health Organization reference values. Fertility and Sterility. 2011;**95**:2711-2714. DOI: 10.1016/j.fertnstert.2011.03.003

[43] Cassuto NG, Hazout A, Hammoud I, Balet R, Bouret D, Barak Y, et al. Correlation between DNA defect and sperm-head morphology. Reproductive Biomedicine Online. 2011;**24**:211-218. DOI: 10.1016/j.rbmo.2011

[44] Vanderzwalmen P, Hiemer A, Rubner P, Bach M, Neyer A, Stecher A, et al. Blastocyst development after sperm selection at high magnification is associate with size and number of nuclear vacuoles. Reproductive Biomedicine Online. 2008;**17**:617-627

[45] Watanabe S, Tanaka A, Fujii S, Mizunuma H, Fukui A, Fukuhara R, et al. An investigation of the potential effect of vacuoles in human sperm on DNA damage using a chromosome assay and the TUNEL assay. Human Reproduction. 2011;**26**:978-986. DOI: 10.1093/humrep/der047

[46] Gatimeln N, Leandri RD, Marino L, Esquerre-Lamare C, Parinaud J. Sperm vacuoles cannot help to differentiate fertile men from infertile men with normal sperm parameter values. Human Reproduction. 2014;**29**:2359-2367. DOI: 10.1093/humrep/deu206

[47] Tanaka A, Nagayoshi M, Tanaka I, Kusunoki H. Human sperm head vacuoles are physiological structures formed during the sperm development and maturation process. Fertility and Sterility. 2012;**98**:315-320. DOI: 10.1016/j.fertnstert.2012.04.034

[48] Bartoov B, Eltes F, Reichart M, Langzam J, Lederman H, Zabludovsky N. Quantitative ultra morphological analysis of human sperm: Fifteen years of experience in the diagnosis and management of male factor infertility. Archives of Andrology. 1999;**43**:13-25

[49] Virro MR, Larson-Cook KL, Evenson DP. Sperm chromatin structure assay (SCSA) parameters are related to fertilization, blastocyst development, and ongoing pregnancy in *in vitro* fertilization and intracytoplasmic sperm injection cycles. Fertility and Sterility. 2004;**81**:1289-1295

[50] Check JH, Graziano V, Cohen R, Krotec J, Check ML. Effect of an abnormal sperm chromatin structural assay (SCSA) on pregnancy outcome following (IVF) with ICSI in previous IVF failures. Archives of Andrology. 2005;**51**:121-124

[51] Berkovitz A, Eltes F, Yaari S, Katz N, Barr I, Ami Fishman A, et al. The morphological normalcy of the sperm nucleus and pregnancy rate of intracytoplasmic injection with morphologically selected sperm. Human Reproduction. 2005;**20**:185-190

[52] Berkovitz A, Eltes F, Ellenbogen E, Peer S, Feldberg D, Bartoov B. Does the presence of nuclear vacuoles in human sperm selected for ICSI affect pregnancy outcome? Human Reproduction. 2006;**21**:1787-1790

[53] Antinori M, Licata E, Dani G, Cerusico C, Versaci C, D'Angelo D, et al. Intracytoplasmic morphologically selected sperm injection: A prospective randomized trial. Reproductive Biomedicine Online. 2008;**16**:835-841

[54] Fekonja N, Strus J, Znidaric MT, Knez K, Bokal EV, Verdenik I, et al. Clinical and structural features of sperm head vacuoles in man induced in the in vitro fertilization program. BioMed Research International. 2014:1-12. Article ID: 927841. DOI: 10.1155/2014/927841

[55] Kacem O, Sifer C, Barraud-Lange V, Ducot B, De Ziegler D, Poirot C, et al. Sperm nuclear vacuoles, as assessed by motile sperm organellar morphological examination, are mostly of acrosomal origin. Reproductive Biomedicine Online. 2010;**20**:132-137. DOI: 10.1016/j.rbmo.2009.10.014

[56] Montjean D, Belloc S, Benkhalifa M, Dalleac A. Menezo Y, Sperm vacuoles are linked to capacitation and acrosomal status. Human Reproduction. 2012;**27**:2927-2932. DOI: 10.1093/humrep/des266

[57] De Vos A, Van de Velde H, Bocken G, Eylenbosch G, Franceus N, Meersdom G, et al. Does intracytoplasmic morphologically selected sperm injection improve embryo development? A randomized sibling-oocyte study. Human Reproduction. 2013;**28**:617-626. DOI: 10.1093/humrep/des435

[58] La Sala GB, Nicoli A, Fornaciari E, Falbo A, Rondini I, Morini D, et al. Intracytoplasmic morphologically selected sperm injection versus conventional intracytoplasmic sperm injection: A randomized controlled trial. Reproductive Biology and Endocrinology. 2015;**13**:97-105. DOI: 10.1186/s12958-015-0096-y

[59] Souza Setti A, Ferreira RC, Paes de Almeida Ferreira Braga D, de Cassia Savio Figueira R, Iaconelli A, Borges E. Intracytoplasmic sperm injection outcome versus intracytoplasmic morphologically selected sperm injection outcome: A meta-analysis. Reproductive Biomedicine Online. 2010;**21**:450-455. DOI: 10.1016/j.rbmo.2010.05.017

[60] Shalom-Paz E, Anabusi S, Michaeli M, Karchovsky-Shoshan E, Rothfarb N, Ellenbogen A. Can intracytoplasmatic morphologically selected sperm injection (IMSI) technique improve outcome in patients with repeated IVF–ICSI failure? A comparative study. Gynecological Endocrinology. 2015;**31**:247-251. DOI: 10.3109/09513590.2014.982085

[61] Wilding M, Coppola G, di Matteo L, Palagiano A, Fusco E, Dale B. Intracytoplasmic injection of morphologically selected spermatozoa (IMSI) improves outcome after assisted reproduction by deselecting physiologically poor quality spermatozoa. Journal of Assisted Reproduction and Genetics. 2011;**28**:253-262. DOI: 10.1007/s10815-010-9505-5

[62] Balaban B, Yakin K, Alatas C, Oktem O, Isiklar A, Urman B. Clinical outcome of intracytoplasmic injection of spermatozoa morphologically selected under high magnification: A prospective randomized study. Reproductive Biomedicine Online. 2011;**22**:472-476. DOI: 10.1016/j.rbmo.2010.11.003

[63] Knez K, Tomazevic T, Zorn B, Vrtacnik-Bokal E, Virant-Klun I. Intracytoplasmic morphologically selected sperm injection improves development and quality of preimplantation embryos in teratozoospermia patients. Reproductive Biomedicine Online. 2012;**25**:168-179. DOI: 10.1016/j.rbmo.2012.03.011

[64] Piette C, de Mouzon J, Bachelot A, Spira A. *In-vitro* fertilization: Influence of women's age on pregnancy rates. Human Reproduction. 1990;**5**:56-59

[65] Figueira Rde C, Braga DP, Setti AS, Iaconelli A, Borges E. Morphological nuclear integrity of sperm cells is associated with preimplantation genetic aneuploidy screening cycle outcomes. Fertility and Sterility. 2011;**95**:990-993. DOI: 10.1016/j.fertnstert.2010.11.018

[66] Kidd SA, Eskenazi B, Wyrobek AJ. Effects of male age semen quality and fertility: A review of the literature. Fertility and Sterility. 2001;**75**:237-248

[67] Silva LF, Oliveira JB, Petersen CG, Mauri AL, Massaro FC, Cavagna M, et al. The effects of male age on sperm analysis by motile sperm organelle morphology examination (MSOME). Reproductive Biology and Endocrinology. 2012;**10**:19. DOI: 10.1186/1477-7827-10-19

6

Sequence of Germ Cells Differentiation During Spermiogenesis of the Amphibian Urodele *Ambystoma dumerilii*

Mari Carmen Uribe and Sergio Gracia-Fernández

Abstract

The spermatogenesis, including the spermiogenesis, in Urodeles contains the meiotic process and the morphological differentiation of the spermatids developing the spermatozoa as in the rest of vertebrates. However, in Urodeles, there are essential differences in the structure of the testis, as a lobular structure; the distribution of the spermatogenic cells, in cephalocaudal progression in the testis; and the cystic condition of the developing spermatogenic cells in synchronous groups bounded by Sertoli cells. All the spermatogenic cells are situated in parallel position with the heads directed to the same side. The big size and elongated morphology of the spermatozoa also characterized this type of spermiogenesis. Spermiation occurs at the caudal portion of the testis to the efferent duct system, which includes the mesonephric nephrones.

Keywords: lobular testis, longitudinal spermatogenesis, spermiogenesis, testicular cysts, Urodeles

1. Introduction

The spermatogenesis of Urodeles occurs in longitudinal course into the testis. The structure of the testis forms abundant longitudinal lobules which contain the germinal cells. The lobules are separated by trabeculae of thin and vascularized connective tissue, which are the continuation of the tunica albuginea. The spermatogonia are situated in the cephalic edge of the testis, and the development of spermatozoa occurs during the way of the spermatogenesis through the testicular lobules to the caudal edge of the testis (**Figure 1A–C**). At the end of the lobules, the spermatozoa are discharged to the deferent duct system [1, 2]. Consequently, the disposition of spermatogenesis in Urodeles is longitudinal, in cephalocaudal progression, where the

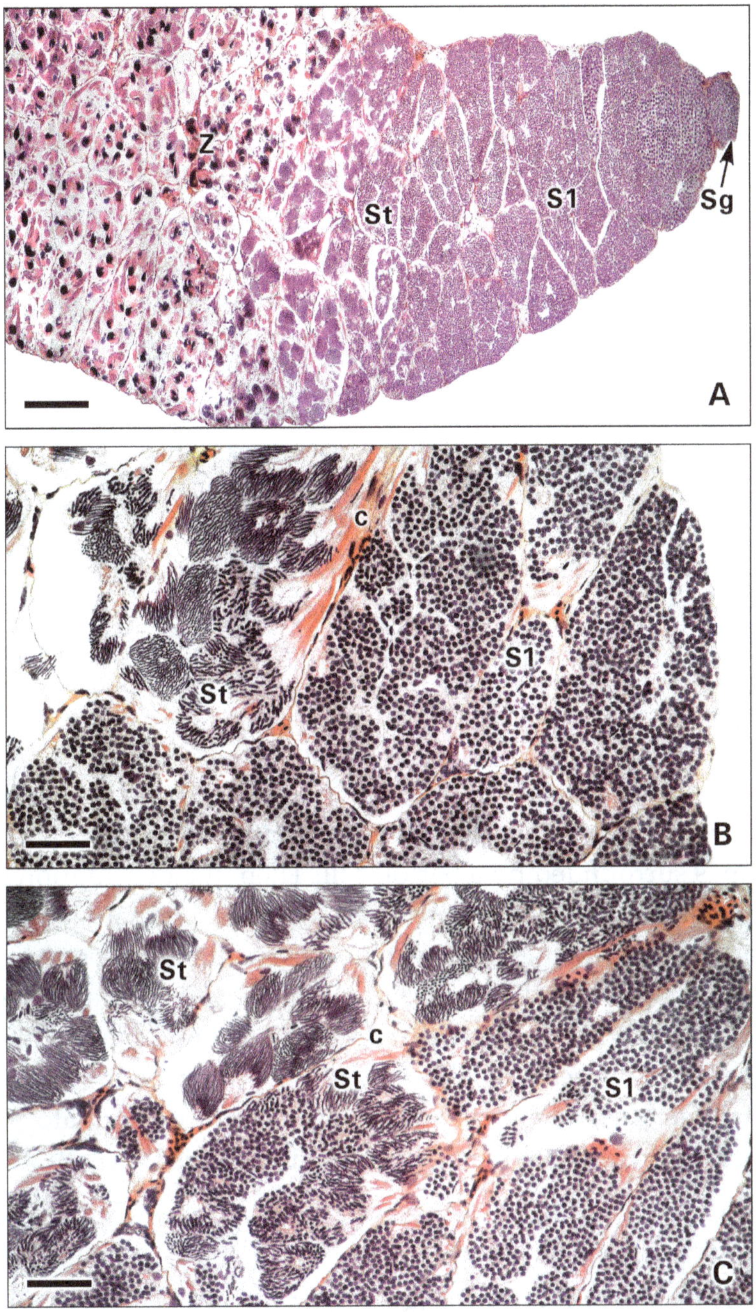

Figure 1. Testis of *Ambystoma dumerilii* in longitudinal sections. Spermatogenesis advancing in successive regions along the cephalocaudal axis of the testis, where the different types of spermatogenic cells are seen. (A) Panoramic morphology of the testis. H-E. Bar = 0.3 mm. (B, C) Testicular lobules containing the spermatogenic cells and surrounded of connective tissue. H-E. Bar = 0.1 mm. Spermatogonia (Sg), primary spermatocytes (S1), spermatids (St), spermatozoa (Z), and interlobular connective tissue (c).

earliest stages are more cephalic and the latest stages are more caudal, in contrast with the tubular structure with radial disposition of the spermatogenesis in the testis of amniotes.

Spermatogenic cells of Urodeles are quite big, compared to amniotes germ cells, as example, the spermatogonia may attain 55 μm in *A. dumerilii* [1, 3] and the spermatozoa may attain 840 μm long in *Necturus maculosus* [4, 5].

For the description of this type of spermiogenesis of Urodeles, we consider convenient detailed illustration in this chapter of the progressive histological changes of the spermatids during the development of the spermatozoa, taking the species *Ambystoma dumerilii* (Ambystomatidae) as a model. The histological sections were stained with hematoxylin-eosin (H-E), Masson's trichrome, periodic acid-Schiff (PAS), and alcian blue. *A. dumerilii* is an endemic species, which habits at the southern edge of the Mexican Plateau in Michoacán State, Mexico, in the Lake Pátzcuaro (260 km^2, moderately shallow to 11 m, and high elevation at 2035 m up sea level). *A. dumerilii* is a neotenic species, because lack metamorphosis, maintaining during all the life cycle as paedomorphic aquatic larva [6].

2. Spermatogenesis in Urodeles

Spermatogenesis in Urodeles was studied by several authors who described stages of germ cell maturation in a variety of species as: in *Desmognathus fusca* [7]; in *Ambystoma tigrinum* [8–10]; in *Trituroides hongkongensis* [11]; in *Necturus maculosus* [12]; in *Salamandrina terdigitata* [13]; in *Salamandra salamandra* [14, 15]; in *A. mexicanum* [16, 17]; Ricote et al. in *Triturus marmoratus* [18]; in *A. dumerilii* [1, 3, 17, 19]; and in *Salamandrella keyserlingii* [20].

The spermatogenic cells of *A. dumerilii*, as in all Urodeles, are in synchronous groups called cysts, where all the cells are at the same stage of development. A cyst is formed when a spermatogonium becomes surrounded by a Sertoli cell. Then, the distribution of cysts in the testicular lobules displays a longitudinal sequence of stages of spermatogenesis, in respect to the cephalocaudal gradient: spermatogonia, primary spermatocytes, secondary spermatocytes, spermatids in spermiogenesis, and spermatozoa. The Sertoli cells are involved in essential functions of the spermatogenesis: they maintain a permeability barrier to the germinal cells into the cyst during all the process of differentiation, determine the endocrine activity that controls the spermatogenesis, and phagocytose degenerating spermatogenic cells, residual bodies, and abnormal spermatozoa during the spermiogenesis [1, 17, 19].

Spermatogonia of *A. dumerilii* are spherical cells with 45–55 μm in diameter (**Figure 2A**). These cells are diploid and have mitotic activity. When spermatogonia initiate the meiotic process become a primary spermatocyte (**Figure 2A–C**).

The primary spermatocytes are also spherical cells; their size is 40–45 μm in diameter. These cells initiate the meiosis; then, their nuclei contain duplicated chromosomes at different stages of prophase I of meiosis exposed clearly in the chromatin changes: leptotene with fine reticular chromatin, zygotene with fine fibrillar pattern of duplicated chromosomes, pachytene with more thick fibrillar pattern of duplicated chromosomes in crossing-over, and diplotene when occurs the separation of homologous duplicated chromosomes, remaining some chiasms (**Figure 3A** and **B**). The primary spermatocytes enter metaphase I, anaphase I, and telophase I (**Figure 3C**), resulting in two secondary spermatocytes.

Secondary spermatocytes are spherical cells and are smaller than primary spermatocytes; they have in average 18–20 μm in diameter. As the result of the first division of meiosis, the secondary

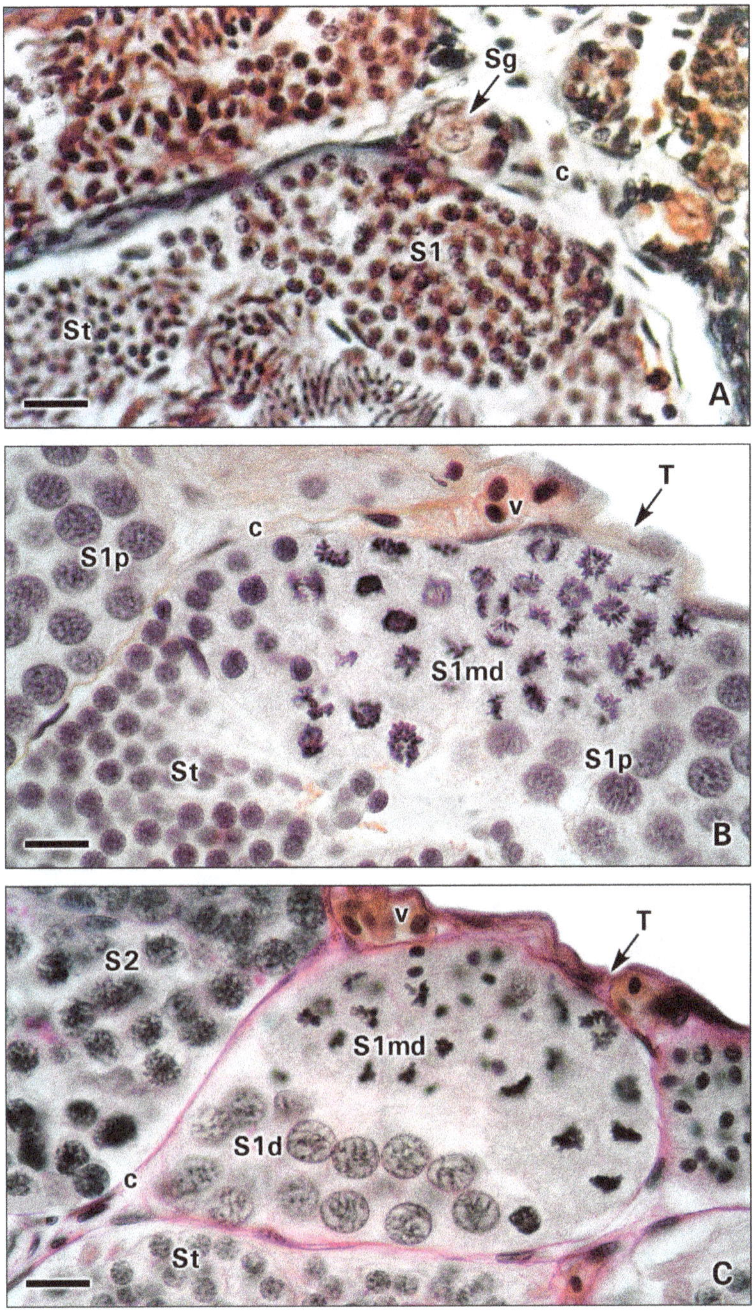

Figure 2. Spermatogenesis in the testis of *Ambystoma dumerilii.* (A) Cephalic region of the testis. Spermatogonia surrounded by connective tissue. Lobules with cysts containing cells in different stages of spermatogenesis. Masson's trichrome. Bar = 30 μm. (B, C) Periphery of the testis in the adjacent region to spermatogonia. Cysts containing primary spermatocytes during the first meiotic prophase, in pachytene, with thick fibrillar chromatin, in diplotene with pairs of chromosomes showing chiasms and during the first meiotic division, secondary spermatocytes and early spermatids. Around the lobules, there is connective tissue. The tunica albuginea with blood vessels surrounds the testis. Spermatogonia (Sg), primary spermatocytes (S1), primary spermatocytes in pachytene (S1p), primary spermatocytes in diplotene (S1d), primary spermatocytes during the first meiotic division (S1md), secondary spermatocytes (S2), spermatids (St), connective tissue (c), tunica albuginea (T), and blood vessels (v). B: H-E, C: PAS. Bar = 20 μm.

spermatocytes contain a haploid, but duplicated, number of chromosomes (**Figure 2C**). These cells are seen less frequent, since they divide during the second part of meiosis after a very short interphase, rapidly giving rise to two spermatids.

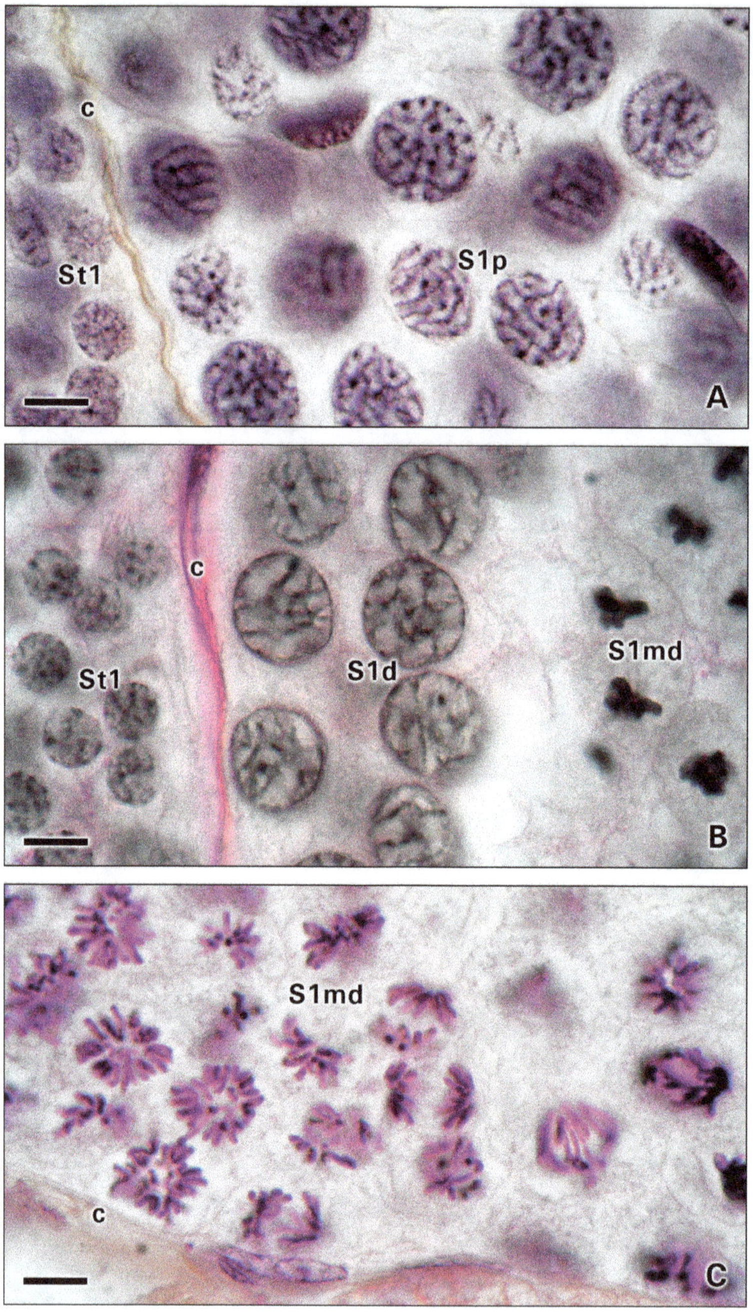

Figure 3. Spermatogenesis in the testis of *Ambystoma dumerilii.* (A) Primary spermatocytes during pachytene and early spermatids. Compare the size of both type of germinal cells. H-E. Bar = 10 µm. (B) Primary spermatocytes during diplotene and early spermatids. Compare the size of both type of germinal cells. PAS. Bar = 10 µm. (C) Primary spermatocytes during the first meiotic division. B: H-E, C: PAS. Bar = 10 µm. Primary spermatocytes in pachytene (S1p), primary spermatocytes in diplotene (S1d), primary spermatocytes during the first meiotic division (S1md), early spermatids (St1), and connective tissue (c).

3. Morphology of spermatids in *A. dumerilii* during spermiogenesis

The spermatids of *A. dumerilii* initiate the spermiogenesis, occurring during a sequence of morphological changes transforming the spermatids into spermatozoa. Early spermatids are spherical in shape and attain a diameter of 14–17 µm; their nuclei contain light fibrillar chromosomes.

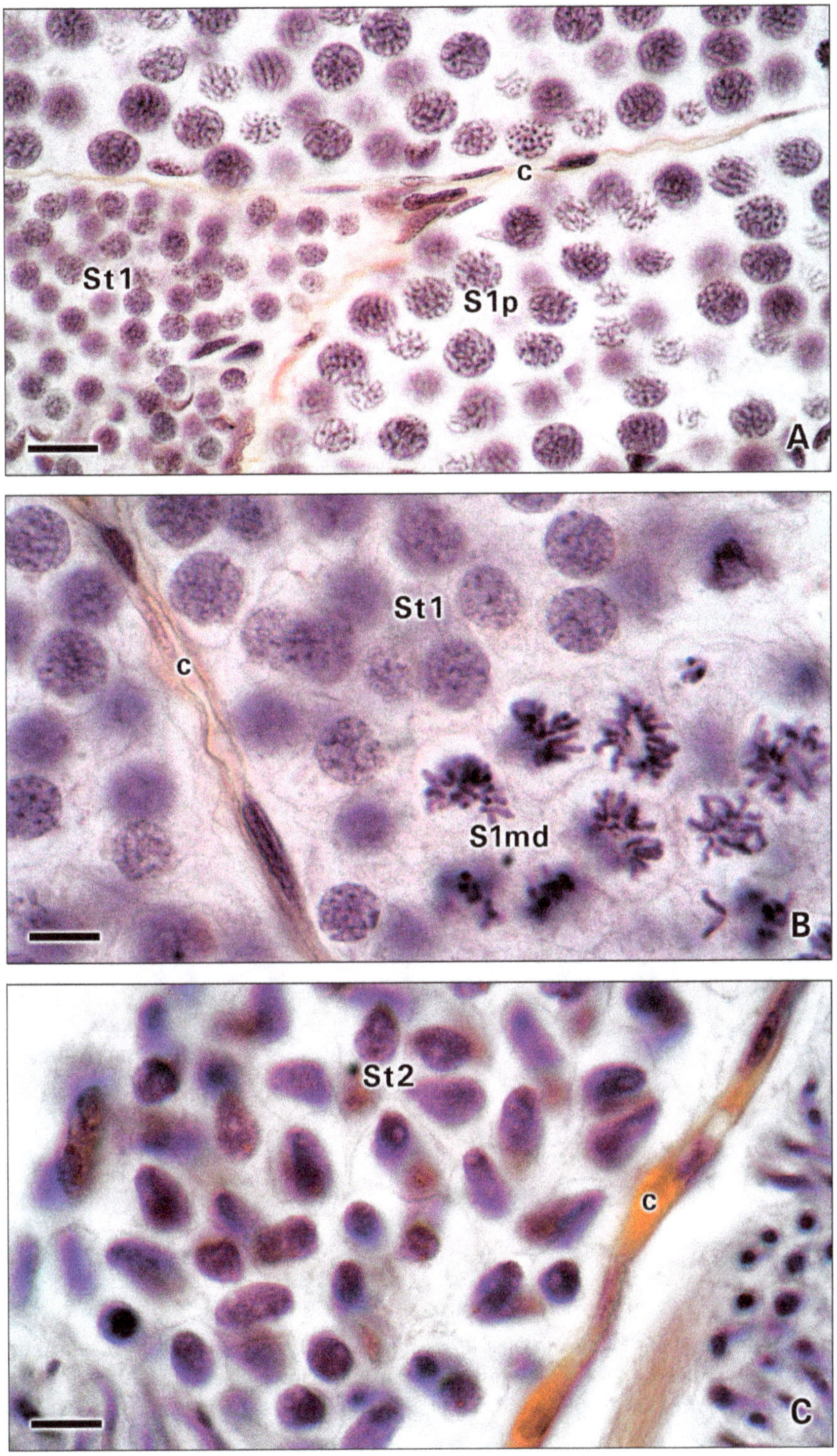

Figure 4. Early spermatids in the testis of *Ambystoma dumerilii*. (A) Primary spermatocytes during pachytene and early spermatids with round nucleus. H-E. Bar = 20 μm. (B) Early spermatids with fine fibrillar chromatin. H-E. Bar = 20 μm. (C) Initial elongation of the spermatids and more compact aspect of the nucleus. H-E. Bar = 20 μm. Early spermatids (St1), (St2) and interlobular connective tissue (c).

The early spermatid nuclei soon are seen as fine granular and progressively come to dense. The early spermatids become progressively elongated and the chromatin shows increasing degree of condensation (**Figure 4A–C**). As spermiogenesis proceeds, the nuclei of spermatids become

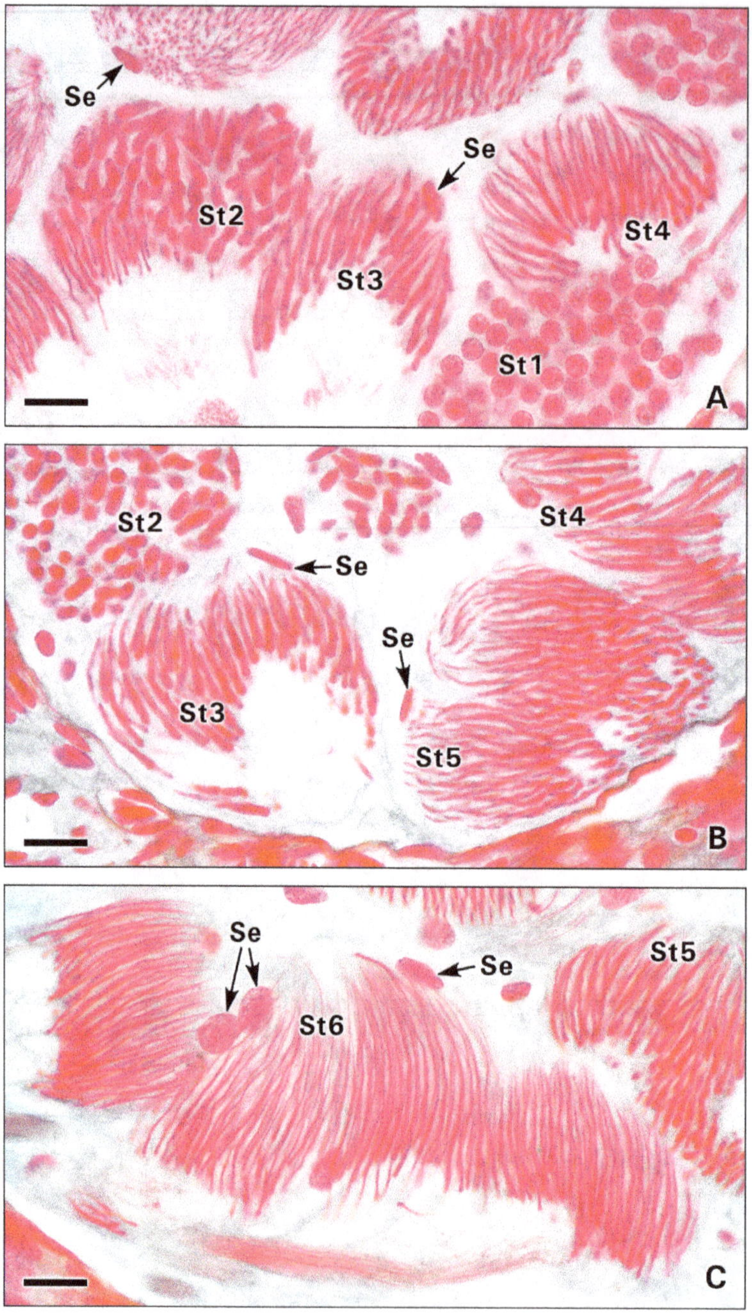

Figure 5. Spermiogenesis in the testis of *Ambystoma dumerilii*. (A–C) Early spermatids, when they are spherical (1). Various cysts present the evident progressive elongation of the spermatids. The nuclei of Sertoli cells are seen around the cysts. Alcian blue. Bar = 20 μm. Early spermatids (St1). Spermatids in elongation (St2), (St3), (St4), (St5), and (St6). Sertoli cells nuclei (Se), connective tissue (c).

larger (**Figures 5A–C** and **6A–C**). The shape of spermatids in spermiogenesis is gradually performing an elongated cell developing head, midpiece, and flagellum. These three parts of the cell are clearly distinguished, additionally to their shape and position in the cell, because their different staining affinity: the head is basophilic; the midpiece is intensely acidophilic; and the flagellum is also acidophilic but less intense than the midpiece. The head of the spermatozoa contains the acrosome and the nucleus, with a narrower cephalic part at the acrosome. All the germinal cells in a cyst maintain the same orientation, with the heads to the same side

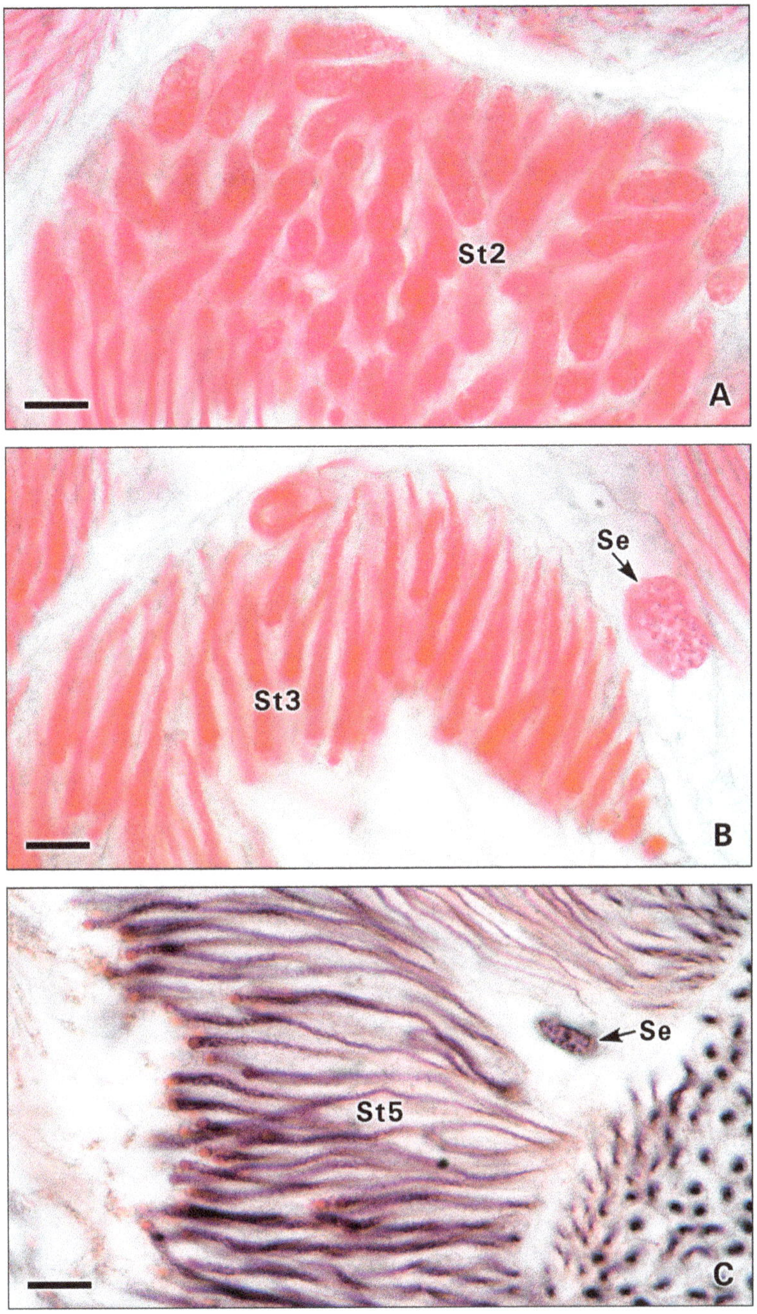

Figure 6. Spermiogenesis in the testis of *Ambystoma dumerilii*. Details of the progressive elongation of the spermatids. (A–C) Cysts contain spermatids during the progressive elongation. Progressive elongation of spermatids (St2), (St3), and (St5). Sertoli cells nuclei (Se). (A, B) Alcian blue. (C) H-E. Bar = 10 μm.

(**Figure 7A–C**). As maturation advances the spermatozoa have a swirl arrangement inside the cyst, keeping their heads oriented in the same direction (**Figure 8A–C**). The large of the spermatozoa may attain 460 μm [1, 6].

The total length of spermatozoa of Urodeles is usually longer than those of other amphibians and other vertebrates. The shortest spermatozoa were reported for *Hynobius nebulosus* with a length of 156 μm, whereas the longest, as we documented before, with a length of 840 μm, was observed in *Necturus maculosus* [4, 5]. The lengths of spermatozoa differ

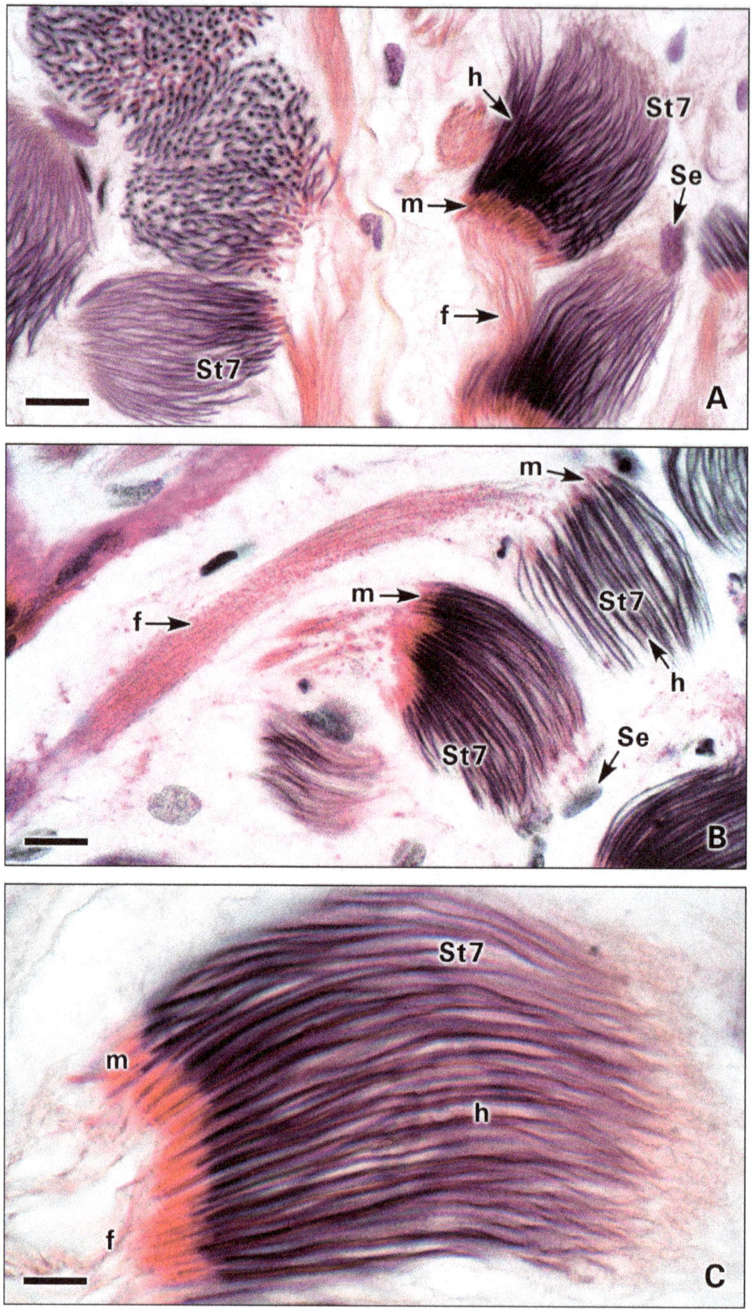

Figure 7. Spermiogenesis in the testis of *Ambystoma dumerilii*. (A–C) The elongation of the late spermatids advances into the cysts. The development of the head, the midpiece, and the flagella is observed by the different staining affinity. The cells conserve the same position, with the heads directed to the same side. (A) H-E. Bar = 20 μm. (B) H-E. Bar = 20 μm. (C) H-E. Bar = 10 μm. Spermatids (St7), head (h), midpiece (m), flagella (f), and Sertoli cells nuclei (Se).

widely in Urodeles as examples are: *Hynobius boulengeri* (197 μm); *Salamandrella keyserlingii* (212 μm) [21]; *Lissotriton italicus* (360 μm) [22]; *Desmognathus aeneus* (388 μm) [23]; *Ambystoma mexicanum* (444 μm) [6]; *Eurycea bislineata* (459 μm), *E. lucifuga* (523 μm), *Pleurodeles dorsalis* (536 μm), *P. dunni* (626 μm) [23]; *Triturus helveticus* (650 μm) [4]; and *Aneides aeneus* (770 μm) [23]. The biological significance of the differences in the lengths of spermatozoa is unknown.

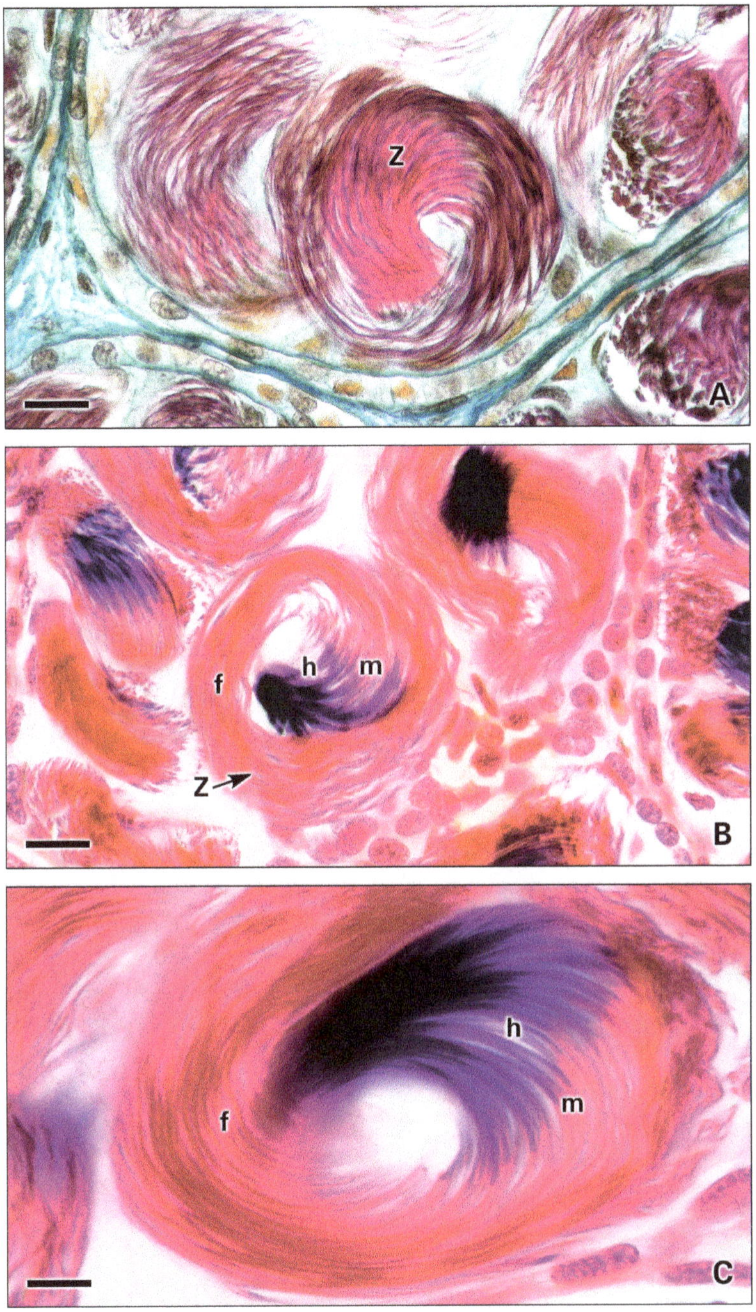

Figure 8. Spermatozoa in the testis of *Ambystoma dumerilii*. (A–C) The cellular maximum elongation is observed in the spermatozoa, and additionally, the spermatozoa screw in where the head is in the interior part and the flagella in the exterior part of this roll, maintaining the cystic condition. (A) Alcian blue. Bar = 20 μm. (B) H-E. Bar = 20 μm. (C) H-E. Bar = 10 μm. Spermatozoa (Z), head (h), midpiece (m), and flagella (f).

4. Spermiation

The region of spermiation is observed at the caudal end of the testis, where the density of cysts with spermatozoa decreases, there are abundant empty cysts containing remnants of Sertoli cells, and few cysts containing spermatozoa, compared with the region before spermiation where there are abundant cysts with spermatozoa (**Figure 9A** and **B**).

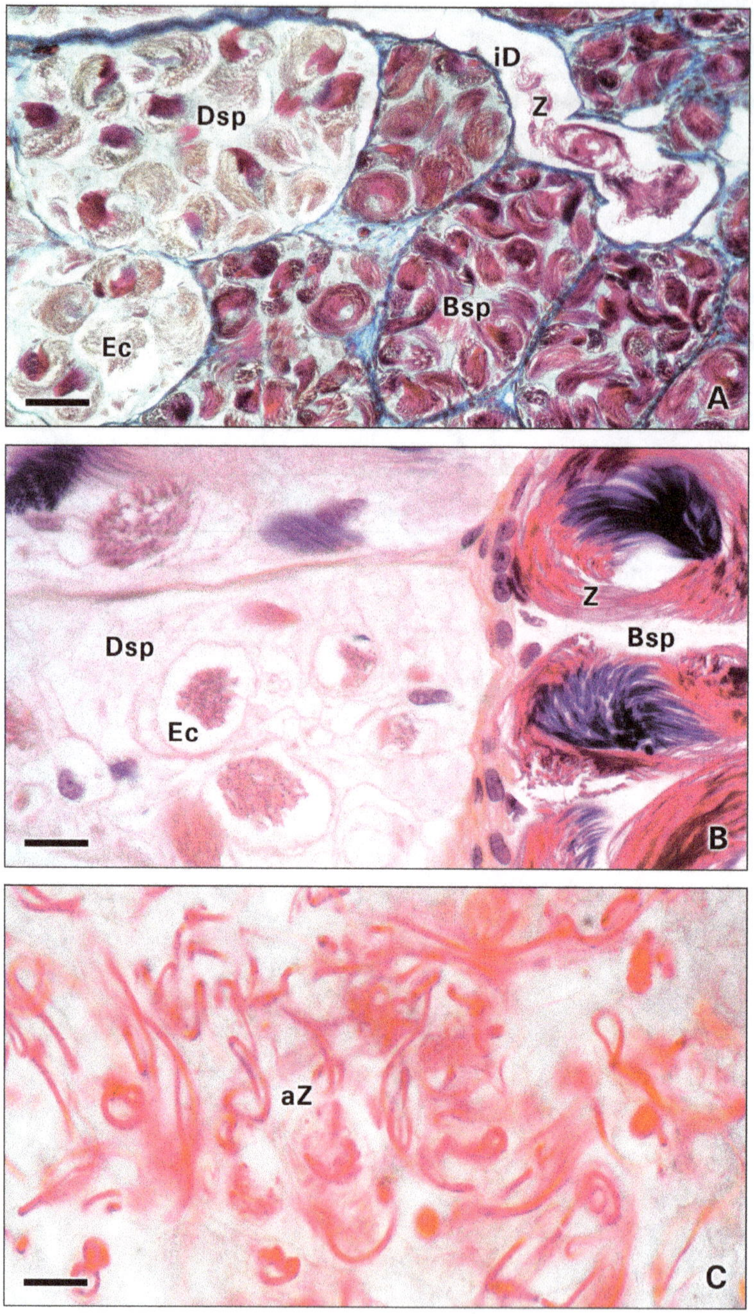

Figure 9. Spermiation in the testis of *Ambystoma dumerilii.* (A, B) Portion of the testis where is seen the limit between the regions before and during spermiation. The region before spermiation contains lobules with abundant cysts with spermatozoa. The region during spermiation contains few cysts with spermatozoa, compared with these seen in the other region and there are also empty cysts, without spermatozoa, containing only the residue of the Sertoli cells. A portion of an intratesticular duct containing spermatozoa is seen. Masson's trichrome. Bar = 0.1 mm. H-E. Bar = 20 μm. (C) During spermiation, abnormal spermatozoa, showing irregular morphology, may remain into the cysts. H-E. Bar = 20 μm. Testicular regions: Before spermiation (BSp) and during spermiation (DSp), spermatozoa (Z), empty cyst (Ec), intratesticular duct (iD), and abnormal spermatozoa (aZ).

Upon the conclusion of the spermiation, when the cysts open and the spermatozoa leave the testis, Sertoli cells remain inside the lobule and undergo morphological changes during their degeneration until they disappear [9, 19, 24]. During the emptying of the cysts, some spermatozoa remain in some of the cysts which show abnormal morphology (**Figure 9C**); these spermatozoa are phagocytized by the Sertoli cells [14].

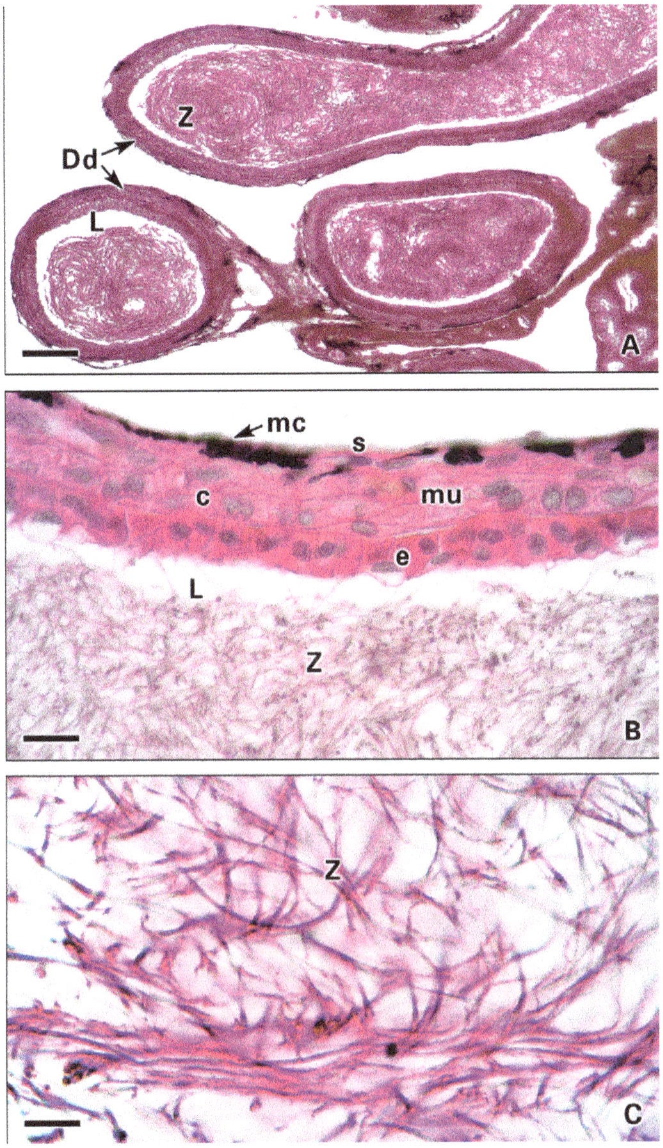

Figure 10. Deferent duct of *Ambystoma dumerilii*. (A) Sections of the large and folded deferent duct containing abundant spermatozoa in the lumen. B: H-E, C: PAS. Bar = 0.1 mm. (B) Detail of the deferent duct lined by cuboidal epithelium, connective tissue, muscle cells, and serosa. Subjacent the serosa, there are melanocytes. B: H-E, C: PAS. Bar = 20 μm. (C) Spermatozoa in the lumen of the deferent duct. B: H-E, C: PAS. Bar = 10 μm. Deferent duct (Dd), spermatozoa (Z), lumen (L), cuboidal epithelium (e), connective tissue (c), muscle cells (mu), serosa (s), and melanocytes (mc).

Throughout spermiation, spermatozoa are progressively released from the cysts to the lobular lumen and then to the efferent duct system [14, 16, 17, 19, 24–26].

Intratesticular ducts (*rete testis*) are embedded in the interlobular connective tissue of the testis (**Figure 9A**). Their lumen is lined with squamous epithelium. The efferent ducts include cephalic mesonephric nephrons, corresponding to the type of mesonephric kidneys of amphibians. The nephronic collecting ducts empty into the vas deferens also called primary urinary duct or Wolffian duct [2]. The Wolffian ducts are the largest of the sperm collecting ducts (**Figure 10A**); their lumen is lined with cuboidal epithelium and subjacent there are connective tissues, smooth muscle cells, and serosa; at the periphery, some melanocytes are dispersed (**Figure 10B** and **C**). In the lumen of the deferent ducts, the spermatozoa are in irregular position (**Figure 10C**); the cystic condition maintained all along the spermatogenesis is ended when the cyst is open at the spermiation, in the testicular lobules, before the entrance to the deferent duct system.

Acknowledgements

We thank Gerardo Gómez-Ríos and Adriana García-Alarcón for processing some histological specimens and valuable discussions during the early progress of this work; we are grateful to Gabino De la Rosa-Cruz for helpful technical assistance with digital photography; and José Antonio Hernández Gómez who kindly prepared the excellent digital figures.

Author details

Mari Carmen Uribe* and Sergio Gracia-Fernández

*Address all correspondence to: mari3uribe3@gmail.com

Department of Compared Biology, Sciences Faculty, Laboratory of Biology of Reproduction, Universidad Nacional Autónoma de México, Mexico City, Mexico

References

[1] Uribe MC, Gómez Ríos G, Brandon RA. Spermatogenesis in the urodele *Ambystoma dumerilii*. Journal of Morphology. 1994;**222**:287-299

[2] Propper CR. Chapter 3. Testicular structure and control of sperm development in amphibians. In: Norris DO, Lopez Kristin H, editors. Amphibians, Hormones and Reproduction in Vertebrates. Vol. 2. Oxford, UK: Ac Press, Elsevier; 2011. pp. 39-53

[3] Uribe MC, Mejía-Roa V. Testicular structure and germ cells morphology in salamanders. Spermatogenesis. 2014;**4**(3):e988090. DOI: 10.4161/21565562.2014.988090

[4] Picheral B. Structural, comparative and functional aspects of spermatozoa in Urodeles. In: Fawcett DW, Bedford JM, editors. The Spermatozoon. Baltimore, Maryland: Urban and Schwarzenberg; 1979. pp. 267-287

[5] Scheltinga DM, Jamieson BGM. The mature spermatozoa. In: Sever D, Volume editor. Jamieson BGM, Series editor. Reproductive Biology and Phylogeny of Urodela. Enfield (NH), USA/Plymouth, UK: Science Publishers; 2003. pp. 203-274

[6] Brandon RA, Martan J, Wortham JWE, Englert DC. The influence of interspecific hybridization on the morphology of the spermatozoa of *Ambystoma* (Caudata, Ambystomatidae). Journal of Reproduction and Fertility. 1974;**41**:275-284

[7] Kingsbury BF. The spermatogenesis of *Desmognathus fusca*. The American Journal of Anatomy. 1901;**1**:99-135

[8] Humphrey RR. The multiple testis in urodeles. The Biological Bulletin. 1922;**43**:45-67 http://dx.doi.org/10.2307/1536690

[9] Carrick R. The spermatogenesis of the axolotl (*Ambystoma tigrinum*). Transactions of the Royal Society of Edinburgh. 1934;**58**:63-76. DOI: 10.1017/S0080456800023048

[10] Norris DO, Norman MF, Pankak MK, Duvall D. Seasonal variation in spermatogenesis, testicular weights, vasa deferentia and androgen levels in neotenic tiger salamander, *Ambystoma tigrinum*. General and Comparative Endocrinology. 1985;**60**:51-57. DOI: 10.1016/0016-6480(85)90291-6 PMID: 4054587

[11] Tso ECF, Lofts B. Seasonal changes in the newt, *Trituroides hongkongenesis* testis. I. A histological and histochemical study. Acta Zoologica-Stockholm. 1977;**58**:1-8. DOI: 10.1111/j.1463-6395.1977.tb00230

[12] Pudney J, Callard GV. Organization of interstitial tissue in the testis of the salamander *Necturus maculosus* (Caudata: Proteidae). Journal of Morphology. 1984;**181**:87-95. DOI: 10.1002/jmor.1051810108 PMID: 6471107

[13] Brizzi R, Calloni C, Vanni S. Spermatogenetic cycle in *Salamandrina terdigitata* (Lacepede, 1788) (Amphibia: Salamandridae). Zeitschrift Fur Mikroskopisch-Anatomische Forschung. 1985;**99**:271-292

[14] Schindelmeiser J, Bergmann M, Greven H. Cellular differentiation in the urodele testis. In: Duncker HR, Fleischer G, editors. Functional Morphology in Vertebrates. Proceedings of the 1st International Symposium on Vertebrate Morphology Giessen 1983 Fortschritte der Zoologie, Band 30; Stuttgart, New York: Gustav Fischer Verlag; 1985. pp. 445-447

[15] Bergmann M, Schindelmeiser J, Greven H. The zone of mature spermatozoa in the testis of *Salamandra salamandra* (L.) (Amphibia, Urodela). Zeitschrift Fur Mikroskopisch-Anatomische Forschung. 1982;**96**:221-234

[16] Armstrong JB. Spermatogenesis. In: Armstrong JB, Malacinski GM, editors. Developmental Biology of the Axolotl. New York: Columbia University Press; 1989. pp. 36-41

[17] Uribe MC. Chapter 3. Spermatogenesis and male reproductive system. Urodela. In: Ogielska M, editor. Reproduction of Amphibians. Enfield, NH, USA/Plymouth, UK: Science Publishers, Inc.; 2009. pp. 100-124

[18] Ricote M, Alfaro JM, Garcia-Tuñon I, Arenas MI, Fraile B, Paniagua R, Royuela M. Control of the annual testicular cycle of the marbled-newt by p53, p21, and Rb gene products. Molecular Reproduction and Development. 2002;**63**:202-209. DOI: 10.1002/mrd.10167 PMID: 12203830

[19] Uribe MC. The testes, spermatogenesis and male reproductive ducts. In: Sever D, Volume editor. Jamieson BGM, Series editor. Reproductive Biology and Phylogeny of Urodela. Enfield (NH), USA/Plymouth, UK: Science Publishers; 2003. pp. 183-202

[20] Yartsev V, Exbrayat JM, Kuranova VN. Spermatogenesis in the Siberian salamander, *Salamandrella keyserlingii* (Caudata: Hynobiidae). Salamandra. 2017;**53**(1):66-76

[21] Kuramoto M. Scanning electron microscopic studies on the spermatozoa of some Japanese salamanders (Hynobiidae, Cryptobranchidae, Salamandridae). Japanese Journal of Herpetology. 1995;**16**:49-58

[22] Sperone E, Bonacci A, Brunelli E, Tripepi S, Jamieson BGM. Male reproductive system in the Italian newt *Lissotriton italicus* (Peracca 1898) (Amphibia, Urodela): Ultrastructural and morphological study with description of spermiogenesis, spermatozoon and spermatophore. Zoomorphology. 2009;**128**:183-195

[23] Wortham Jr JWE, Brandon RA, Martan RA. Comparative morphology of some plethodontid salamander spermatozoa. Copeia. 1977;(4):666-680

[24] Norris DO. Vertebrate Endocrinology. New York: Academic Press; 1997. p. 634

[25] Lofts B. Amphibians. In: Lamming GE, editor. Marshall's Physiology of Reproduction. Vol. 1. Reproductive Cycles of Vertebrates. Edinburgh: Churchill Livingstone; 1984. pp. 127-105

[26] Bergmann M. The morphology of the testis in *Salamandra salamandra* (L.). In: Greven H Thiesmeier HB, editors. Mertensiella. Supplement zu Salamandra. Proceedings of the Symposium Biology of Salamandra and Mertensiella Nummer 4; Bonn; 1994. pp. 75-82

7

Advanced Label-Free Optical Methods for Spermatozoa Quality Assessment and Selection

Annalisa De Angelis, Maria Antonietta Ferrara,
Giuseppe Coppola and Anna Chiara De Luca

Abstract

Current *in vitro* fertilization (IVF) techniques require a severe selection of sperm, generally based on concentration, morphology, motility, and DNA integrity. Since routinely separation methods may damage the viability of the sperm cell, there is a growing interest in providing a method for noninvasively analyzing spermatozoa taking into account all those parameters. This chapter first reviews the state-of-the-art of label-free sperm cell imaging for IVF, highlighting the limitations of the used techniques. Then, our innovative approach combining Raman spectroscopy and digital holography will be described and its advantages detailed. These include the ability to perform a simultaneous and correlative morphological and biochemical analysis of sperm cells, without labeling, in a fast and reliable way. Finally, the difficulty in reaching clinical use will be discussed, as well as the possible solutions offered by new technological improvements.

Keywords: Raman spectroscopy, digital holography, sperm morphology, label-free analysis, sex-sorting

1. Introduction

It has been estimated that about 15–20% of couples worldwide have infertility problems or impaired fecundity. Approximately 40–50% of these cases are due to male infertility, which could be indirectly measured through the assessment of the sperm production and quality. According to WHO's criteria [1], indeed, men with low sperm concentration (oligospermia), poor sperm motility (asthenospermia), and abnormal sperm morphology (teratospermia) are considered to have male infertility factors. The revised WHO's parameters and the corresponding lower reference limits for semen analyses are reported in **Table 1**.

Infertile couple usually resort to assisted reproduction techniques (ART), chosen by the clinician according to the degree (soft, moderate, or severe) and kind (male and/or female) of

Parameter	Reference value	95% confidence index
Sperm volume	1.5 mL	1.4–1.7
Sperm concentration	15 million sperm/mL	12–16
Total sperm number	39 million sperm per ejaculate	33–46
Morphology	4% normal forms	3–4
Vitality	58% live	55–63
Progressive motility	32%	31–34
Total motility (progressive + nonprogressive)	40%	38–42

Table 1. WHO's parameters for semen analysis (2010).

infertility. For soft/moderate infertility, usually homologous intrauterine insemination (HIUI) or *in vitro* fertilization (IVF) is carried out. HIUI consists in transferring a small volume of selected and isolated motile and morphologically normal spermatozoa directly into the uterus a few hours before the ovulation. IVF is used after continued failures of HIUI due, for example, to an impervious uterine tube, and the fertilization of the oocytes takes place outside the woman body.

In case of severe male infertility, the intracytoplasmic sperm injection (ICSI) is preferred. In this technique, a single spermatozoon is directly injected into an oocyte, bypassing the physiological selection naturally performed by the female tract. Although ICSI has drastically reduced the number of viable sperm required for fertilization, giving hope of conception to extremely severe cases of oligospermia, the rate of successful pregnancy still remains low (<30%), due to the lack of accurate and reliable methods for selecting the spermatozoon that able to fertilize the oocyte.

The first selection is based on motility and morphology. The sperm cells preparation procedure includes a density gradient centrifugation (morphology-based selection) followed by swim-up method (motility-based selection) in order to mimic the physiological selection of the spermatozoa made by the female genital tract. In most laboratories, the sperm quality assessment is relied on the expertise and the subjective skills of the operator. To increase precision and reproducibility, numerous automated computer-aided sperm analysis (CASA) systems have been introduced, and they can automatically view multiple fields in a shallow specimen chamber to capture images of 500 to >2000 sperm in <2 minutes [2]. By using CASA, it is also possible to retrieve some morphometrical parameters, such as ellipticity and regularity, whereas the measurement of the acrosome area generally requires staining.

Moreover, CASA has difficulty in distinguishing spermatozoa from particulate debris, leading to some extent of inaccuracy. In addition, several studies have shown that the correlation between male fertility and the percentage of morphologically normal or motile sperm cells in semen sample is relatively low [3, 4]. Indeed, in infertile men, a high percentage of spermatozoa with a normal morphology or motility could have a damaged DNA, and therefore, they are, in principle, incapable to fertilize the oocyte [4, 5].

Sperm DNA integrity is generally assessed by biochemical methods such as terminal deoxynucleotidyl transferase dUTP nick end labeling (TUNEL) assay [6], comet assay [7], sperm chromatin dispersion (SCD) test [8], or sperm chromatin structural assay (SCSA) [9], which assess the quality of DNA bases, chromatin, and altered protein in sperm nuclei using specific stains. Indeed, all currently employed tests to determine DNA integrity are of limited clinical utility as they are invasive and destructive, rendering the sample unusable for IVF [6–11].

All these methods mentioned above, only based on assessing morphology or motility, are inadequate to select the fertile spermatozoon as the selection techniques have to be noninvasive, safe, highly discriminative, and relatively easy to perform. Moreover, they should simultaneously assess three conditions: normal morphology, motility, and DNA integrity.

Recently, several techniques are emerging for label-free selection of viable spermatozoa. In this chapter, we focus on two of them: Raman-based spectroscopy and phase contrast imaging. Raman spectroscopy (RS) investigates the biochemical and physiological state of a sample by detecting the inelastic light scattering, without labeling or long preparation procedures [12]. Phase contrast imaging includes basic microscopies (bright-field) [13] and more advanced ones (interferometric microscopies) [14–17], such as digital holography. These methods exploit the phase delay of light when passing through a sample. Then, these light delays are converted into intensity changes and recorded on a camera as holograms containing the information suited for morphological sperm cell reconstructions.

The physical principles and the technical instrumentation of Raman and holographic techniques will be separately described in Sections 2 and 3, respectively, also highlighting some relevant results in sperm cells analysis. In Section 4, we will report on our recent achievements using the two techniques in a multimodal analysis setting. Indeed, both the techniques are based on intrinsic optical properties of the sample and may offer the unique advantage to simultaneously acquire the holographic and Raman data assessing single spermatozoa on the base of their morphological and biochemical parameters and their motility. The complete analysis is performed by the same optical system, with a strong impact on costs and times for the analysis. This aspect makes the proposed approaches very promising for clinical applications; however, at present, they are only in experimental stages and specific recommendations for routine procedures cannot be made. At the end of this chapter, the difficulty in reaching clinical use will be discussed, as well as the possible solutions offered by new technological improvements.

2. Label-free biochemical sperm analysis

2.1. Basic principles of Raman spectroscopy

Raman spectroscopy is an optical technique based on the scattering of the light interacting with a sample. Light scattering originates from the elastic or inelastic collision between an incident photon and a molecule of the sample. When the collision occurs, the molecule undergoes an excitation to a virtual state followed by a nearly simultaneous de-excitation towards the initial energy level (elastic) or a vibrational level different from the initial one

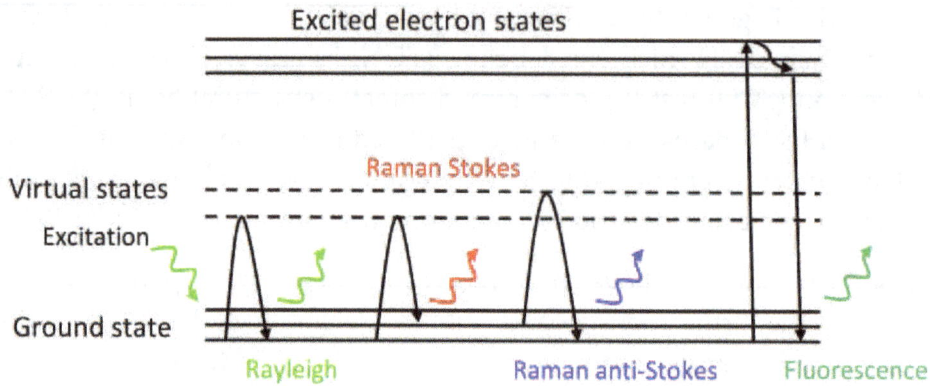

Figure 1. Jablonski diagram representing quantum energy transitions for Rayleigh, Raman scattering (Stokes and anti-Stokes), and fluorescence emission.

(inelastic) (**Figure 1**). The virtual state is an energy level created only when photons interact with electrons and its energy is determined by the frequency itself of the incident photons. When molecules return back to their initial energy state, photons are emitted (scattered). In the elastic process, named Rayleigh scattering, the emitted photons have the same energy of the incident ones. Whereas in the inelastic scattering, there are two possibilities (**Figure 1**): 1. molecules decay from the virtual state to an excited vibrational level emitting photons with a lower energy than the incident ones (Stokes scattering) and 2. when molecules in a vibrational state were excited in a virtual state, they can decay in the ground state, producing photons with energy higher than the incident ones (anti-Stokes scattering). Since the number of molecules in an excited state decreases very fast, anti-Stokes scattering is much less probable than the Stokes scattering (typically by a factor around 1000). For this reason, Raman analysis is usually limited to the observation of the Stokes scattering.

The energy difference between the initial and final vibrational levels (Raman shift) expressed in wavenumbers (cm^{-1}) is given through the relation:

$$\hbar v = \hbar\left(\frac{1}{\lambda_{inc}} - \frac{1}{\lambda_{scat}}\right) \quad (1)$$

in which λ_{inc} and λ_{scat} are the wavelengths of the incident and Raman scattered photons, respectively. Therefore, the energy (or frequency) shifts in the scattered radiation provide a direct measure of the vibrational frequencies of the molecule (v). Since different molecules are characterized by defined vibrational modes, by collecting the photons scattered at different frequencies allows reconstructing a sort of "chemical fingerprint" of the sample.

Therefore, RS turns out to be an extremely powerful tool for interdisciplinary researches, involving physicists, chemists, and biologists, as it allows the characterization of molecules based on properties of chemical bonds. It is a noninvasive and nondestructive technique providing molecular-level information, allowing the investigation of functional groups, bonding types, and molecular conformations.

From an experimental point of view, to observe a Raman spectrum, it is required to suppress the light scattered at the same frequency of the incident radiation (Rayleigh scattering), often more intense than the Raman scattering. Using the notch filter, disperse the spectral components of the light by means of the diffraction grating and image the light onto the detector (high sensitive charge-coupled device (CCD) camera).

In a confocal configuration (micro-RS), a spatial resolution of ~300 nm in the transverse x-y plane and of ~1.2 μm in the axial direction can be achieved. Moreover, for extended samples, it is possible to acquire the Raman spectra on a two- or three-dimensional array of points, scanning the sample with a step comparable with the spatial resolution (Raman imaging). In this way, 2D images (or 3D profiles) are obtained, reporting the spatial variation of a given Raman parameter. This parameter is usually the intensity of a particular Raman band or sometimes it derives from a more complicated analysis of the whole Raman spectrum [18, 19].

2.2. Raman spectroscopy analysis of sperm cells quality

Interestingly, due to the cited characteristics, RS has been successfully employed for the study of several living/fixed cells with subcellular resolution [18]. The first Raman-based single cell analyses were conducted just on individual living salmon sperm cells due to their relative simple structure [20]. Since this pioneer study, no other Raman experiments on sperm cells have been reported until the 2009 when Huser and colleagues [21] examined the spectra obtained from human spermatozoa with different nuclear shapes (box 1 in **Figure 2**) in order to determine if there was a correlation between DNA-protein complex in sperm chromatin and the morphology of the nucleus. RS results showed that while the DNA packaging of normal and abnormal shaped nuclei was different, the nature and the efficiency of DNA packaging in normal head spermatozoa appeared to vary greatly [21]. Therefore, by selecting sperm cells solely based on morphology, a fraction of the normal considered sperm cells used for *in vitro* fertilization will contain improperly packaged DNA, thus resulting infertile. In this study, fixed membrane-free cells were used in order to minimize the potentially interfering contributions from membrane proteins.

The results of this study are also relevant from an epigenetic point of view. Indeed, they show the possibility to use RS for detecting epigenetic alterations (DNA packaging and spatial conformation, methylation and histone modification) in those spermatozoa that, if used in assisted reproductive techniques, may increase the incidence of imprinting disorders and have a deleterious impact on embryonic development [21, 22].

In other studies, RS was applied on whole and fixed sperm cells in order to demonstrate the efficiency of the technique in identifying DNA-damaged sperm cells (box 2 and panels A and Z in the box 3 of **Figure 2**). Usually, the DNA fragmentation as a consequence of oxidative stress is induced by UV radiation [23, 24] or Fenton's treatment [25]. All the studies found that the PO_2 backbone of DNA was significantly affected by the exposure to radiation or treatment, and thus, its corresponding Raman band could represent a significant biomarker of DNA fragmentation [23–25]. Mallidis et al. previously identified characteristic spectral changes indicative of nuclear DNA damage of single fixed human spermatozoa and using Raman mapping, they localized the most damaged sites [24].

In the following study [25], the same group determines the possibility to use Raman microspectroscopy for identifying different levels of sperm nuclear DNA damage induced by oxidative

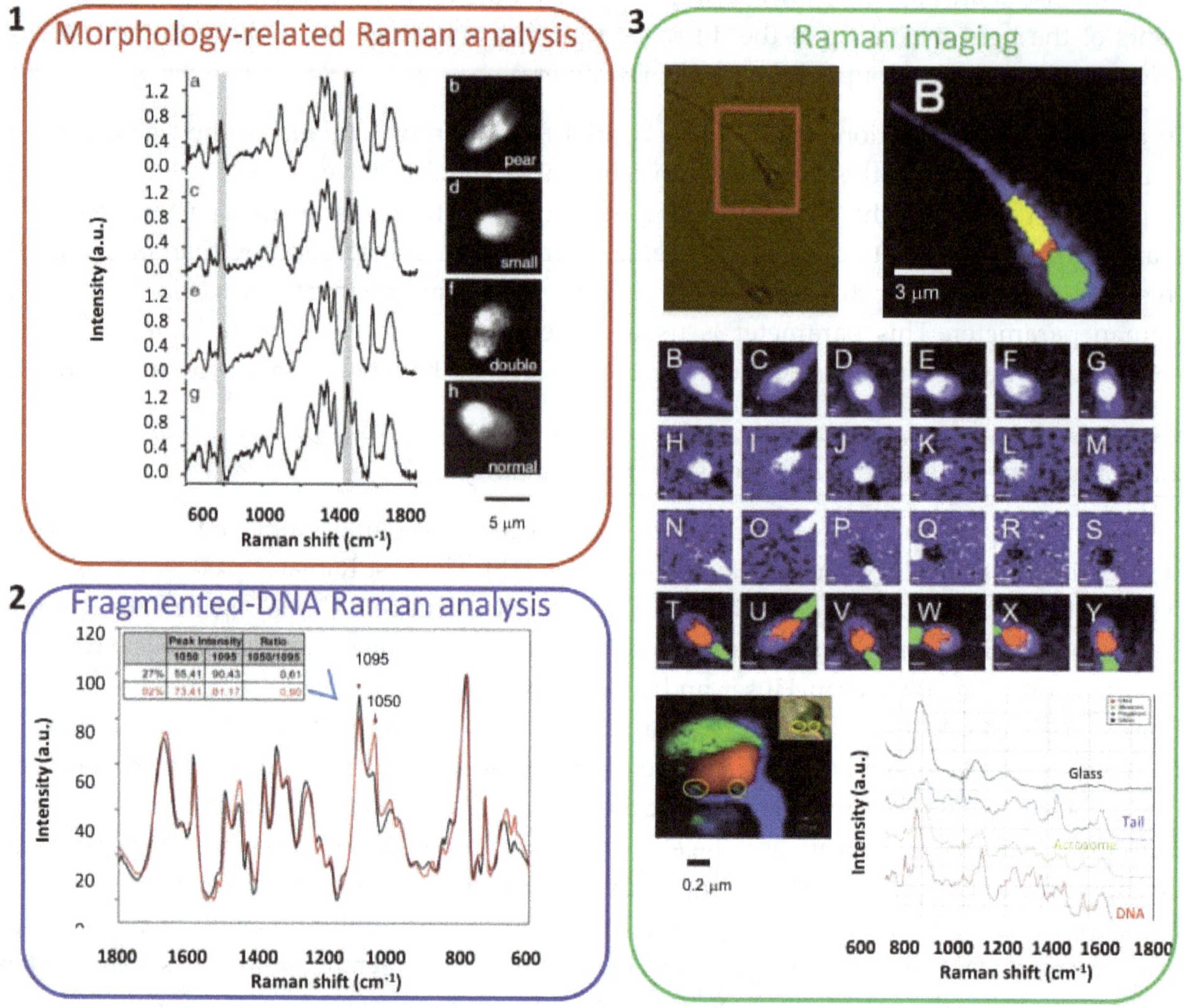

Figure 2. Overview of the most representative studies on Raman spectroscopy and imaging for the label-free analysis of sperm cells. Box 1: the highlighted variations in peak intensities in the Raman spectra correspond to different sperm head shapes [21]. Box 2: the peaks at 1095 and 1050 cm^{-1} represent biomarkers of fragmented DNA in the sperm nucleus [24, 25]. Box 3: panel A shows the chemical Raman reconstruction of distinct sperm regions [23]; panels B–Y represent the biochemical composition of individual immobilized, living human sperm cells [26]; and panel Z shows the efficiency of Raman imaging in revealing small irregularities in the sperm head such as vacuoles (yellow circles) distinguishable based solely on the presence of differing spectra [24].

stress and corroborated the findings using an established assay and an alternative but complementary spectroscopic technique (Fourier-transform infrared (FTIR) spectroscopy). The results of this last work confirm that RS is able to reveal different levels of oxidative DNA fragmentation, especially associated to alterations within the 1050–1095 cm^{-1} spectral range (Raman spectra in the box 2 of **Figure 2**), which includes the band associated with the DNA phosphate backbone, changes that were confirmed by similar shifts in the corresponding FTIR peaks (not shown) [25]. Also, the Raman bands associated to protein and lipid content (1400–1600 cm^{-1}) showed some alterations induced by UV radiation, consistent with protein denaturation and lipid peroxidation that are well-known markers of oxidative damage [27]. Raman-based identification of DNA-damaged sperm cells linearly correlated with the findings from the flow cytometric analysis of DNA fragmentation, which represents the most statistically robust, reproducible, and standardized procedure available for the determination of sperm nDNA damage [28].

In 2015, Edengeiser et al. [26] analyzed spermatozoa under near-physiological conditions using confocal Raman microspectroscopy. The spermatozoa are immobilized on pre-treated object slides. More in detail, CaF_2 slides were coated with concanavalin A and overlaid with preheated Ringer's solution just before putting a drop of isolated spermatozoa which, after the analysis, can be easily removed from the substrate. The study demonstrated for the first time the possibility to image and analyze several tens to hundreds individual cells with a rate of one cell per minute with submicrometer resolution (panels B–Y in the box 3 of **Figure 2**). This opens up possibilities to investigate different physical and biochemical parameters under physiological conditions, leaving the assessed spermatozoa functional.

3. Quantitative phase imaging for sperm analysis

3.1. Basic principles of quantitative phase microscopy

Quantitative phase microscopy (QPM) is a label-free imaging technique, which allows reconstructing both the amplitude and the phase information of an optical field that passes through the sample, and it is particularly interesting in case of transparent biological cells. Respect to differential interference contrast (DIC) microscopy [29] or Nomarski/Zernike's phase contrast [30], the QPM gives a quantitative measure of the optical path difference (OPD) at each point in the sample. OPD in each position (x, y) of the acquisition plane is defined as the refractive index variation across the cell thickness, $t(x, y)$:

$$OPD(x,y) = t(x,y)(n_c - n_s) \tag{2}$$

where n_c and n_s are the refractive index of the cell and the surrounding medium (assumed to be homogeneous), respectively. The resulting OPD map of the cell is reconstructed by recording the interference fringes pattern, the so called "hologram," of two superimposed coherent beams, one that interacts with an object under test and another that does not come in contact with the object and acts as a reference beam, and calculating the phase difference between them [31]. If the hologram is acquired by a digital sensor array, typically a charge-coupled device (CCD) or a complementary metal-oxide semiconductor (CMOS) device, digital holographic microscopy (DHM) technique is implemented. A typical interferometric setup for DHM is reported in **Figure 3**.

The acquired hologram is then mathematically analyzed, allowing obtaining the complex field of the object beam that can be reconstructed at different distances, too. Therefore, numerical refocusing of a digital hologram, that is a 2D image, at different object planes, without any z-scan of the optical system, allows to retrieve a 3D quantitative imaging [31]. This makes digital holography a very powerful method for metrology applications, particularly attractive in the field of biology as it is noninvasive, noncontact, and label-free, allowing the characterization of live specimen.

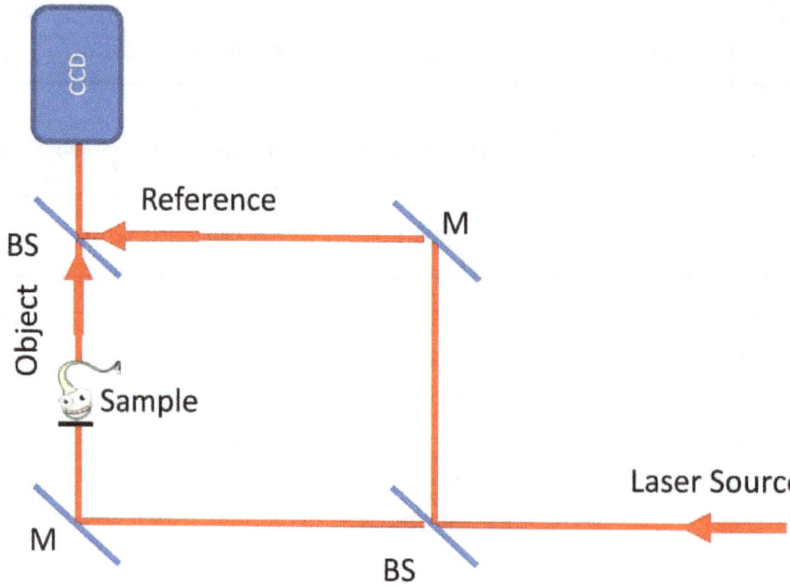

Figure 3. Typical interferometric setup for digital holography microscopy. BS: beam splitter, M: mirror. Reference and object beams are highlighted.

In DHM, in addition to the hologram of the sample under investigation, a second hologram is acquired on a reference region near to the object in order to numerically compensate all the aberrations due to the optical components, comprising the defocusing due to the microscope objective. An "off-axis" configuration is generally adopted to avoid a spatial overlapping of the real and conjugate images due to the holographic reconstruction, leading to the separation of first diffraction order from the entire spatial frequency spectrum. Thus, the spectrum of the sample (object field defined as $S(x,y) = |S(x,y)|e^{i\varphi(x,y)}$, with $|S(x,y)|$ and $\varphi(x,y)$ amplitude and phase, respectively) can be retrieved except for a constant [32]. Then, it is possible to propagate the optical wavefront at different distances from the plane of acquisition applying the Fourier formulation of the Fresnel-Kirchhoff diffraction formula [33, 34]. This reconstruction can be obtained by means of the operator algebra proposed by J. Shamir [35], where Fresnel diffraction is described by replacing the Fresnel-Kirchhoff integral, the lens transfer factor, and other operations by operators. The resulting propagated object field $S_{prop}(\xi,\eta)$ is expressed as a function of the initial object field $S(x,y)$ and can be written as [36, 37]:

$$S_{prop}(\nu,\mu) = \exp(ikd) \times \left\{\Im^{-1}\left[\exp\left(-\frac{ikd\lambda^2}{2}(p^2+q^2)\right)\right]\cdot\Im(S(x,y))\right\} \tag{3}$$

being $\Im[f(x)]$ the Fourier transform of the function $f(x)$, $k = \frac{2\pi n}{\lambda}$ (with n refractive index of the medium), p and q spatial frequencies defined as $p = \frac{\nu}{\lambda d}$ and $q = \frac{\mu}{\lambda d}$, and d the reconstruction distance. For digital reconstruction, Eq. (3) is applied in a discrete form:

$$S_{prop}(m,n) = \exp(ikd)\left\{\Im_D^{-1}\left[-\frac{ikd\lambda^2}{2N^2d^2}(U^2+V^2)\right]\cdot\Im_D(S(h,j))\right\} \tag{4}$$

where N is the number of pixels in both directions and m, n, U, V, h, and j are integer numbers varying from 0 to $N-1$.

Intensity and phase distributions can be reconstructed by $S_{prop}(m, n)$ according to the following equations:

$$I_{prop}(m,n) = \left|S_{prop}(m,n)\right|^2; \tag{5}$$

$$\varphi_{prop}(m,n) = \arctan\frac{\mathrm{Im}\left[S_{prop}(m,n)\right]}{\mathrm{Re}\left[S_{prop}(m,n)\right]}. \tag{6}$$

The phase $\varphi_{prop}(m, n)$ includes information about the morphological profile of the object under investigation; in fact, it is related to the *OPD*:

$$OPD(m,n) = \frac{\lambda}{2\pi}\varphi_{prop}(m,n). \tag{7}$$

The relation between the *OPD* and the thickness of the cell *t* is given by Eq. (2).

3.2. Digital holography microscopy for sperm cells assessment

Digital holography (DH) allows retrieving a fully 3D image of the sample, thus offering new prospects for the analysis of sperm cells in a noninvasive, quantitative, and label-free way. Sperm cells were acquired by a digital holographic microscope for the first time in 2008 by Mico et al. [38].

The potential of applying this technique for label-free sperm assessment was recently confirmed by Shaked's group. Indeed, they demonstrated that DHM allows obtaining equivalent information about key morphological parameters of fixed human spermatozoa to that obtained by bright field microscopy (BFM) imaging of stained sperm cells [39].

Additionally, the opportunity to have information about the third dimension in the sperm analysis can offer a better understanding of this kind of cell and of male infertility [40]. Furthermore, since this technique allows obtaining quantitative information and numerical analysis, estimation area or profiles in a given direction may be carried out. Such kind of analysis can help to study the male infertility and its possible relation with the abnormal morphology [41, 42].

DH has been mainly employed to study the morphology of human sperm cells in order to verify the integrity of their structures and to evaluate their kinematic parameters and concentration. This approach allows to visualize the morphology of abnormal sperm and to analyze in 3D some typical defects such as cytoplasmic droplet along the tail, bent tail, and acrosome broken, as reported in the box 1 of **Figure 4** [42].

Additionally, a quantitative study of vacuoles has been performed by DH. In particular, it was demonstrated that the profile of the normal spermatozoon results higher than that of the spermatozoon with vacuoles, whereas their 2D dimensions (such as area and axes length) are similar [43]. The difference in height denotes a reduced volume in spermatozoon with vacuoles respect to the normal spermatozoon; this difference could be ascribed to a modification of the inner structure of the sperm head with loss of material (see box 1 in **Figure 4**).

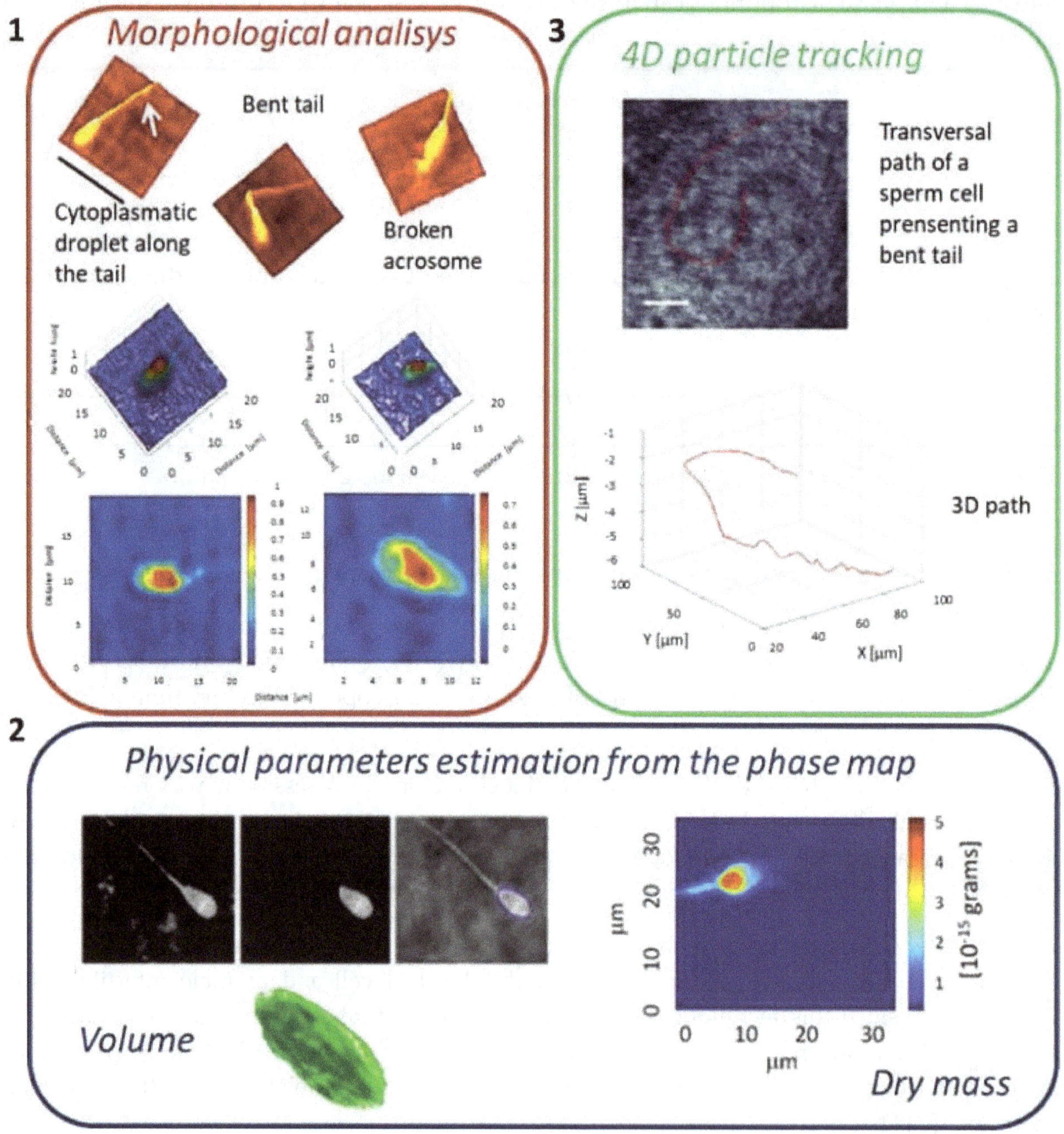

Figure 4. Some potentialities of DHM. Box 1: morphological analysis of semen carried out by DHM; top panels: sperm cells with distinct morphological defects; center and bottom panels: difference in height denotes a reduced volume in spermatozoon head with vacuoles respect to the normal spermatozoon [41, 43]. Box 2: examples of some physical parameters obtained by DHM [31, 44]. Box 3: 4D tracking of clinical sperm samples [45].

In 2013, Merola et al. [44] provided an evaluation of the biovolume of spermatozoa (about 55 μm^3). The authors used optical tweezers to trap and rotate the cells; meanwhile, they flow through a microchannel, enabling recording digital holograms of the sperm at different angles and the production of a tomographic 3D model, as showed in the box 2 of **Figure 4**.

Another important semen parameter, the dry mass of the cell (i.e. the average mass of the proteins, carbohydrates, lipids, and so on within the cell), can be obtained by DHM. Indeed, the *OPD* of the cell linearly depends on the axially averaged refractive index of the cell relative to the surrounding medium, for a given thickness *t* [45]. Thus, considering that the human spermatozoa head can be divided in the cell nucleus and the acrosome, which differ in the composition and concentration of proteins, nucleic acids, and other components, Balberg et al. evaluated the dry mass of the cell by starting by the knowledge of the *OPD* [31]. In particular, the authors measured the dry mass of separate cellular compartments in the *OPD* maps of unlabeled human spermatozoa, as reported in the box 2 of **Figure 4**.

Finally, the movements of living spermatozoa have been tracked applying an automatic 4D tracking (movements in the 3D spatial directions over time) of the swimming samples in [46]. The results are showed in the box 3 of **Figure 4**, where an anomalous spermatozoa behavior, known as "bent tail," is highlighted. A collection of several holograms at a fixed distance between the sample and the microscope objective was acquired. In order to simultaneously track multiple spermatozoa, a proximity criterion has been included into the algorithm. In particular, by means of this approach, the position in the $(n + 1)$th frame has been searched in a reasonable neighborhood of the nth frame position.

Therefore, DH could be seen as a breakthrough that can renew the sperm analysis in the spermatology laboratories, encouraging researchers in the field of sperm cell biology to consider using DH as a standard method for their characterization studies.

4. Combined optical approach for the noninvasive analysis of single spermatozoa

As seen in the previous sections, Raman spectroscopy and quantitative phase microscopies have been separately developed for assessing spermatozoa from a biochemical and morphological perspective, respectively. The two photonic techniques, employing intrinsic contrast mechanisms, allow noninvasively selecting the fertile spermatozoon according to its normal morphology as well as its DNA integrity. Kang et al. [47] first proposed a combined system where quantitative phase microscopy and Raman imaging allowed correlating morphological parameters with molecular information, i.e. the red blood cell thickness was correlated to the hemoglobin distribution. Huang and colleagues in 2014 published a study that evaluated the possibility to combine micro-Raman spectroscopy with image analysis for label-free identification of normal spermatozoa [48]. Recently, our group proposed a similar system, which combines Raman spectroscopy/imaging and digital holography microscopy as a potential tool to rapidly and objectively identify the healthy spermatozoa [36, 49, 50].

4.1. The optical setup

The setup used in our works for the simultaneous Raman and holographic analysis essentially consists of a Raman microscope coupled to an interferometer (**Figure 5**) [36, 49, 50]. We used two different laser sources: a green laser at 532 nm for the Raman excitation and a long coherence (>100 m) red laser at 660 nm for the holographic experiments. The red laser beam was split into two beams: the object beam passing through the sample and the reference beam

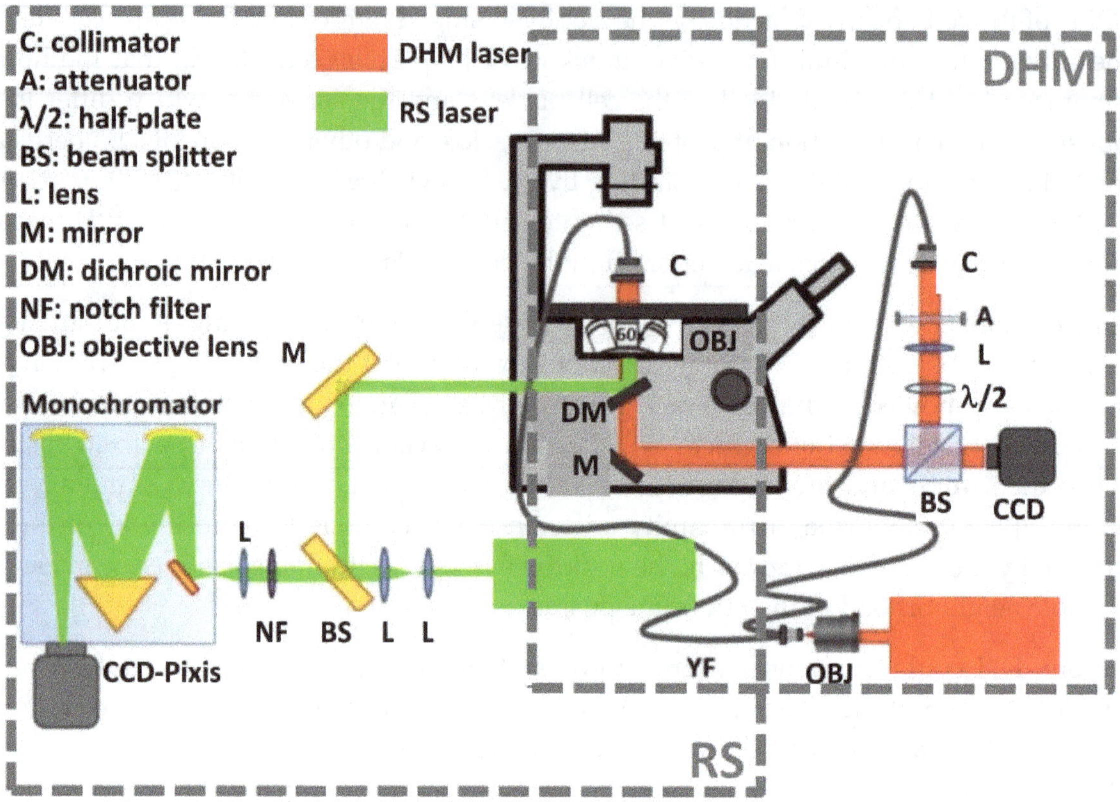

Figure 5. Experimental set up of the combined Raman and holographic system used in our works [36, 49, 50].

that directly goes to the detector. Importantly, the reference beam was controllable in intensity and polarization enabling us to improve signal intensity and contrast. The collimated object beam of the holographic pathway is recombined to the reference beam by a beam splitter (BS). The recombined beams are filtered and sent to the CCD camera (CCD1) for the holograms recording.

The green light is focused on the sample by a high numerical aperture objective lens. The high N.A. of the objective and the wavelength chosen for the Raman beam allows to reaching spatial resolutions on the order of less than 0.5 μm, particularly suitable for cell imaging application. The back-scattered light from the sample is collected by the same objective lens (OBJ) and separated from the holographic radiation by a long pass dichroic mirror (DM) reflecting wavelength below 600 nm. The scattered light, consisting of Rayleigh and Raman radiation, is filtered through a dichroic beam splitter (BS45) that rejects the Rayleigh light at 532 nm. The Raman signal is further filtered using a laser-blocking filter (NF0) to eliminate the residual Rayleigh scattering and then focused onto the entrance slit of a monochromator. The Raman signal is finally detected using a cooled CCD camera (CCD2).

4.2. Morphological and biochemical analysis of single sperm cells

In this paragraph, some of the most interesting results we have obtained by applying the Raman/holographic microscope for the sperm cell characterization will be discussed. Our investigations mainly focused on:

1. correlative analysis of morphological and biochemical alterations [49];
2. morphological and biochemical analysis of photo-damaged spermatozoa [36];
3. sex classification of bovine spermatozoa [49, 51].

With the aim of demonstrating the potential applicability of the proposed multimodal imaging approach in identifying the fertile spermatozoa for IVF, we have first performed a qualitative Raman/holographic analysis of single sperm cells [49].

Raman imaging can be performed scanning the laser over a region of interest of the sperm cell or on the entire cells, acquiring in that way a point-by-point spectrum. Similar spectral features correspond to similar molecular structures; consequently, we can identify separate regions of the spermatozoon (acrosome, nucleus, and tail) according to their different chemical composition (**Figure 6a** and **b**). Pseudo-color Raman map of the sperm is shown in **Figure 6b**, in which each color is arbitrarily associated to specific Raman spectral patterns. Therefore, the Raman map delineates not only the distribution of DNA and protein in the nucleus, acrosome and tail but also detects, in a label-free manner, small biochemical discrepancies correlated with the presence of morphological defects, highlighted by digital holography (**Figure 6c**). We found that the peculiar protuberance in the region of the spermatozoon connecting the head to the tail, the so-called middle piece, well correlated with the biochemical alteration detected in the Raman map. Indeed, by analyzing the typical Raman bands of the spectra acquired in that specific cell region, it was possible to correlate the morphological alteration to an increased amount of proteins in the middle-piece region, where mitochondria are localized [49].

Recently, we applied the multimodal imaging tool for the online evaluation of the damages induced by green laser radiation for studying in which dose and how it affects the irradiated sperm cells [36]. Severe spermatozoa variations associated with a topological redistribution of the sample and a gradual decrease in the Raman signal intensity were detected in a label-free configuration (**Figure 7a–c**). Importantly, at laser fluences (30 MJ/cm^2) where no morphological alterations were detected by digital holography, high specific spectral variations were monitored to evaluate the cell photodegradation. More specifically, Raman analysis provided precise information on the most affected biochemical structures, finding that DNA phosphate

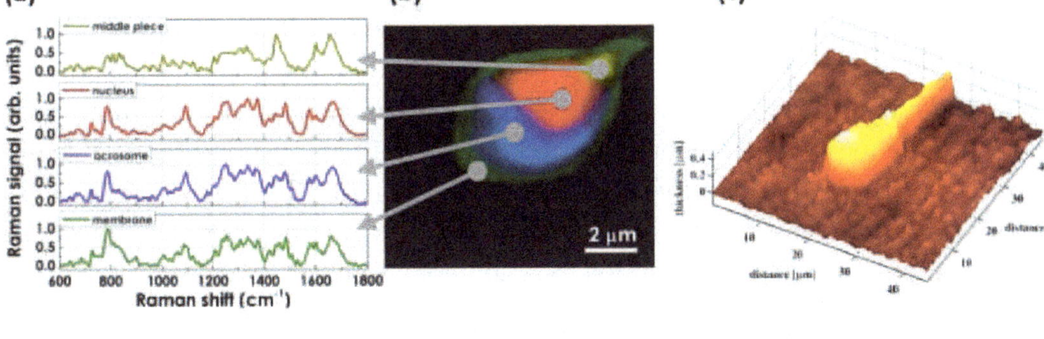

Figure 6. (a) Raman spectra and (b) false-color Raman map of different regions of the sperm cell head: middle piece (yellow), nucleus (red), acrosome (blue), and membrane (green). (c) 3D digital holographic reconstruction of the sperm cell morphology [49].

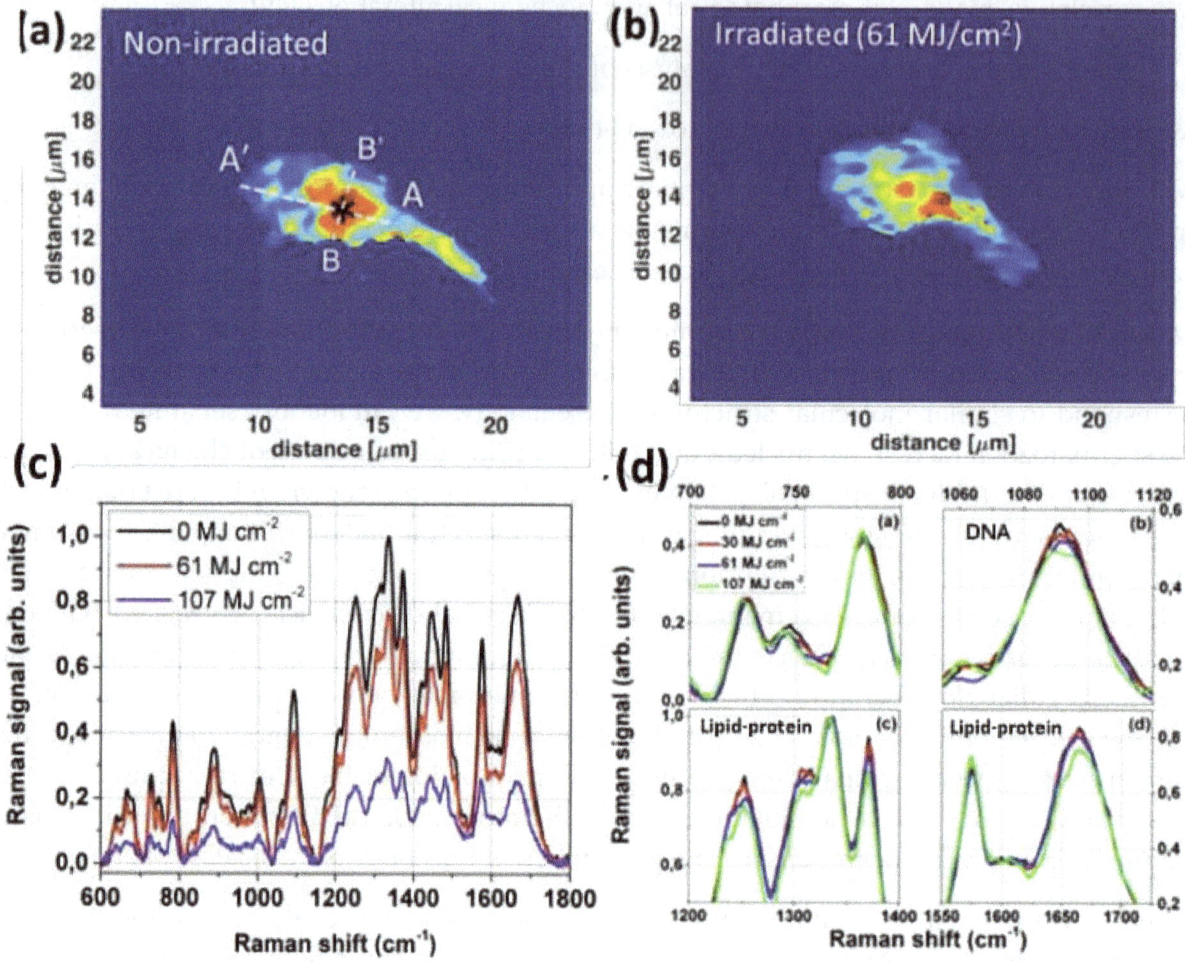

Figure 7. (Top) Reconstructed phase map of the (a) nonirradiated and (b) irradiated region of interest at the focus plane. The star (*) indicates the cell position where the Raman spectrum is acquired that corresponds to the irradiated area. (c) Raman spectra of the sperm cell at three different selected laser fluences (0, 61 and 107 MJ/cm^2). (d) Zoom of four selected Raman spectra acquired at laser fluences of 0, 30, 61 and 107 MJ/cm^2 in the spectral region between 700–800 cm^{-1}, 1050–1120 cm^{-1}, 1200–1400 cm^{-1} and 1550–1720 cm^{-1} [36].

backbone (900–1100 cm^{-1}) and lipids and proteins (1200–1400 cm^{-1}) are very sensitive to photoxidative denaturation (**Figure 7d**) [36].

To test the biochemical/morphological ability of the proposed multimodal approach, we additionally tested bovine sperm cells. The sex preselection of the offspring reveals a high significant impact on animal production management as well as genetic improvement programs. Since a noninvasive method for sex predetermination in animals is still not available, we used our multimodal approach for identifying and separating X and Y-bearing sperm cells. The key parameters estimated in our works [49, 51], on hundreds bovine spermatozoa of different bulls, were the Raman bands correlated to DNA content and head volume.

Indeed, specific peaks related to the vibrational modes of the DNA bases (726 and 785 cm^{-1}) can be used to sort X- and Y-bovine sperm cells (**Figure 8a** and **b**). However, additional significant spectral variations can be observed in the Raman bands mainly associated with the presence of lipids and proteins (1400–1600 cm^{-1}, **Figure 8a** and **b**), due to the different composition of the

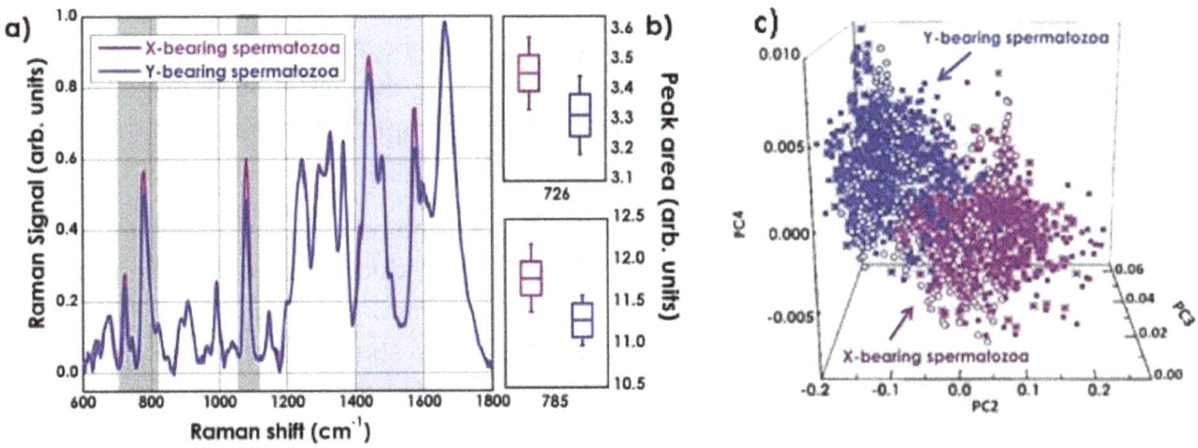

Figure 8. (a) Average Raman spectra of 900 X- (purple line) and 900 Y- (blue line) sperm cell spectra acquired in the "fingerprint" spectral region. (b) Measured peak area of the bands at 726 and 785 cm^{-1}, highlighting the different DNA content measured for X and Y sperm cells, $\Delta A = 4.2 \pm 0.9\%$. (c) PCA score plots of PC2, PC3 and PC4 showing the separation of data corresponding to X- and Y- sperm cells [49, 51].

sex-associated membrane proteins in X- and Y-bearing sperm cells. In order to quantify the efficiency and the accuracy of the Raman spectroscopy in discriminating the two sperm cell populations, we have analyzed the data using a multivariate statistical method, known as principal component analysis, that allows to visualizing the separation of the two classes of cells into two well distinct clusters (**Figure 8c**), only on the base of the differences in their Raman fingerprint. The sorting accuracy resulted of 90.6%, which is comparable to the accuracy (90–94%) achievable with standard sorting techniques such as fluorescence-activated cell sorting (FACS).

Then, the spectroscopic results have been correlated with the morphological analysis, where the sperm head volume has been evaluated by applying the Otsu's method [51] on the holographic phase map, a procedure generally used to indirectly measure morphological properties of the region under investigation (results not reported, see [49, 51]). As the main differences between X and Y chromosomes are the size (X chromosome is bigger than Y one) and the total DNA content, these major differences can be reflected in the head sperm volume, representing therefore a fast and automated way to identify the chromosome type [49, 51].

Therefore, by combining holographic with Raman microscopy provides label-free, quantitative morphological and chemical information from unfixed sperm cells. The combination offers an excellent system for a complete, morphological and physiological, monitoring of the sperm cell quality.

5. Towards clinical applications: a demanding path

Despite the feasibility of Raman spectroscopy and holography microscopies has been successfully demonstrated in many medical and biological applications [14, 16, 30, 52–55], there is still a significant lack of translation and implementation of such innovative techniques into clinical practice. Indeed, while thanks to the technological advances the capability and information achievable are quickly expanding, there are some concerns to consider [56].

The Raman signals are generally low and often obscured by the presence of the cell autofluorescence. However, the fluorescence-free detection can be achieved using instruments working in the near-IR region of the spectrum, also reducing the cell photodamage. Alternatively, modulating or multiwavelengths approaches can be employed to eliminate the fluorescence background [57–59].

Another crucial aspect for translational applications is the time required to collect the spectral data and reconstruct the Raman images. Indeed, for reproductive medicine applications, performing experiment in real-time is crucial. Recently, several approaches have been proposed providing a faster imaging modality and allowing investigation of several sperm cells simultaneously such as the Coherent anti-Stokes Raman scattering (CARS) and surface-enhanced Raman scattering (SERS) imaging [60, 61] or the use of structured illumination [62, 63]. Moreover, in our specific case, the sample is moving while measuring. This represents another problem that researchers are trying to overcome using the laser trapping capability [64, 65], slide functionalization procedures [25, 66], or microfluidic devices [67, 68].

A further obstacle to the clinical success of these new methods is the complexity in interpreting the results. Indeed, the newer instruments for Raman/holographic imaging are fast, efficient, and reliable; however, they require specialized operators. An useful system should be easier to use, providing clear and automated answers to biomedical problems instead of spectra or holograms. The ongoing implementation of computer-assisted diagnosis algorithms is helping the interpretation of the holographic images, while further work on the creation of larger Raman database is still required.

The economical aspect has also to be considered. Raman spectroscopy and digital holography use precise equipment. If we consider that a holographic imaging system is sensitive to optical pathway differences on the nanoscale and has to be isolated to any kinds of vibrations for avoiding artifacts, we can well image that the precision required in the construction of such devices is more expansive than that of conventional microscopes currently in clinical use.

The path to clinical implementation of innovative multimodal imaging techniques for sperm cell assessment passes through the following milestones: 1. identification of the medical problem and the need for a new technique; 2. experimental tests of the technique, showing the proof of principle and the feasibility of the specific application; 3. closely collaboration between researchers and clinicians for evaluating the clinical relevance of the information the new technique provides; 4. optimisation of the technique for the specific application in order to improve its sensibility, specificity and robustness; 5. clinical trials; 6. industrial implementation of the system for making it clinician and patient friendly; and 7. Clinical implementation.

The proof of principle of Raman spectroscopy and holographic imaging as sperm selection techniques has been successfully demonstrated. Their use for detecting epigenetic alterations, including DNA packaging and spatial conformation, methylation, and histone modification, that could seriously affect the embryonic development has been showed [21]. Researches in this field are currently focusing on the points 3 and 4, as highlighted in this chapter. Our efforts aim to assess the feasibility and the reliability of the two techniques before initiating the clinical trials, filling in such a way the gap between experimentation and clinical implementation.

Author details

Annalisa De Angelis[1]*, Maria Antonietta Ferrara[2], Giuseppe Coppola[2] and Anna Chiara De Luca[1]

*Address all correspondence to: a.deangelis@ibp.cnr.it

1 Institute of Protein Biochemistry - National Research Council, Naples, Italy

2 Institute for Microelectronics and Microsystems - National Research Council, Naples, Italy

References

[1] Cooper TG, Noonan E, von Eckardstein S, Auger J, Baker HWG, Behre HM, et al. World Health Organization reference values for human semen characteristics. Human Reproduction Update. 2009;**00**(0):1-15

[2] Mortimer ST. CASA—Practical aspects. Journal of Andrology. 2000;**21**(4):515-524

[3] Hirano Y, Shibahara H, Obara H, Suzuki T, Takamizawa S, Yamaguchi C, et al. Andrology: Relationships between sperm motility characteristics assessed by the computer-aided sperm analysis (CASA) and fertilization rates in vitro. Journal of Assisted Reproduction and Genetics. 2001;**18**(4):215-220

[4] Zaini A, Jennings MG, Baker HWG. Are conventional sperm morphology and motility assessments of predictive value in subfertile men? International Journal of Andrology. 1985 Dicembre;**8**(6):427-435

[5] Avendaño C, Oehninger S. DNA fragmentation in morphologically normal spermatozoa: How much should we be concerned in the ICSI era? Journal of Andrology. 2011 Jul 8;**32** (4):356-363

[6] Sharma R, Masaki J, Agarwal A. Sperm DNA fragmentation analysis using the TUNEL assay. In: Spermatogenesis: Methods and Protocols. 2013;**927**:121-136

[7] Simon L, Lutton D, McManus J, Lewis SE. Sperm DNA damage measured by the alkaline Comet assay as an independent predictor of male infertility and in vitro fertilization success. Fertility and Sterility. 2011;**95**(2):652-657

[8] Fernández JL, Muriel L, Goyanes V, Segrelles E, Gosálvez J, Enciso M, et al. Simple determination of human sperm DNA fragmentation with an improved sperm chromatin dispersion test. Fertility and Sterility. 2005;**84**(4):833-842

[9] Evenson DP. Sperm chromatin structure assay (SCSA®). In: Spermatogenesis: Methods and Protocols. 2013;**927**:147-164

[10] Sánchez V, Wistuba J, Mallidis C. Semen analysis: Update on clinical value, current needs and future perspectives. Reproduction. 2013;**146**(6):R249-R258

[11] Henkel R, Kierspel E, Hajimohammad M, Stalf T, Hoogendijk C, Mehnert C, et al. DNA fragmentation of spermatozoa and assisted reproduction technology. Reproductive Biomedicine Online. 2003;**7**(4):477-484

[12] Notingher I. Raman spectroscopy cell-based biosensors. Sensors. 2007;**7**(8):1343-1358

[13] Chang L, LoBiondo JG. Setup of micromanipulator for sperm selection and injection for IMSI: Configuring the microscope for intracytoplasmic morphology-selected sperm injection (IMSI). In: Agarwal A, Borges Jr E, Setti A. (eds) Non-Invasive Sperm Selection for In Vitro Fertilization. Springer, New York, NY; 2015. p. 91-103 https://doi.org/10.1007/978-1-4939-1411-1_9

[14] Haifler M, Girshovitz P, Band G, Dardikman G, Madjar I, Shaked NT. Interferometric phase microscopy for label-free morphological evaluation of sperm cells. Fertility and Sterility. 2015 Luglio;**104**(1):43-47.e2

[15] Coppola G, Caprio GD, Wilding M, Ferraro P, Esposito G, Matteo LD, et al. Digital holographic microscopy for the evaluation of human sperm structure. Zygote. 2014 Nov;**22**(4):446-454

[16] Gianaroli L, Magli MC, Ferraretti AP, Crippa A, Lappi M, Capitani S, et al. Birefringence characteristics in sperm heads allow for the selection of reacted spermatozoa for intracytoplasmic sperm injection. Fertility and Sterility. 2010;**93**(3):807-813

[17] De Angelis A, Ferrara MA, Di Caprio G, Managò S, Sirleto L, Coppola G, et al. A combined holographic and Raman microscopy approach for the assessment of spermatozoa. In: Fotonica AEIT Italian Conference on Photonics Technologies, 6-8 May 2015; Turin, Italy: IET Digital Library; 2015. p. 1- 4

[18] Puppels GJ, de Mul FFM, Otto C, Greve J, Robert-Nicoud M, Arndt-Jovin DJ, et al. Studying single living cells and chromosomes by confocal Raman microspectroscopy. Nature. 1990 Sep 20;**347**(6290):301-303

[19] Majzner K, Kaczor A, Kachamakova-Trojanowska N, Fedorowicz A, Chlopicki S, Baranska M. 3D confocal Raman imaging of endothelial cells and vascular wall: Perspectives in analytical spectroscopy of biomedical research. The Analyst. 2013;**138**(2):603-610

[20] Kubasek WL, Wang Y, Thomas GA, Patapoff TW, Schoenwaelder KH, Van der Sande JH, et al. Raman spectra of the model B-DNA oligomer d (CGCGAATTCGCG) 2 and of the DNA in living salmon sperm show that both have very similar B-type conformations. Biochemistry (Moscow). 1986;**25**(23):7440-7445

[21] Huser T, Orme CA, Hollars CW, Corzett MH, Balhorn R. Raman spectroscopy of DNA packaging in individual human sperm cells distinguishes normal from abnormal cells. Journal of Biophotonics. 2009;**2**(5):322

[22] Rajender S, Avery K, Agarwal A. Epigenetics, spermatogenesis and male infertility. Mutation Research. 2011;**727**(3):62-71

[23] Meister K, Schmidt DA, Bründermann E, Havenith M. Confocal Raman microspectroscopy as an analytical tool to assess the mitochondrial status in human spermatozoa. The Analyst. 2010;**135**(6):1370-1374

[24] Mallidis C, Wistuba J, Bleisteiner B, Damm OS, Gross P, Wübbeling F, et al. In situ visualization of damaged DNA in human sperm by Raman microspectroscopy. Human Reproduction. 2011;**26**(7):1641-1649

[25] Sánchez V, Redmann K, Wistuba J, Wübbeling F, Burger M, Oldenhof H, et al. Oxidative DNA damage in human sperm can be detected by Raman microspectroscopy. Fertility and Sterility. 2012;**98**(5):1124-1129

[26] Edengeiser E, Meister K, Bründermann E, Büning S, Ebbinghaus S, Havenith M. Non-invasive chemical assessment of living human spermatozoa. RSC Advances. 2015;**5**(14): 10424-10429

[27] Barry H, Okezie IA. DNA and Free Radicals. England: Ellis Horwood Limited; 1993

[28] Shamsi MB, Imam SN, Dada R. Sperm DNA integrity assays: Diagnostic and prognostic challenges and implications in management of infertility. Journal of Assisted Reproduction and Genetics. 2011;**28**(11):1073-1085

[29] Arnison MR, Larkin KG, Sheppard CJ, Smith NI, Cogswell CJ. Linear phase imaging using differential interference contrast microscopy. Journal of Microscopy. 2004;**214**(1):7-12

[30] Zernike F. Phase contrast, a new method for the microscopic observation of transparent objects. Physica. 1942;**9**(7):686-698

[31] Balberg M, Levi M, Kalinowski K, Barnea I, Mirsky SK, Shaked NT. Localized measurements of physical parameters within human sperm cells obtained with wide-field interferometry. Journal of Biophotonics. 2017 Gennaio;n/a-n/a

[32] Schnars U, Jüptner W. Direct recording of holograms by a CCD target and numerical reconstruction. Applied Optics. 1994;**33**(2):179-181

[33] Yu L, Cai L. Iterative algorithm with a constraint condition for numerical reconstruction of a three-dimensional object from its hologram. JOSA A. 2001;**18**(5):1033-1045

[34] Goodman JW. Introduction to Fourier Optics. Roberts and Company Publishers. 3rd ed. Greenwood Village, CO; 2005. 520 p

[35] Nazarathy M, Shamir J. Fourier optics described by operator algebra. JOSA. 1980;**70**(2): 150-159

[36] Ferrara MA, De Angelis A, De Luca AC, Coppola G, Dale B, Coppola G. Simultaneous holographic microscopy and Raman spectroscopy monitoring of human spermatozoa photodegradation. IEEE Journal of Selected Topics in Quantum Electronics. 2016;**22**(3):1-8

[37] Ferrara MA, Dardano P, De Stefano L, Rea I, Coppola G, Rendina I, et al. Optical properties of diatom nanostructured biosilica in *Arachnoidiscus* sp: Micro-optics from mother nature. PLoS One. 2014;**9**(7):e103750

[38] Mico V, Zalevsky Z, Ferreira C, García J. Superresolution digital holographic microscopy for three-dimensional samples. Optics Express. 2008;**16**(23):19260-19270

[39] Haifler M, Girshovitz P, Band G, Dardikman G, Madjar I, Shaked NT. Interferometric phase microscopy for label-free morphological evaluation of sperm cells. Fertility and Sterility. 2015;**104**(1):43-47

[40] Guerrero A, Carneiro J, Pimentel A, Wood CD, Corkidi G, Darszon A. Strategies for locating the female gamete: The importance of measuring sperm trajectories in three spatial dimensions. MHR: Basic Science of Reproductive Medicine. 2011;**17**(8):511-523

[41] Di Caprio G, Gioffre MA, Saffioti N, Grilli S, Ferraro P, Puglisi R, et al. Quantitative label-free animal sperm imaging by means of digital holographic microscopy. IEEE Journal of Selected Topics in Quantum Electronics. 2010;**16**(4):833-840

[42] Di Caprio G, Ferrara MA, Miccio L, Merola F, Memmolo P, Ferraro P, et al. Holographic imaging of unlabelled sperm cells for semen analysis: A review. Journal of Biophotonics. 2015;**8**:779-789

[43] Coppola G, Di Caprio G, Wilding M, Ferraro P, Esposito G, Di Matteo L, et al. Digital holographic microscopy for the evaluation of human sperm structure. Zygote. 2014; **22**(4):446-454

[44] Merola F, Miccio L, Memmolo P, Di Caprio G, Galli A, Puglisi R, et al. Digital holography as a method for 3D imaging and estimating the biovolume of motile cells. Lab on a Chip. 2013;**13**(23):4512-4516

[45] Shaked NT, Satterwhite LL, Rinehart MT, Wax A. Quantitative analysis of biological cells using digital holographic microscopy. In: Joseph Rosen, editor. Holography, Research and Technologies. InTech; 2011. p. 219-236

[46] Di Caprio G, El Mallahi A, Ferraro P, Dale R, Coppola G, Dale B, et al. 4D tracking of clinical seminal samples for quantitative characterization of motility parameters. Biomedical Optics Express. 2014;**5**(3):690-700

[47] Kang JW, Lue N, Kong C-R, Barman I, Dingari NC, Goldfless SJ, et al. Combined confocal Raman and quantitative phase microscopy system for biomedical diagnosis. Biomedical Optics Express. 2011;**2**(9):2484-2492

[48] Huang Z, Chen G, Chen X, Wang J, Chen J, Lu P, et al. Rapid and label-free identification of normal spermatozoa based on image analysis and micro-Raman spectroscopy. Journal of Biophotonics. 2014;**7**(9):671-675

[49] Ferrara MA, Di Caprio G, Managò S, De Angelis A, Sirleto L, Coppola G, et al. Label-free imaging and biochemical characterization of bovine sperm cells. Biosensors. 2015;**5**(2):141-157

[50] De Angelis A, Managò S, Ferrara MA, Napolitano M, Coppola G, De Luca AC. Combined Raman spectroscopy and digital holographic microscopy for sperm cell quality analysis. Journal of Spectroscopy. 2017;**2017**:1-14

[51] De Luca AC, Managó S, Ferrara MA, Rendina I, Sirleto L, Puglisi R, et al. Non-invasive sex assessment in bovine semen by Raman spectroscopy. Laser Physics Letters. 2014;**11**(5):055604

[52] Otsu N. A threshold selection method from gray-level histograms. Automatica. 1975;**11** (285–296):23-27

[53] Harz M, Rösch P, Popp J. Vibrational spectroscopy—A powerful tool for the rapid identification of microbial cells at the single-cell level. Cytometry. Part A. 2009;**75**(2):104-113

[54] Li M, Xu J, Romero-Gonzalez M, Banwart SA, Huang WE. Single cell Raman spectroscopy for cell sorting and imaging. Current Opinion in Biotechnology. 2012;**23**(1):56-63

[55] Managò S, Valente C, Mirabelli P, Circolo D, Basile F, Corda D, et al. A reliable Raman-spectroscopy-based approach for diagnosis, classification and follow-up of B-cell acute lymphoblastic leukemia. Scientific Reports. 2016;**6**:24821

[56] Webb SJ. Laser-Raman spectroscopy of living cells. Physics Reports. 1980;**60**(4):201-224

[57] Canetta E, Mazilu M, De Luca AC, Carruthers AE, Dholakia K, Neilson S, et al. Modulated Raman spectroscopy for enhanced identification of bladder tumor cells in urine samples. Journal of Biomedical Optics. 2011;**16**(3):037002-037002

[58] De Luca AC, Mazilu M, Riches A, Herrington CS, Dholakia K. Online fluorescence suppression in modulated Raman spectroscopy. Analytical Chemistry. 2009;**82**(2):738-745

[59] De Luca AC, Dholakia K, Mazilu M. Modulated Raman spectroscopy for enhanced cancer diagnosis at the cellular level. Sensors. 2015;**15**(6):13680-13704

[60] Li L, Wang H, Cheng J-X. Quantitative coherent anti-Stokes Raman scattering imaging of lipid distribution in coexisting domains. Biophysical Journal. 2005;**89**(5):3480-3490

[61] Zito G, Rusciano G, Pesce G, Dochshanov A, Sasso A. Surface-enhanced Raman imaging of cell membrane by a highly homogeneous and isotropic silver nanostructure. Nanoscale. 2015;**7**(18):8593-8606

[62] De Luca AC, Reader-Harris P, Mazilu M, Mariggio S, Corda D, Di Falco A. Reproducible surface-enhanced Raman quantification of biomarkers in multicomponent mixtures. ACS Nano. 2014;**8**(3):2575-2583

[63] Kosmeier S, Zolotovskaya S, De Luca AC, Riches A, Herrington CS, Dholakia K, et al. Nonredundant Raman imaging using optical eigenmodes. Optica. 2014;**1**(4):257-263

[64] De Luca AC, Kosmeier S, Dholakia K, Mazilu M. Optical eigenmode imaging. Physical Review A. 2011 Aug 15;**84**(2):021803

[65] Di Caprio G, Ferrara MA, Miccio L, Merola F, Memmolo P, Ferraro P, et al. Holographic imaging of unlabelled sperm cells for semen analysis: A review. Journal of Biophotonics. 2015 Oct 1;**8**(10):779-789

[66] De Luca AC, Rusciano G, Ciancia R, Martinelli V, Pesce G, Rotoli B, et al. Spectroscopical and mechanical characterization of normal and thalassemic red blood cells by Raman tweezers. Optics Express. 2008;**16**(11):7943-7957

[67] Frimat J-P, Bronkhorst M, de Wagenaar B, Bomer JG, Van der Heijden F, Van den Berg A, et al. Make it spin: Individual trapping of sperm for analysis and recovery using micro-contact printing. Lab on a Chip. 2014;**14**(15):2635-2641

[68] De Wagenaar B, Berendsen JTW, Bomer JG, Olthuis W, van den Berg A, Segerink LI. Microfluidic single sperm entrapment and analysis. Lab on a Chip. 2015;**15**(5):1294-1301

8

In Vitro Spermatogenesis: Past, Present, and Future

DMAB Dissanayake

Abstract

The study of culturing spermatogonial stem cells (SSCs) dates back to the 1950s. However, regeneration of complete spermatogenesis process *in vitro* is still a greater challenge. Studying spermatogenesis *in vitro* is significant in elucidating germ cell biology, and the knowledge may be useful for genetic manipulations of defective germ cells or producing transgenic animals, fertility preservation, and treatment of infertility. Fertility preservation would be more beneficial for adult and prepubescent patients who develop sterility due to gonadotoxins. Discovering of the stepwise stages in spermatogenesis and various forms of arrests at specific stages would help in the diagnosis of especially, idiopathic infertility and deciding treatment options. Different techniques have been tried to differentiate stem cells into germ cells over decades. A larger number of studies has used genetically manipulated stem cells to achieve differentiated germ cells. In contrast, differentiation of stem cells directly into SSCs bypassing the step into primordial germ cells (PGCs) to minimize time frame and employing techniques involved in least genetic manipulations are other important techniques to increase utilization within a clinical setting. As the use of transfected cell lines disqualifies the putative gametes obtained for clinical applications, trying to generate patient-specific germ cell with least genetic manipulations will be more effective in future applications, especially for patients with pre-pubertal cancer and azoospermic men who desire to become biological fathers.

Keywords: spermatogonial stem cells, germ cells, 3D culture, sperm, infertility

1. Introduction

Treatment of male infertility is always a challenge. Understanding correct pathological processes is difficult and time consuming as different etiologies may be responsible for a given semen parameter abnormality. It has been estimated that 8% of men in reproductive ages seek medical reproductive assistance [1]. Among half of subfertile couples, male factor is the causative or contributory factor and according to our experience around 12% of subfertile men are severe oligozoospermics or azoospermics. In majority of azoospermia cases, especially in non-obstructive azoospermics, the etiologies are genetically manipulated, and treatment with foci of sperm using assisted reproductive technologies (ART) may carry a greater chance of genetic diseases in the outcome. *In vitro* matured sperm are a greater hope for those men to attain the biological fatherhood.

Spermatozoa are not only act as a vehicle for delivering paternal DNA to the oocyte, but also robustly contribute to epigenetic processes in embryogenesis. Sperm DNA and the chromatin structure as a unit, drive genes toward activation or silencing upon delivery to the egg [1]. For better performance, it has to undergo several rounds of morphological, biochemical, physiological, and epigenetic changes during spermatogenesis. Even after leaving the testis, sperm is subjected to further maturation in the epididymis, and is not fully competent to do the deterministic task until mixing with accessory gland secretions and activating several proteins, cytokines and signaling pathways. All those processes are interrelated with the stability of DNA it carries.

Modeling spermatogenesis will ease the study of complex biological interactions *in vitro*, in relation to gametogenesis and fertilization (i.e., epigenetic processes, transcription, translation variations, activation or silence of signaling pathways, etc.). In addition, the modeling will helps to elaborate genetic disorders or other pathological conditions and to discover new drugs (fertility drugs or contraceptive drugs). Rapid development of the field of bioinformatics is immensely useful toward this progress. However, the use of artificial gametes for fertility treatment is far from the vicinity considering the questions still to be answered.

One of the technical challenges in the study of spermatogenesis is lack of a proper *in vitro* model to recapitulate the process [2]. Recent development of techniques and technologies such as different cell culture systems gene cloning/transgenic animals, gene expression, gene silencing, mass spectrometry and microarray, etc., has immensely been contributed to identify a plethora of endogenous and exogenous factors in the regulation of this process. Compiling all these data in a proper order, for example, grouping expressed genes, proteins, and metabolites into functional categories may allow in recapitulating spermatogenesis process and better understanding of the underlying mechanisms of normal and abnormal pathways [3].

Attempts to make gametes outside the body (*in vitro*) or outside its niche (*ex vivo*) have been ongoing for more than a century [4], and there is a rapid escalation of research in the past decade. Main approaches in achieving this goal include (a) autologous or allogenic testicular transplantation of SSCs, stem cells or differentiated putative germ cells from other sources; (b) auto or xeno-grafting of testicular tissues, SSCs, differentiated putative germ cells into other parts of the body, for example, under the skin; (c) *in vitro* culture of SSCs, stem cells or differentiated putative germ cells with testicular tissues/cells (organ culture systems) or without testicular tissues; (d) sperm cloning, etc. Two main barriers encountered in the *in vitro* spermatogenesis process are; haploidization of stem cells or progression beyond pachytene stage, and inability to further differentiation of the few round spermatids obtained by culture, especially up to formation of tail.

2. Understanding the natural process of spermatogenesis

2.1 Models to describe spermatogenesis

Spermatogonial stem cells represent a very rare population of germ cells consisting about 0.03% (20,000–35,000) in adult mouse testes [5] or even lesser 2000–3000 [6]. Self-renewal of SSCs and spermatogenesis are described using different models. Among them, more detailed studies have been done with mouse. The "A-single" (A_s) model originally proposed by Huckins et al., and according to them two types of SSCs are present in the seminiferous tubules; Type A and Type B. Type A—SSCs are more primitive due to absence of heterochromatin, while Type B cells are more differentiated as their nuclear heterochromatin content is high. Type A spermatogonia are subdivided into three groups according to their topological arrangements in the seminiferous tubule; A-single (A_s), A-paired (A_{pr}), and A-aligned (A_{al}). Division of A_s spermatogonia leads either to produce individual two new cells (self-renewing cells) or connected two cells by intercytoplasmic bridges (A_{pr}). Further divisions of A_{pr} lead to formation of A_{al} or chains of 4, 8, 16, and occasionally 32 cells. A_s represents the stem cell pool and same characteristics may remain among few A_{pr} cells as well. Larger chains of A_{al} (8, 16, 32) differentiate toward the Type A1 spermatogonia and then give rise to A2, A3, A4, Intermediate and B, respectively. These differentiated spermatogonia divide in a synchronize manner and found at specific stages of the seminiferous epithelial cycle. B spermatogonia differentiate into spermatocytes, and they undergo further divisions by meiosis to produce secondary spermatocytes and haploid spermatids, respectively. Single A_{pr} cell passes eight mitotic steps resulting 1024 spermatocytes, and total 4096 haploid spermatids from subsequent meiotic division. Spermatids are subjected to 16 steps of morphological changes to become mature spermatozoa [7–9].

There are two other models to describe SSCs self-renewal: A0/A1 model and A-dark and A-pale model. In A0/A1 model normal spermatogenesis is maintained by an "active" pool of SSCs (A1) and other quiescent "reserve" pool of SSCs (A0) is mobilized only following an insult to spermatogenesis [10]. In higher primates and humans two types of morphologically distinct SSCs are described, A_{dark} and A_{pale}. Observing biological functions of two cell types, A_{pale} is considered as progenitor cells and A_{dark} as true stem cells. A_{dark} represents only 1% of spermatogonia population, and stay dormant or divide very rarely if only progenitor cells have been destroyed. A_{pale} proliferate at defined periods during each cycle of the seminiferous epithelium and differentiate into B spermatogonia while leaving sufficient amount A_{pale} as functional reserve. In primates, single A_{pale} involve 5 mitotic divisions producing 32 spermatocytes and finally 128 spermatids. Amount of clonal expansion is very low in humans, and only 16 haploid cells are produced through 2 mitotic and meiotic divisions as depicted in **Figure 1** [11]. Due to low number of haploid cells produced by a single cell, both humans and primates maintain a population of progenitor cells (A_{pale}) as a replenishment reserve. This is to minimize mitotic activity of true stem cells and preserve their genetic stability. Thus, the role of SSCs is to regenerate and sustain a cycling cell lineage, while progenitor population which is lacking regenerative capacity contributes to steady-state conditions [12]. There is no consensus on SSCs self-renewal in aforementioned models; whether it is through symmetrical (produce two stem cells or two interconnected cells destined to differentiate) or asymmetrical (produce one stem cell and other cell committed to differentiate). Using a mouse model, Wu

Mouse	A_{singl}	A_{pair}	A_{align}	A1	A2	A3	A4	Int	B	Spc
No. of cells	1	2	4/8/16	16	32	64	128	256	512	1024
Rhesus monkey	A_{dark}	***A_{pale}***	B1	B2	B3	B4	Spc			
No. of cells	1	***1***	2	4	8	16	32			
Human	A_{dark}	***A_{pale}***	B	Spc						
No. of cells	1	***1***	2	4						

Figure 1. Pre-meiotic steps of spermatogenesis (SSCs to pre-leptotene spermatocytes) in different species of mammals. Spermatogonial stem cells Undifferentiated spermatogonia *Progenitor cells*. Int – intermediate, Spc - spermatocytes.

et al. support the theory of asymmetrical division. Furthermore, they have proposed that fate decision of mammalian SSCs bifurcation is autonomous and stochastic [13].

Spermiogenesis is the process of transformation of spherical, haploid spermatids (n) to sperm-like mature spermatids. Human spermatid develops into a mature sperm through a series of 12 steps and it takes about 5 weeks. It is assumed that nuclear condensation during this process shuts RNA synthesis, and proteins required in the period (mainly protamine) are produced by stored mRNAs derived from the diploid phase of spermatogenesis [14]. Contrary to this suggestion, supportive evidences are emerging on the minor activity of transcription in haploid spermatids as well [15]. Spermiation is the last process involving breakage of the structures and bonds anchoring mature spermatids to Sertoli cells in order to release spermatozoa into the tubule lumen. Peristaltic waves created by peritubular smooth muscle cells help to move spermatozoa and testicular fluids through the seminiferous tubules to the epididymis [16]. This ~10–16 days migration through epididymis helps sperm to attain motility and natural fertilization capacity up to a certain extent [17, 18]. The total motility and fertilizability is gained only after mixing with accessory sex gland secretions [19].

2.2. Regulatory mechanisms of natural spermatogenesis

Number of sperm produced per day by testes (daily sperm production, DSP) is a tool for quantitative assessment of spermatogenesis. DSP can decrease with reduced amount of true stem cells present, failure to produce committed A_{pale} cells, changes in niche environment due to multitude of causes, age (DSP is low in very young and older men), etc. [20]. However, even in the normal spermatogenic procedure germ cells may degenerate at various levels; pre-leptotene and leptotene spermatocytes in older men, and pachytene/diplotene spermatocytes across all ages. This would be a mechanism of eliminating cells with genetic abnormalities [21]. Other possible reason is to maintain the ratio of Sertoli cells to germ cells, as one Sertoli cell can assist only to a specific number of cells. Furthermore, there is no fine regulation of formation of spermatocytes in different areas of tubules, resulting unequal distribution of those cells. The apoptosis mainly involving the *BCL-2* family of apoptosis regulating proteins helps to maintain an equal density of spermatocytes along the seminiferous tubule [22, 23].

In normal seminiferous epithelium, there is a well balance between SSCs self-renewal and differentiation. Loss of the equilibriums may cause either germ cell tumor or infertility subsequent to SSCs depletion. However, in specific situations, such as toxicity-induced spermatocytes destruction, this balance may be shifted toward differentiation over proliferation. One of the main regulators identified in the SSCs self-renewal is glial cell line-derived neurotrophic factor (GDNF) secreted by Sertoli cells [24]; whereas, well-known differentiation factors are stem cell factor (SCF) secreted by Sertoli cells and biologically active derivative of vitamin A; retinoic acid (RA).

2.3. Markers expression during spermatogenesis

Knowledge on cytological markers expressed or suppressed at different stages of spermatogenesis is a key factor on rapid development of *in vitro* spermatogenesis strategies. Several cytological markers such as genes, transcription factors, cytokines, growth factors, enzymes, other proteins and micro RNAs (miRNAs), etc., have been studied at distinct phases of spermatogenesis pathway from embryonic germ cells allocation to postnatal spermatogenesis process which is broadly divided into three phases; proliferation, differentiation, and spermiogenesis. Some of them are surface antigens found in different regions of the sperm and others are intracellular; in the nucleus or cytoplasm. Knowledge on the expression of stage-specific cytological markers is vital on studying germ cells biology, normal and abnormal pathways of spermatogenesis and deciding corrective measures. Proper process of spermatogenesis requires precise coordination of multitude of genes. Stage-specific surface markers may be involved in differentiation process at least part by interaction with Sertoli cells [25]. Surface antigens are extensively used for tracking subset of germ cells at specific differentiation stages, but the process is hampered as very few markers have been identified so far. Although most of these markers expressed on SSCs and early stages of differentiation, little or none of these antigens remaining on the head or tail of the sperm [26]. Majority of markers have characterized with animal germ cells, specifically using rat and mouse germ cells, and very few of them have tested in humans. We assume that the presence and behavior of majority of these genes are more or less similar between animals and humans.

2.3.1. PGCs, SSCs, and spermatogonial progenitor cells (SPCs) markers

The chemokine receptor type 4 receptor (*CXCR4*) and *DDX4* or mouse vasa homolog (*MVH*) genes are first expressed during migratory phase of PGCs, and *MVH* expression is continued until post-meiotic germ cells are formed. Decreased proliferative capacity of PGCs and defective spermatogenesis has been observed in *MVH* null mice. *PIWI*, *Fragilis*, *SSEA1*, and *STELLA* are other genes expressed in different levels in migratory PGSc. *Fragilis* is considered to be important for the migration of PGCs toward the genital ridges [27, 28]. B-lymphocyte-induced maturation protein-1 gene (*BLIMP1*) is involved in the initial specification of PGCs. Germ cells positive for *BLIMP1* proliferate continuously, and this process can be helpful to express other PGCs markers such as *Fragilis* and *STELLA*. A network of transcription factors are involved in maintaining embryonic properties of stem cells. *SALL4* is a member of Spalt-like transcription factor family, highly expressed in multiple embryonic tissues including PGCs and gonocytes. It is also involved in SPCs differentiation. Promyelocytic Leukemia Zinc Finger (*PLZF* or

ZBTB16) shows lower expression levels in embryonic germ cells and its peak in postnatal SPCs. It helps to maintain the properties of SPCs and also detected in early stages of SSCs differentiation. *SALL4* and *PLZF* physically interact and mutually oppose one another's localization to cognate chromatin domains depending on their relative expression levels at distinct stages of germ cells development. c-KIT, the transmembrane tyrosine kinase receptor for stem cell factor (SCF), also known as KIT ligand (KL) is essential to the proliferation and survival of differentiating spermatogonia, and its expression directly repressed by *PLZF*. At the time of differentiation, *SALL4* level increases with suppression of *PLZF* facilitating to expression of *c-KIT* [29]. *GPR125*, an orphan adhesion-type G-protein-coupled receptor, is another gene exclusively expressed in SPCs and SSCs, and not in differentiated spermatocytes. *GPR125* positive cells can be cultured in undifferentiated state with remarkable increase in their number [30]. A gene named transcriptional repressor inhibitor of differentiation 4 (*ID4*) was recently identified using a transgenic mouse model and it was highly expressed in most gonocytes, a subpopulation of SSCs, and a minor subset of pachytene spermatocytes [12]. But, they conclude the appearance of *ID4* in pachytene stage may be nonspecific, and proposed that *ID4* positive subpopulation may be a heterogeneous population of SPCs and SSCs in mouse. Another subset of rare and highly proliferative A_{single} spermatogonia has been characterized in mouse by expression of the paired box transcription factor (*PAX7*). Using cell lineage tracing studies they have confirmed that *PAX7* cells function as bona fide stem cells [31]. The marker is co-expressed with well characterized other spermatogonial markers such as, c-*KIT, PLZF, FOXO 1, RET*, and *GFRα1*. *PAX7* was reported perfectly conserved in 11 different species, and it is resistant to chemo and radiotherapy insults [32]. GDNF seems to stimulate SSCs self-renewal by signaling through *Ret* and *GFRα1* receptors system, and overexpression causes to an increase of undifferentiated spermatogonia in the testis [24]. POU family transcription factor 1 or octamer-binding transforming factor4 (*POU5F1/OCT4*) is expressed throughout the PGCs migration and later on in SSCs and differentiation male germ cells up to pachytene stage [5]. *Oct4* is rather considered as a pluripotency marker and expression is inhibited when RA binds to the responsive site, allowing the cells for differentiation. Many other markers expressed by SSCs and SPCs have described such as, *TERT, POU3F1, RBM, HSP90x, NGN3, NANOS2* & *3, SOHLH1* & *2*, integrin alpha chain 6 (*ITGA6 /α6-Integrin/CD49f*), *LIN28, UTF1, CDH1, ITGB1* (*β1-Integrin/CD29*), *EPCAM* (*CD326*), *CD9, CD24* and *THY1* (*CD90*). *LIN28* and *EPCAM* are increasingly expressed in malignant germ cell tumors indicating their role as maintenance of cells in undifferentiated state. The *NANOS2* is also reported to block germ cells differentiation and lack of the gene induces progressive loss of germ cells in the postnatal testis [24, 28, 33–35]. New four marker genes specifically found in mouse PGCs and SSCs, but not in somatic cells were described as, *FKBP6, MOV10l1, 4930432K21Rik*, and *TEX13* recently [36].

The above markers have been described using different techniques and most of them may have conserved among closely related animals during evolution. Results from RT-PCR analysis of freshly isolated human spermatogonia indicated that they are positive for *GPR125, GFRα1, PLZF*, ubiquitin carboxyl-terminal esterase L1 (*UCHL1*), and *RET* transcripts [37]. Using immunofluorescence and colorimetric staining it has been shown that human spermatogonia on the basement membrane express *UTF1, SALL4, ZBTB16, GFRα1, UCHL1, GPR125, LIN28, EXOSC10, FGFR3, DSG2, CBL, SSX2, OCT2, OCT4a/b, TERT, NANOG, ENO2*, and *PCNA* (a proliferation marker). Not like in rodents, *GPR125* is expressed only in subset of SSCs in humans. SSCs expressing, epithelial cell adhesion molecule (*EPCAM*), *THY1* and *ITGA6* have been enriched using fluorescence-activated cell sorting (FACS) and magnetic-activated cell sorting (MACS) techniques [38–41].

2.3.2. *Differentiation markers*

These markers can be categorized according to the timing of meiotic cycle; pre-meiotic, meiotic, and post-meiotic markers.

2.3.2.1. *Pre-meiotic*

c-KIT is an early differentiation marker highly expressed in A_{al} spermatocytes onward. c-KIT and its ligand SCF or KL are involved in growth and survival of germ cells. Interaction between the *SCF* positive Sertoli cells and the *c-KIT* positive germ cells are helpful for the progression through meiosis. Cytochrome p450 family 26, sub family b, polypeptide1 (*CYP26b1*) gene is increasingly expressed in pre-meiotic germ cells. It may prevent spermatocytes enter into meiosis by blocking the action RA, which is one of the key signaling molecule that helps to induce meiosis by binding through nuclear RA receptors. Stimulated by retinoic acid 8 (*STRA 8*) is the major responsive gene for RA induction and prominently expressed in pre-meiotic cells. At the same time RA receptors are expressed from type A spermatogonia to pre-leptotene spermatocytes in mice. Similarly, growth factor KL increases the percentage of meiotic entry in cultured spermatogonia concomitantly with an upregulation of *STRA8*. Activation of phosphatidyl inositol 3 kinase (*PI3K*) signaling appears to be important in meiotic initiation of germ cells [33, 42, 43].

XT-1 is an adhesion related surface antigen found on differentiation spermatocytes in mouse testes. It is first detectable and uniformly distributed on leptotene spermatocytes, and later localized on the base of the head, tail and cytoplasmic lobe of the elongating spermatids [26]. Bone morphogenetic protein4 (BMP4) is an early differentiation marker, mainly activate through cell adhesion pathways and also upregulate *c-KIT* expression. It is prominently expressed in pachytene stage spermatocytes, and downstream proteins, SMAD1, 5, 8 are phosphorylated during BMP4-induced differentiation [17, 33]. SMAD1, 4, and 5 proteins are found in SSCs to round spermatids, while SMAD7 is found in differentiating spermatogonia up to round spermatids. SMAD8 is detected from spermatocytes to elongating spermatids [44]. Deleted in azoospermia-like gene (*DAZL*), *VASA, BLIMP1, STELLA* are also considered as pre-meiotic early germ cells differentiation markers [34]. Highest expression of *DAZL* is found in pachytene spermatocytes, and is assisted in the translation of MVH in the males. *Cyclin D2* is another gene expressed around epithelial stage VIII when the A_{al} spermatogonia differentiate into A_1 stage [23].

2.3.2.2. *Meiotic*

Specific markers well defined for meiotic germ cells are synaptonemal complex protein 3 (*SCP3*) gene and dosage suppressor of mck1 homolog (*DMC1*). Both SCP2 and SCP3 are components of the lateral element of the synaptonemal complexes and are associated with the centromeres in meiotic metaphase I cells. Another antigen named testicular differentiation antigen 95 (TDA95), residing on zygotene and early pachytene spermatocytes has been defined using two monoclonal antibodies, CA12 and BC7. TDA95 may be one of the cell adhesion molecules between

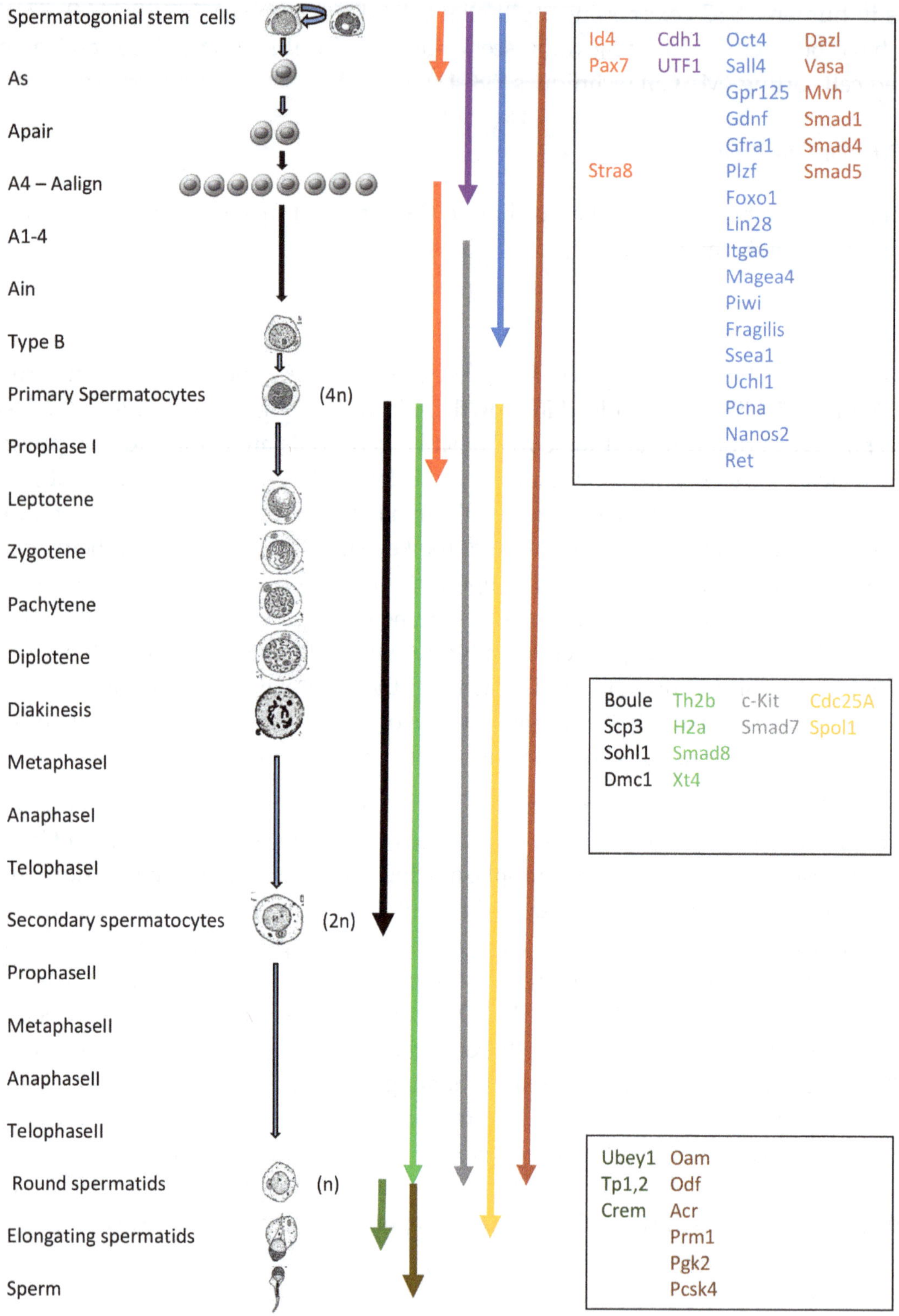

Figure 2. Stage-specific germ cell markers compiled from different sources. Most of them are germ cell specific and some of the markers are common to both germ cell and few types of somatic lineage cells. These markers are significant in solid identification of germ cells at different phases of development.

spermatocytes and Sertoli cells, and plays an essential role during early meiotic prophase of spermatogenesis. *SCP1, CREST,* and *Tesmin* are other markers present in human pachytene spermatocytes. *Tesmin* expression coincides with meiotic entry of germ cells [25, 37]. *BOULE* is a candidate meiotic regulator gene conserved among different species from drosophila to human, and deficient animals are infertile due to meiotic arrest in their male germ cells. The protein is detectable from pro-metaphase of first meiotic division to diplotene spermatocytes in humans and up to early spermatids in mice [45]. Similar expression pattern showed another meiotic promoter protein CDC25A, which was found in 1^{ry} and 11^{ry} spermatocytes and in some species up to elongating spermatids. Variations of three different isoforms of *BOULE* (*BOULE1, 2, & 3*) during spermatogenesis were described in humans [46]. *SPO11* (a type II topoisomerase), *H2A, TH2b* are other few genes, needed for meiotic recombination [43, 47].

2.3.2.3. *Post-meiotic*

Expression of acrosin (*ACR*), transition protein 1 & 2 (*TNP1, 2*), ubiquitin-activating enzyme (*UBE1Y*), Kinesin light chain proteins (*KLC3*) and protamine1 & 2 (*PRM1, 2*) genes has been reported in post-meiotic cells [37]. *ACR* gene is transcribed in the diploid stage, and translationally expressed in the post-meiotic haploid cells. Hence, proacrosin is first localized in the cytoplasm of round spermatids. PRM1 and PRM2 are small and highly basic proteins that are reported to be transcribed in round and elongating spermatids. KLC3 is a testis specific protein and acts as an anchor protein for binding mitochondria to outer dense fibers of sperm tail. During the spermiogenesis, somatic histones are replaced with testis specific nuclear proteins, termed as transition proteins (TNP1 & TNP2), and subsequently TNPs are replaced with PRMs. Formation of extensive disulfide cross links between PRMs results in condensation of nuclear proteins and repression of transcriptional activity [48]. Alteration of *PRM* expression has been reported to affect human male fertility. For example, high susceptibility to DNA damage was reported with diminished levels [49]. Bone morphogenetic family proteins BMP8a and BMP8b receptors are expressed in male germ cells in a bimodal manner. First, low levels of transcripts are found in spermatogonia and primary spermatocytes, and subsequently higher levels are expressed in round spermatids. BMP8b is most important in initiation and maintenance of spermatogenesis [50]. **Figure 2** depicts stage-specific expression of few selected markers commonly found in literature.

3. Attempts to differentiate spermatozoa outside the niche (*in vitro, in vivo,* and *ex vivo*)

Understanding the components of SSCs niche and their interactions with each other are vital aspects in regeneration of spermatogenesis *in vitro*. The *in vivo* niche of mammalian SSCs is comprised of Sertoli cells, peritubular cells, and a complex array of matrix proteins. The normal SSC pool is maintained throughout adulthood, through signals provided by adhesion molecules and other cell surface receptors. SSCs are exposed to signals from both tubular lumen and the interstitial space sides of the basement membrane. Fate of SSCs is regulated mainly by Sertoli cells, inter-tubular blood vessels, and surrounding Leydig cells also have a role [51]. Steady state of germ cell niche can be disturbed by physiological changes of individual components by intrinsic or external factors. Regeneration of sperm has been difficult due to incomplete understanding of complex interactions within the niche environment, and germ cell-specific events such as, meiosis, chromatin re-modeling/repackaging, flagellum development and transcriptional reprogramming, etc. [52]. However, some recent advancements in sciences, such as construction of "omics" databases involving genomics, proteomics, and metabolomics have immensely contributed to rapid development of germ cell biology. Studies have shown that thousands of genes are successively expressed or suppressed leading to changes in biochemical composition in germ cells along the spermatogenesis pathway. Epigenetic reprogramming of genes and post transcriptional modifications of proteins are further favored this process. In addition, miRNAs play a significant role in regulating germ cells differentiation [37]. Based on the available data scientists have developed *in vitro* culture systems to induce male germ cells development from different types of stem cells. The improved culture systems facilitate to study the distinct pattern of gene expression in germ cells at various developmental stages.

Recapitulation of spermatogenesis completely or as in part, outside its niche is essential to understand the series of biological events associated with this complex process. The techniques can be utilized to study the germ cell biology (mitosis, meiosis, morphogenesis, initiation of motility, etc.) toxicological studies, fertility preservation, production of transgenic sperm, and have the potential for new therapeutic approaches in male infertility [53]. Continuous attempts have been made using pre-existing immature germ cells or various sources of stem or somatic cells as the starting source for *in vitro* derived gametes with satisfactory results [54]. However, same weight can be given for the doubts still have to be clarified. The strategies are broadly categorized into three aspects; development of different culture systems, haploidization, and differentiation of germ or somatic cells, and autologous or xenologous transplantation of germ or putative germ cells.

Methods to isolate SSCs from testicular tissue and differentiate into haploid cells or further to sperm, with feeder or feeder free conditions have been explored in different studies. Enrichment of SSCs *in vitro* facilitates dissection of germ cells biology, because SSCs represent a very rare population of germ cells consisting about 0.03% (20,000–35,000) in adult mouse testes [5] or even lesser 2000–3000 [6]. Early attempt to germ cell culture (in which whole segment of seminiferous tubules were maintained in culture) goes back to 1964 [55]. The first human SSC culture was reported in 1998 using a crude extract of testicular tissue, and the efficacy has now been improved with varying techniques [56]. Digested testicular tissues from obstructive azoospermic men cultured with high concentrations of follicle-stimulating hormone (FSH) and testosterone continued the *in vitro* reduction of germ cell ploidy with rapid morphological changes toward spermiogenesis. Two different mechanisms are possibly involved in endocrine regulation of the above process, and they would be, prevention of Sertoli cells apoptosis by testosterone and stimulation of the spermiogenesis by FSH [57]. Following a simple two enzymatic digestion protocol *OCT4*$^+$ SSCs were isolated from human testis with 87% purity. SSCs colonies were able to culture for around 1 month on a Sertoli cells feeder layer [40]. In another study, *THY1*$^+$ mouse SSCs have been cultured in the presence of Sertoli cells, hormones (FSH/testosterone) and vitamins (RA/vit.E/C), either with a mix of three components or with individual components. After 7 days of culture spermatid-like cells expressing post-meiotic markers were prominent in mixed supplement group compared to individual supplements [47]. Addition of FSH to bovine SSCs culture has proven the increased colonization capacity of spermatogonia [58].

Differential plating is the simplest technique isolating germ cells from digested testicular tissues. However, a highly purified SSCs population is expected only from sorting of cells using combination of surface markers. The array of potential markers reported for isolating SSCs are *GPR125, ITGA6, CD9,* or *GFRα1* [51]. Culturing of SSCs isolated using differential plating technique from testicular tissue of cancer patients, in laminin or gelatin coated wells (feeder free conditions) and serum free culture media supplemented with human GDNF, bFGF, EGF and LIF resulted in the increase of GPR125⁺ cells from 2 to 70% [59]. In another study, human adult SSCs were able to culture in laminin coated plates, up to 28 weeks with 18,000-fold increased in number in the presence of LIF, bFGF, GDNF, and EGF [60]. In contrast, SSCs underwent massive apoptosis in feeder free conditions, but testicular somatic cells together with GDNF supported the propagation of SSCs more than 1 year [51].

Maintaining the spatial arrangement of testicular cells seems to be important in the process of regulation and completion of spermatogenesis. The goal may be achieved by arranging germ and somatic cells in three-dimensional (3D) culture systems by formation of embryoid bodies (EBs) or culturing the cells in soft agar or methyl cellulose [61]. Two culture systems are depicted in **Figures 3** and **4**. The studies have been highlighted that, low temperature (equal to testicular temperature), endocrine factors, and supporting somatic cells are prerequisites to be considered in *in vitro* spermatogenesis. Supportive mechanisms provided by somatic cells to develop germ cells are controversial. Presence of somatic cells, but not necessarily the direct contact is suggested for *in vitro* proliferation of male germ cells in one study [61] In contrast, significance of direct cell to cell contact between Sertoli cells and stem cells has been emphasized for successful germ cells formation from Warton's jelly-derived mesenchymal stem cells [62]. Reasons of such kind of variations, whether due to the source of cells used for differentiation of germ cells or specific stage of supporting along the differentiation process, should further be investigated.

Transmeiotic differentiation is one of the critical step in the spermatogenesis pathway, and it is inducible employing bio-mechanical or chemical methods such as, simulated gravity, KL, or RA. *c-KIT*⁺ spermatogonia cultured under simulated microgravity for 48 h entered into meiosis even in the absence of exogenous supplements or Sertoli cells. Microgravity may act as an inducer or accelerator in the progression of meiosis [43]. Co-culture with testicular somatic cells, induction with RA and BMP4 are other well documented methods for meiotic initiation of SSCs. Mouse embryonic stem cells (ESCs) are reported to enter early meiosis when co-cultured with Sertoli cells compared to culture provided with RA. Sertoli cells provide RA for germ cells in two ways; by direct delivery of RA and delivery of retinol via membrane receptor *STRA6* [63]. Rate of germ cells formation and meiotic entry may also vary in

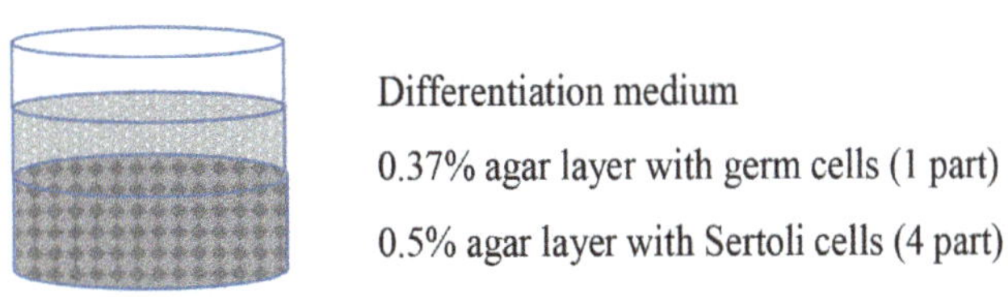

Figure 3. Schematic of soft agar 3D culture system.

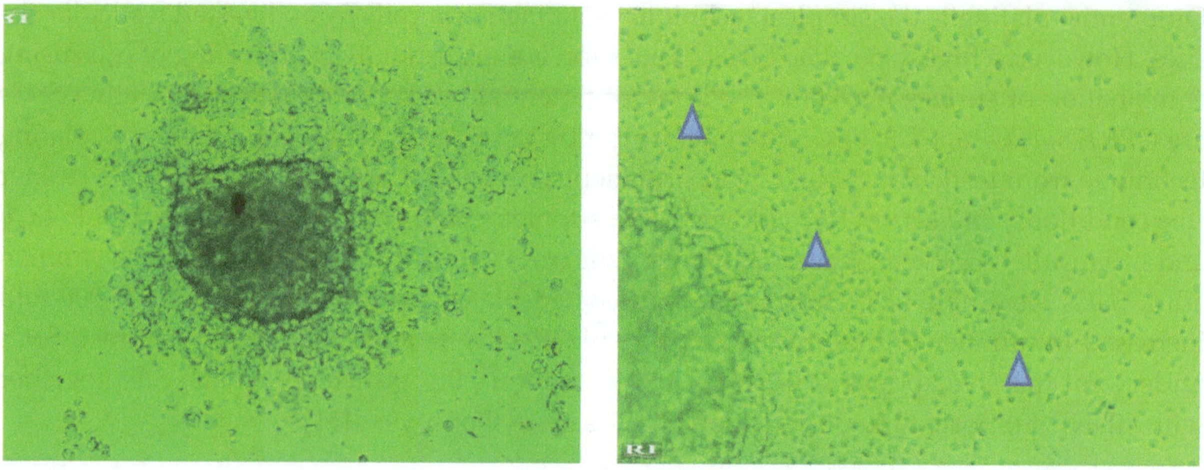

Figure 4. SSCs co-cultured with Sertoli cells in embryoid bodies culture system. A—initial culture (day 5) showing spermatocytes and spermatids like stages. B—late phase of culture (day 14), few sperms with normal morphology are observed (arrow heads).

different culture systems, and with the source of cells used. For example, 3% of bone marrow mesenchymal stem cells (MSCs) were differentiated into germ cells when treated with RA [64]. Another study achieved around 20% of germ cells after co-culturing human ESCs with fetal gonadal stromal cells [65]. Mouse-induced pluripotent stem cells (iPSCs) treated with BMP4 led to formation of 41% primordial germ cells like cells [66]. However, very limited or pseudoentry of meiosis was noted by many studies. Around 3–5% of haploid cells were present in FACS sorted cells after induction of mouse SSCs in differentiation medium [67]. Similarly, 1–5% of post-meiotic cells were emerged when hESCs derived embryoid bodies (EBs) were treated with mouse testes conditioned medium supplemented with RA and BMP4 [68]. In contrast, 20% of haploid cells were observed in BMP4-induced human IPCs culture, and around 70% was positive for acrosin after sorting for 1 N cells [69]. Cell organization in EBs may reflect more of the arrangement of embryonic gonadal ridge [64], and correct erasure of imprinting genes was observed with EBs culture system [70]. It has been reported that, testosterone causes to increase in *STRA8* mRNA levels (pre-meiotic marker) when cells were treated with both RA and testosterone [71]. The spontaneous differentiation of stem cells into haploid state may also be possible in appropriate culture conditions with a very low efficiency, amounting around 2% in human iPSCs culture [69]. Spontaneous differentiation may increase with prolongation of culture, and due to inducing factors contained in culture medium. For example, media supplemented with 10% fetal bovine serum contain approximately 3.6×10^{-8} M of RA [72]. However, spontaneous differentiation of ESCs into germ line is generally low and inefficient with majority of germ cells undergoing degeneration [71].

Most of data have produced from very short period of cultures (2–30 days), indicating germ cell differentiation proceed an unusual speed *in vitro*. It is not clear how the timing went shorten, and it has been suggested that in the absence of environmental cues, germ cells may develop according to an intrinsic clock [73]. However, establishing a standard culture system of SSCs is difficult due to many reasons. Inherent variability between cells of different species leads to inconclusive results. For example, feeder cells and serum in culture may positively be affected on some cell lines, but not on others. Batch to batch variations of serum and positive or negative impact of unknown factors added by both feeder cells and serum are also concern [56]. Many authors emphasize the requirement of refined culture system eliminating serum and feeder cells to better understanding of individual cellular and molecular interactions.

The *in vitro* maturation of available germ cells has a little value considering the therapeutic aspects of infertile men especially for men with non-obstructive azoospermia. To overcome this situation, ESCs derived gametes were tested as a first line remedial step by scientific community. Initial attempts were least successful due to unresponsiveness of cells for specific media or culture conditions [74]. However, encouraging models have been described later on by different authors, not only for ESCs but also for other multipotent cell types including iPSCs and somatic stem cells. Two main approaches for this are (a) direct differentiation of stem cells into germ cell lineage using exogenous factors; (b) transfection of stem cells with marked or fluorescent proteins linked to specific gene promoters, such as *STRA8* and *PRM1* [75]. These methods can be employed as monolayer adherent cell culture or three-dimensional embryoid bodies, with or without feeder cells. Optimum time point for obtaining germ-like cells from human pluripotent stem cells (PSCs) was recorded day 10, while day 7 cultures yielded lower numbers and day 15 not indicated a significant increase [67]. It is reported that germ cell formation in EB culture system seems to faster than in monolayer culture system [76]. Given the priority for direct differentiation method is more acceptable as gene transfection method disqualifies in clinical applications. However, the gene transfection and iPSCs systems may provide the necessary information on the behavior of related genes in germ cell development. Whatever the method employed, the imprinting regulation of gametes obtained from concerned methods has to be further validated, if ever they are to be used for clinical applications [73].

The possibility of using PGCs and germ line stem cells (GSCs) in transplantation studies to restore fertility has been studied with varying degrees of success [65]. Grafting or transplantation of gonadal fragments, germ cells or genetically modified germ cells and transmeiotic pluripotent stem cells onto immune compromised animals is an alternative strategy to investigate germ cell development. Successful autologous-transplantation of spermatogonial stem cells has achieved in a wide range of species so far [77]. Autologous cryopreserved testicular tissue grafting is an option for preserving genetic materials in endangered species and immature cancer patients. Success of homing ability of grafts may depend on various factors such as, age of collecting graft (immature is the better), low GnRH level (suppressed spermatogenesis with more primitive cells), method of cryopreservation, etc. [78]. Homing ability of SSCs from different species including human, to basement membrane of seminiferous tubules of nude mice has been proven by many authors [60]. The niche for spermatogonial proliferation appears to be generally similar among different species, because proliferation is undisturbed between cross-species after xenotransplantation of spermatogonia. However, the niche for spermatogonial differentiation is thought to work through a species-specific mechanism [78].

The most advanced progress in meiosis and qualified male gametes may be obtained following transplantation of *in vitro* derived PGCs or GSCs into the testis. The ability to develop more mature germ cells from PGCs like cells derived from mouse iPSCs has shown after

Source of cells	Method used	Observations	References
BM stem cells from *STRA8-EGFP* transgenic mouse line	Induced with RA (10 μm) for 10 days. and EGFP positive cells were sorted using FACS	3% cells differentiated into male germ cells assessed by *OCT4, Fragilis, STELLA, MVH, RNF17, DAZLl, c-KIT, PIWIL2, RBM, STRA8, TEX 18*. But arrested at pre-meiotic stage	Nyernia et al. [64]
hESCs (HSF1, HSF6 and H9) and hIPS	Co-cultured with human fetal gonadal stromal cells for 14 days	20% germ cells with triple positive markers (*cKIT, SSEA1* & *PLAP or VASA*). Repression of *HOX* genes and imprint erasure by day 7. No report of meiosis	Park et al. [65]
hESCs (H1) and iPSCs (HFF1)	Cultured in mouse SSCs differentiation medium for 10 days and haploid cells were confirmed after sorting by FACS	*UTF1, PLZF* and *CDH* positive spermatogonia, *HIWIi* and *HILL*-positive spermatocytes, and *ACR, TP1* and *PRM1* expressing haploid cells (3.9–4.5%) were observed. Unimpaired uniparental genomic imprints on two loci: *H19* and *IGF2*	Easley et al. [67]
iPSCs (iHUF4/IMR90) hESCs (H9/HSF1)	Induced with BMP-4, 7, and 8b for 14 days in feeder free conditions Transduced with *VASA-GFP* reporter	Increased *Vasa* and *DAZL* expression. 4–6% GFP positive cells within 14 days. Increased number of meiotic cells in *DAZL* overexpressed cells	Panula et al. [69]
STRA8-EGFP transfected Mouse ESC line (C57BL6)	Co-cultured with Sertoli cells or RA (on gelatin coated plates)	*DAZL, SYCP3, PRM* expression in both groups after 12 days of induction. Number of colonies and positive cells were high in Sertoli cell group	Miryounesi et al. [63]
hESC lines (Shef1–6 & H7)	EBs were induced with RA, Bmp4 and neonatal mouse testis conditioned medium for 14 days	Progressive elevation of both spermatogenesis and oogenesis markers. Effect was prominent with RA treatment. 1–5% post-meiotic cells & few with the beginning of flagellum formation	Aflatoonian et al. [68]
Mouse C2C12 myoblast cells	*STRA8*-positive C2C12 myoblasts were treated with 10 μM all-trans-RA for 8 days	Pre-meiosis, meiosis and post-meiosis gene markers were expressed. Few cells exhibited spherical morphology with tail tike structure. But the cells were diploid indicating arrest at pre-meiotic stage	Jia et al. [35]
Pre-meiotic male germ cells from immature mouse	Cells were cultured in gel matrices (soft agar or methyl cellulose) with the support of somatic cells and gonadotropins for 40 days	Morphologically normal but immotile spermatozoa	Stukenborg et al. [61]

Source of cells	Method used	Observations	References
Stella-GFP+ ES cells	Cells were cultured in Ham's F12/IMDM medium with BMP4 as adherent or EBs culture systems	Cells in both cultures, predominantly in EBs were differentiated, into primordial germ cells with correct gene expression patterns. Correct pattern of parental imprint erasure was confirmed (*PEG3 and IGF2R*)	Wei et al. [70]
Porcine skin-derived somatic stem cells	Induced with porcine follicular fluid for 50 days	Large, round PGCs like cells with 0.25% positive for alkaline phosphatase (AP). Cells were positive for *c-KIT, OCT4, VASA, STELLA, DAZL*. 99% of CpG sites were unmethylated in *DMR1* of PGCs	Linher et al. [86]
Human ESCs (HSF-6 & H-9)	50–250 cell colonies were cultured on mouse primary embryonic fibroblast in ESCs growth medium for 7d. The cells were co-cultured with putative Sertoli cells	AP & *CXCR4, c-KIT* positive primordial germ cells arose. Electron microscopic pictures showed large round nucleus with numerous mitochondria	Bucay et al. [87]
Mouse SSCs from 7d old male	3D agar culture system consisting 0.5 agar and 25% FCS in lower layer and 0.37 agar and 20% FCS in upper layer. Culture continued for 30d with PRMI media	Different stages of spermatogenesis were observed with increasing meiotic and post-meiotic markers with time. Average 15 spermatozoa per well of 24 well plate were present	Elhija et al. [88]
Laminin binding spermatogonia from Sprague-Dawley rats	Cells were cultured in gelatin coated wells with a serum free formulated medium for 120 days. Other supplements were GDNF and FGF	Cultured SSCs effectively regenerated spermatogenesis in testes of busulfan-treated recipient rats	Wu et al. [89]
Immature spermatogenic cells isolated from non-obstructive azoospermic men	3D culture in a collagen gel matrix with somatic cells. The media supplemented with RA and rFSH	More round and elongating spermatids emerged at day 12 of culture. *PRM2* + ve cells and haploid cells were increased with time	Lee et al. [90]
in vitro generated germ cell line from teratocarcinoma cells (F9)	TC cells were transfected with *Stra8-EGFP* fusion construct and positive cells were induced with RA. FACS sorted germ-like cells were transplanted.	Mature sperm after 7 months of transplantation in recipient mice testes. Performance of ICSI confirmed the oocytes activating capacity of these sperm	Nayernia et al. [91]
TESE dissociated *CD49f* positive cells from azoospermic men	Cells were cultured with Sertoli cells and culture media containing RA, GDNF, FSH & testosterone for 15 days	Progression of meiosis up to day 5. Correct gene expression pattern (*SCP3* and *CREST* and haploid cells were obtained	Riboldi et al. [92]

Source of cells	Method used	Observations	References
Human Wharton's jelly-derived MSCs	MSCs were co-cultured with mitotic inactivated newborn mouse Sertoli cells for 3 weeks	Typically round germ-like cells were appeared with time. The cells were positive for early germ cell specific *STELLA* & *VASA* and male germ cells specific *DAZL* markers	Xie et al. [62]
Human testicular tissues from first and second trimester fetuses	Testis tissues were inserted subcutaneously into mice. Mice with second-trimester xenografts were randomly given hCG injection	Completed the normal seminiferous cord formation. Induction of steroidogenesis was observed with hCG treatment. Germ cells differentiation was confirmed by decreasing *OCT4* and increasing *Vasa* expressing cells	Mitchell et al. [93]
MSCs from human umbilical cord Wharton's jelly	Cells were induced with 2×10^{-6} M RA and 10 ng/ml BMP4 in DMEM for 7–14 days	Small number of germ cells expressing *SCP3* and *VASA* were formed	Hua et al. [94]
Mouse ESCs	ESCs derived PGCs like cells were cultured with testicular somatic ells in the presence of Knockout serum, RA, BMP 2, 4, 7, Activin A, FSH, Testosterone and bovine pituitary extract for 14 days. Resultant spermatids like cells were used for ICSI	Confirmed meiosis in 84% of colonies and erasure of genetic imprinting. ICSI procedure using spermatids like cells produced viable and fertile offspring	Zhou et al. [95]

Table 1. A summary of selected studies designed to differentiate male germ cells from different sources of stem cells.

transplantation into testis of infertile mice [66]. Nayernia et al. reported 300–500-fold increase in spermatogonial population after transplantation of mouse bone marrow (BM) derived SSCs into germ cells depleted recipient mice, but the cells were arrested at pre-meiotic stage [64]. A similar study has shown that transplanted green fluorescence protein positive (GFP^+) mouse BM cells can differentiate into both somatic and germ cell lineages in a favorable testicular niche [79]. Transplanted adipose tissue-derived MSCs could induce spermatogenesis in busulfan-treated recipient rats in another study [80]. Toyooka et al. cultured *Mvh* knock-in GFP or *Lac-Z* mouse embryoid bodies with *BMP 4,8* expressing embryonic trophoblast cells, and they could achieve morphologically normal sperm after transplantation of *MVH* overexpressing cells under the testis capsules of nude mice [81]. Use of combination of gene transfection and subsequent germ cells transplantation techniques could results live sperm (with reduced motility) and offspring after intracytoplasmic sperm injection (ICSI) in mice. Though the newborns died within few months due to imprinting defects, this finding paves the way to promising *in vitro*- and/or *ex vivo*-derived functional gametes in the future [82]. Additional treatment with hormones (hCG) after stem cell transplantation may be a powerful tool for increasing the efficiency of transplantation [83]. It is suggested that FSH and testosterone favor the survival of germ cells by regulating both intrinsic and the extrinsic apoptotic pathways. Furthermore, FSH is needed to initiation of meiosis and androgen is necessary for the completion of meiosis and spermiogenesis [84].

Adult somatic cells induction (SCI) and sperm cloning (male genome cloning) are recent advancements and future directions for generating clinically applicable germ cells from stem cells. In SCI technique, somatic cell nucleus is injected into enucleated oocyte and cells are cultured further to produce two separated chromosome sets. Thus, the immature oocyte helps somatic cell to become haploid. The resultant cells are genetically identical and immune-compatible with the donor of the somatic cells. In case of severe oligozoospermia, a single viable sperm from testicular biopsy sample can be used for replicating its genome. Here, a single sperm is injected into enucleated oocyte and allows it to become a haploid embryo dividing through parthenogenesis process. Resulting blastomeric cells may be used for further *in vitro* maturation or direct injection into oocyte. These new techniques still remain in experimented animal models with low efficiency [85]. The contribution by various authors for development of this field is summarized in **Table 1**.

4. Conclusion

Among the different models used in *in vitro* spermatogenesis better results have been achieved through 3D culture systems. Formation of EBs using germ and Sertoli cells seems to be more efficient and resemble the testicular niche environment compared to soft agar culture system. Although this system is well supported for the proliferation and differentiation of putative germ cells obtained from somatic stem cells up to the spermatids state there is no firm evidence to conclude the support for an efficient spermiogenesis process. Complete spermatogenesis has been achieved by transplanting stem cells or putative germ cells into testes in few studies, but with lower efficiency. Clinical applications of xeno or autologous transplantation studies among humans, and between humans and animals are still far away due to ethical and safety related issues. Similarly, use of autologous stem cells for differentiation of germ cells and infertility treatment may have little value for the patients with cancer or genetic diseases, as there is a possibility to re-infuse cancer cells or passing genetic abnormalities to offspring. However, *in vitro* maturation of germ cells may be immensely helpful for men with maturation arrest or azoospermia due to non-genetic causes.

Abbreviations

AP	alkaline phosphatase
ART	assisted reproductive technologies
bFGF	basic fibroblast growth factor
BM	bone marrow
DMEM	Dulbecco's modified eagle medium
DSP	daily sperm production
EBs	embryoid bodies
EGF	epidermal growth factor

EGFP	enhanced green fluorescence protein
ESCs	embryonic stem cells
FACS	fluorescence-activated cell sorting
FCS	fetal calf serum
GDNF	glial cell line-derived neurotrophic factor
GSCs	germline stem cells
ICSI	intra cytoplasmic sperm injection
iPSCs	induced pluripotent stem cells
LIF	leukemia inhibitory factor
MACS	magnetic-activated cell sorting
miRNA	microRNA
MSCs	mesenchymal stem cells
PGCs	primordial germ cells
RA	retinoic acid
SPCs	spermatogonial progenitor cells
SSCs	spermatogonial stem cells
TESE	testicular sperm extraction
3D culture	three-dimensional culture

Author details

DMAB Dissanayake

Address all correspondence to: anuradissa@kln.ac.lk

Department of Obstetrics and Gynaecology, Faculty of Medicine Ragama, University of Kelaniya, Sri Lanka

References

[1] Esteves SC, Agarwal A. The azoospermic male: Current knowledge and future perspectives. Clinics. 2013;**68**:1-4

[2] Songa HW, Wilkinson MF. *In vitro* spermatogenesis. Spermatogenesis. 2012;**2**:38-244

[3] Hamada AJ, Esteves SC, Agarwal A. A comprehensive review of genetics and genetic testing in azoospermia. Clinics. 2013;**68**:39-60

[4] Gohbara A, Katagiri K, Sato T, Kubota Y, Kagechika H, Araki Y, Araki Y, Ogawa T. *In vitro* murine spermatogenesis in an organ culture system. Biology of Reproduction. 2010;**83**: 261-267

[5] Ketkar AA, Reddy KVR. Expression pattern of OCT-4 and PLZF transcription factors during the early events of spermatogenesis in mice. Journal of Cell Science and Therapy. 2012;**3**. DOI: 10.4172/2157-7013.1000120

[6] Caires K, Broady J, McLean D. Maintaining the male germline: Regulation of spermatogonial stem cells. Journal of Endocrinology. 2010;**205**:133-145

[7] Huckins C. The spermatogonial stem cell population in adult rats. Cell and Tissue Kinetics. 1971;**4**:313-334

[8] Moens PB, Hugenholtz AD. The arrangement of germ cells in the rat seminiferous tubule: An electron microscope study. Journal of Cell Science. 1975;**19**:487-507

[9] Phillips BT, Gassei K, Orwig KE. Spermatogonial stem cell regulation and spermatogenesis. Philosophical Transactions of the Royal Society. 2010;**365**:1663-1678

[10] Hermann BP, Phillips BT, Orwig KE. The elusive spermatogonial stem cell marker? Biology of Reproduction. 2011;**85**:221-223

[11] Ehmcke J, Wistuba J, Schlatt S. Spermatogonial stem cells: Questions, models and perspectives. Human Reproduction Update. 2006;**12**:275-282

[12] Chan F, Oatley MJ, Kaucher AV, Yang QE, Bieberich CJ, Shashikant CH, Oatley JM. Functional and molecular features of the Id4+ germline stem cell population in mouse testes. Genes & Development. 2014;**28**:1351-1362

[13] Wu Z, Falciatori I, Molyneux LA, Richardson TE, Chapman KM, Hamra FK. Spermatogonial culture medium: An effective and efficient nutrient mixture for culturing rat spermatogonial stem cells. Biology of Reproduction. 2009;**81**:77-86

[14] Nayernia K, Adham I, Kremllng H, Reim K, Schlicker M, Schluter G, Engel W. Stage and developmental specific gene expression during mammalian spermatogenesis. The International Journal of Developmental Biology. 1996;**40**:379-383

[15] Dadoune JP, Siffroi JP, Alfonsi MF. Transcription in haploid male germ cells. International Review of Cytology. 2004;**237**:1-56

[16] Egger GF, Witter K. Peritubular contractile cells in testis and epididymis of the dog, *Canis lupus familiaris*. Acta Veterinaria Brono. 2009;**78**:3-11

[17] Hu J, Chenb YX, Wanga D, Qia X, Lia TG, Haoa J, Mishinac Y, Garbersa DL, Zhaoa GQ. Developmental expression and function of Bmp4 in spermatogenesis and in maintaining epididymal integrity. Developmental Biology. 2004;**276**:158-171

[18] Whelly S, Johnson S, Powell J, Borchardt C, Hastert MC, Cornwall GA. Nonpathological extracellular amyloid is present during normal epididymal sperm maturation. PLoS One. 2012;**7**:1371-1378

[19] Cooper HW, Bausek N. Evolution and spermatogenesis. Philosophical Transactions of the Royal Society B. 2010;**365**:1465-1480

[20] Chenoweth PJ, Lorton SP, editors. Animal Andrology: Theories and Applications. 1st ed. Croydon: CAB International; 2014. pp. 11-33

[21] Li XC, Barringer BC, Barbash BA. The pachytene checkpoint and its relationship to evolutionary patterns of polyploidization and hybrid sterility. Heredity. 2009;**102**:24-30

[22] Amann RP. The cycle of the seminiferous epithelium in humans: A need to revisit? Journal of Andrology. 2008;**29**:469-487

[23] Rooij DG. Proliferation and differentiation of spermatogonial stem cells. Reproduction. 2001;**121**:347-354

[24] Iwamori N. Regulation of spermatogonial stem cell compartment in the mouse testis. Fukuoka Acta Medica. 2014;**105**:1-10

[25] Koshimizu U, Watanabe D, Sawada K, Nishimune YA. Novel stage-specific differentiation antigen is expressed on mouse testicular germ cells during early meiotic prophase. Biology of Reproduction. 1993;**49**:875-884

[26] Bechtol KB. Characterization of a cell-surface differentiation antigen of mouse spermatogenesis: Timing and localization of expression by immunohistochemistry using a monoclonal antibody. Journal of Embryology and Experimental Morphology. 1984;**81**:93-104

[27] West FD, Rios MIR, Abraham S, Rao RR, Natrajan MS, Bacanamwo M, Stice SL. KIT ligand and bone morphogenetic protein signaling enhances human embryonic stem cell to germ-like cell differentiation. Human Reproduction. 2010;**25**:168-178

[28] Kaplan OL. *In vivo* and *in vitro* differentiation of male germ cells in the mouse. Reproduction. 2004;**128**:147-152

[29] Hobbs RM, Fagoonee S, Papa A, Webster K, Altruda F, Nishinakamura R, Chai L, Pandolfi PP. Functional antagonism between Sall4 and Plzf defines germline progenitors. Cell Stem Cell. 2012;**10**:284-298

[30] Seandel M, James D, Shmelkov SV, Falciatori I, Kim J, Chavala S, Scherr DS, Zhang F, Torres R, Gale NW, Yancopoulos GD, Murphy A, Valenzuela DM, Hobbs RM, Pandolfi PP, Rafii S. Generation of functional multipotent adult stem cells from GPR125+ germline progenitors. Nature. 2007;**20**:346-350

[31] Aloisio GM, Nakada Y, Saatcioglu HD, Peña CG, Baker MD, Tarnawa ED, Mukherjee J, Manjunath H, Bugde A, Sengupta AL, Amatruda JF, Cuevas I, Hamra FK, Castrillon DH. PAX7 expression defines germline stem cells in the adult testis. Journal of Clinical Investigations. 2014;**124**:3929-3944

[32] Kumar TR. The quest for male germline stem cell markers: PAX7 gets ID'd. The Journal of Clinical Investigation. 2014;**124**:4219-4222

[33] Carlomagno G, van Bragt MPA, Korver CM, Repping S, de Rooij DG, Van Pelt AMM. BMP4-induced differentiation of a rat spermatogonial stem cell line causes changes in its cell adhesion properties. Biology of Reproduction. 2010;**83**:742-749

[34] Kee K, Angeles VT, Flores M, Nguyen HN, Pera RAR. Human DAZL, DAZ and BOULE genes modulate primordial germ cell and haploid gamete formation. Nature. 2009;**462**: 222-225

[35] Jia W, Cheng D, Chen S, Lei L, Wang H. Retinoic acid induces myoblasts transdifferentiation into premeiotic Stra8-positive cells. Cell Biology International. 2011;**35**:365-372

[36] Sabour D, Arauzo-Bravo MJ, Hubner K, Ko K, Greber B, Gentile L, Stehling M, Scholer HR. Identification of genes specific to mouse primordial germ cells through dynamic global gene expression. Human Molecular Genetics. 2010;**20**:115-125

[37] Liu Y, Niu M, Yao C, Hai T, Yuan O, Liu Y, Guo Y, Li Z, He Z. Fractionation of human spermatogenic cells using STA-PUT gravity sedimentation and their miRNA profiling. Scientific Reports. 2015;**5**. DOI: 10.1038/srep08084

[38] Bhartiya SD, Kasiviswanathan S, Unni SK, Pethe P, Dhabalia JV, Patwardhan S, Tongaonkar HB. Newer insights into premeiotic development of germ cells in adult human testis using Oct-4 as a stem cell marker. Journal of Histochemistry & Cytochemistry. 2010; **58**:1093-1106

[39] He Z, Kokkinaki M, Jiang J, Dobrinski I, Isolation DM. Characterization, and culture of human spermatogonia. Biology of Reproduction. 2010;**82**:363-372

[40] Liu S, Tang Z, Xiong T, Tang W. Isolation and characterization of human spermatogonial stem cells. Reproductive Biology and Endocrinology. 2011;**9**:141-149

[41] Valli H, Sukhwani M, Dovey SL, Peters KA, Donohue J, Castro CA, Chu T, Marshall GR, Orwig KE. Fluorescence and magnetic activated cell sorting strategies to isolate and enrich human spermatogonial stem cells. Fertility and Sterility. 2014;**102**:566-580

[42] Bowles J, Koopman P. Retinoic acid, meiosis and germ cell fate in mammals. Development. 2007;**134**:3401-3411

[43] Pellegrini M, Siena SD, Claps G, Cesare SD, Dolci S, Rossi P, Geremia R, Grimaldi P. Microgravity promotes differentiation and meiotic entry of postnatal mouse male germ cells. PLoS One. 2010;**5**:1371-1380

[44] Itman C, Loveland KL. SMAD expression in the testis: An insight into BMP regulation of spermatogenesis. Developmental Dynamics. 2008;**237**:97-111

[45] Luetjens CM, Xu EY, Pera RAR, Kamischke A, Nieschlag E, Gromoll J. Association of meiotic arrest with lack of BOULE protein expression in infertile men. The Journal of Clinical Endocrinology & Metabolism. 1993;**89**:1926-1933

[46] Kostova E, Yeung CH, Luetjens CM, Brune M, Nieschlag E, Gromoll J. Association of three isoforms of the meiotic BOULE gene with spermatogenic failure in infertile men. Molecular Human Reproduction. 2007;**13**:85-93

[47] Zanganeh BM, Rastegar T, Roudkenar MH, Kashani IR, Amidi F, Abolhasani F, Barbarestani M. Co-culture of spermatogonial stem cells with sertoli cells in the presence

of testosterone and FSH improved differentiation via up-regulation of post meiotic genes. Acta Medica Iranica. 2013;**51**:1-11

[48] Peschon JJ, Behringer RR, Brinster RL, Palmiter RD. Spermatid-specific expression of protamine 1 in transgenic mice. Developmental Biology. 1987;**84**:5316-5319

[49] Ravel C, Bastaraud SC, Houate BE, Berthaut I, Verstraete L, De Larouziere V, Lourenc D, Dumaine A, Antoine JM, Mandelbaum J, Siffroi JP, Mc Elreavey K. Mutations in the protamine 1 gene associated with male infertility. Molecular Human Reproduction. 2007; **13**:461-464

[50] Zhao GQ, Liaw L, Hogan BLM. Bone morphogenetic protein 8A plays a role in the maintenance of spermatogenesis and the integrity of the epididymis. Development. 1998;**125**: 1103-1112

[51] Seandel M, Falciatori I, Shmelkov SV, Kim J, James D, Rafii S. Spermatogonial progenitors marked by GPR125. Cell Cycle. 2008;**15**:135-140

[52] Calvel P, Rolland AD, Je'gou B, Pineau C. Testicular post genomics: Targeting the regulation of spermatogenesis. Philosophical Transactions of the Royal Society B. 2010; **365**:1481-1500

[53] West FD, Shirazi R, Mardanpour P, Ozcan S, Dinc G, Hodges DH, Lichaei HRS, Nayernia K. *In Vitro* derived gametes from stem cells. Seminars in Reproductive Medicine. 2013;**31**:33-38

[54] Aponte PM, Schlatt S, de Franca LR. Biotechnological approaches to the treatment of aspermatogenic men. Clinics. 2013;**68**:157-167

[55] Steinberger A, Steinberger E, Perloff WH. Mammalian testes in organ tubules. Experimental Cell Research. 1964;**36**:19-27

[56] Nagano MC. Techniques for culturing spermatogonial stem cells continue to improve. Biology of Reproduction. 2011;**84**:5-6

[57] Tesarik J, Guido M, Mendoza C, Greco E. Human spermatogenesis *in vitro*: Respective effects of follicle-stimulating hormone and testosterone on meiosis, spermiogenesis, and sertoli cell apoptosis. The Journal of Clinical Endocrinology and Metabolism. 1998; **83**:4467-4473

[58] Sani RN, Tajik P, Yousefi MH, Movahedin M, Panahi BQ, Shafiei S, Hamedani MA. Follicle stimulating hormone increases spermatogonial stem cell colonization during *in vitro* co-culture. Veterinary Research Forum. 2012;**4**:37-41

[59] Goharbakhsh L, Mohazzab A, Salehkhou S, Heidari M, Zarnani AH, Parivar K, Akhondi MM. Isolation and culture of human spermatogonial stem cells derived from testis biopsy. Avicenna Journal of Medical Biotechnology. 2013;**5**:54-61

[60] Ardekani HS, Mizrak SC, van Daalen SKM, Korver CM, Gajadien HLR, Koruji M, Hovingh S, de Reijke TM, de la Rosette JJMCH, van der Veen F, de Rooij DG, Repping S, van Pelt AMMM. Propagation of human spermatogonial stem cells *in vitro*. Journal of American Medical Association. 2009;**302**:2127-2134

[61] Stukenborg JB, Schlatt S, Simoni M, Yeung CH, Elhija MA, Luetjens CM, Huleihel M, Wistuba J. New horizons for *in vitro* spermatogenesis? An update on novel three-dimensional culture systems as tools for meiotic and post-meiotic differentiation of testicular germ cells. Molecular Human Reproduction. 2009;**15**:521-529

[62] Xie L, Lin L, Tang Q, Li W, Huang T, Huo X, Liu X, Jiang J, He G, Ma L. Sertoli cell-mediated differentiation of male germ cell-like cells from human umbilical cord Wharton's jelly-derived mesenchymal stem cells in an *in vitro* co-culture system. European Journal of Medical Research. 2015;**20**. DOI: 10.1186/s40001-014-0080-6

[63] Miryounesi M, Nayernia K, Dianatpour M, Mansouri F, Modarressi MH. Co-culture of mouse embryonic stem cells with Sertoli cells promote *in vitro* generation of germ cells. Iranian Journal of Basic Medical Science. 2013;**16**:779-783

[64] Nayernia K, Lee JH, Drusenheimer N, Nolte J, Wulf G, Dressel R, Gromoll J, Engel W. Derivation of male germ cells from bone marrow stem cells. Laboratory Investigation. 2006;**86**:654-663

[65] Park TS, Galic Z, Conway AE, Lindgren A, Van Handel BJ, Magnusson M, Richter L, Teitell MA, Mikkola HKA, Lowry WE, Plath K, Clark AT. Derivation of primordial germ cells from human embryonic and induced pluripotent stem cells is significantly improved by co-culture with human fetal gonadal cells. Cells. 2009;**27**:783-795

[66] Li Y, Wang X, Feng X, Liao L, Zhang D, Cui X, Gao F, Han C. Generation of male germ cells from mouse induced pluripotent stem cells *in vitro*. Stem Cell Research. 2014;**12**: 517-530

[67] Easley CA, Phillips BT, McGuire MM, Barringer JM, Valli H, Hermann BP, Simerly CR, Rajkovic A, Miki T, Orwig KE, Schatten GP. Direct differentiation of human pluripotent stem cells into haploid spermatogenic cells. Cell Reports. 2012;**27**:440-446

[68] Aflatoonian B, Ruban L, Jones M, Aflatoonian R, Fazeli A, Moore HD. *In vitro* post-meiotic germ cell development from human embryonic stem cells. Human Reproduction. 2009;**24**:3150-3159

[69] Panula S, Medrano JV, Kee K, Bergström R, Nguyen HN, Byers B, Wilson KD, Wu JC, Simon C, Hovatta O, Pera RAR. Human germ cell differentiation from fetal- and adult-derived induced pluripotent stem cells. Human Molecular Genetics. 2011;**20**:752-762

[70] Wei W, Qing T, Ye X, Liu H, Zhang D, Yang W, Deng H. Primordial germ cell specification from embryonic stem cells, PLoS ONE. 2008;3, doi; org/10.1371/journal.pone.0004013

[71] Silva C, Wood JR, Salvador L, Kostetskii I, Williams CJ, Strauss JF. Expression profile of male germ cell-associated genes in mouse embryonic stem cell cultures treated with all-trans retinoic acid and testosterone. Molecular Reproduction and Development. 2009;**76**:11-21

[72] Fuchs E, Green H. Regulation of terminal differentiation of cultured human keratinocytes by vitamin A. Cell. 1981;**25**:617-625

[73] Aflatoonian B, Moore H. Germ cells from mouse and human embryonic stem cells. Reproduction. 2006;**132**:699-707

[74] Childs AJ, Saunders PTK, Anderson RA. Modelling germ cell development *in vitro*. Molecular Human Reproduction. 2008;**14**:501-511

[75] Mari AIM, Kaplan OL, Medrano LV, Pellicer A, Simon C. Differentiation of germ cells and gametes from stem cells. Human Reproduction Update. 2009;**15**:379-390

[76] Zhou GB, Meng QG, li N. *In vitro* derivation of germ cells from embryonic stem cells in mammals. Molecular Reproduction & Development. 2010;**77**:586-594

[77] Kubota H, Brinster RL. Technology insight: *in vitro* culture of spermatogonial stem cells and their potential therapeutic uses. Endocrinology & Metabolism. 2006;**2**:99-108

[78] Sato Y, Taniguchi M, Otoi T. tudying spermatogenesis by using in vivo and *in vitro* models: Advantages and disadvantages of these models for practical use. Journal of Veterinary Science and Technology. 2012:3. DOI: 10.4172/2157-7579.1000115

[79] Lue Y, Erkkila K, Liu PY, Ma K, Wang C, Hikim AS, Swerdloff RS. Fate of bone marrow stem cells transplanted into the testis. The American Journal of Pathology. 2007; **170**:899-908

[80] Mehrabani D, Hassanshahi MA, Tamadon A, Zare S, Keshavarz S, Rahmanifar F, Dianatpour M, Khodabandeh Z, Jahromi IR, Tanideh N, Ramzi M, Aqababa H, Hoseinabadi OK. Adipose tissue-derived mesenchymal stem cells repair germinal cells of seminiferous tubules of busulfan-induced azoospermic rats. Journal of Human Reproductive Sciences. 2015;**8**:103-110

[81] Toyooka Y, Tsunekawa N, Akasu R, Noce T. Embryonic stem cells can form germ cells *in vitro*. PNAS. 2003;**100**:11457-11462

[82] Nayernia K, Nolte J, Michelmann HW, Lee JH, Rathsack K, Drusenheimer N, Dev A, Wulf G, Ehrmann IE, Elliott DJ, Okpanyi V, Zechner U, Haaf T, Meinhardt A, Engel W. *In vitro*-differentiated embryonic stem cells give rise to male gametes that can generate offspring mice. Developmental Cell. 2006b;**11**:125-132

[83] Akhondi MM, Najar RA, Tehrani MJ, Sadeghi MR, Zarnani AH, Rabbani H, Salehkhou S, Eini L, Hoseinzadeh F, Heidari M. The effect of human chorionic gonadotropin treatment on recipient mouse germ cell proliferation following spermatogonial stem cell transplantation of neonatal donor mice. Avicenna Journal of Medical Biotechnology. 2010;**2**:23-35

[84] Ruwanpura SM, McLachlan RI, Meachem SJ. Hormonal regulation of male germ cell development. Journal of Endocrinology. 2010;**205**:117-131

[85] Pelosi E, Forabosco A, Schlessinger D. Germ cell formation from embryonic stem cells and the use of somatic cell nuclei in oocytes. Annals of the New York Academy of Science. 2011;**1221**:18-26

[86] Linher K, Dyce P, Li J. Primordial germ cell-like cells differentiated *in vitro* from skin-derived stem cells. PLoS ONE. 2009:4. DOI: 10.1371/journal.pone.0008263

[87] Bucay N, Yebra M, Cirulli V, Afrikanova I, Kaido T, Hayek A, Montgomery AMP. A novel approach for the derivation of putative primordial germ cells and Sertoli cells from human embryonic stem cells. Stem Cells. 2009;**27**:68-77

[88] Elhija MA, Lunenfeld E, Schlatt S, Huleihel M. Differentiation of murine male germ cells to spermatozoa in a soft agar culture system. Asian Journal of Andrology. 2012;**14**:285-293

[89] Wu Z, Phelps KL, Bugde A, Molyneux LA, Denard B, Li WH, Süel GM, Garbers DL. Capacity for stochastic self-renewal and differentiation in mammalian spermatogonial stem cells. The Journal of Cell Biology. 2009;**187**:513-524

[90] Lee JH, Gye MC, Choi KW, Hong JY, Lee YB, Park DW, Lee SJ, Min CK. *In vitro* differentiation of germ cells from non-obstructive azoospermic patients using three dimensional culture in a collagen gel matrix. Fertility Sterility. 2007;**87**:824-833

[91] Nayernia K, Li M, Jaroszynski L, Khusainov R, Wulf G, Schwandt I, Korabiowska M, Michelmann HW, Meinhardt A, Engel W. Stem cell based therapeutical approach of male infertility by teratocarcinoma derived germ cells. Human Molecular Genetics. 2004;**13**:1451-1460

[92] Riboldi M, Rubio C, Pellicer A, Gil-Salom M, Simon C. *In vitro* production of haploid cells after co-culture of CD49fD with Sertoli cells from testicular sperm extraction in non-obstructive azoospermic patients. Fertility and Sterility. 2012;**98**:580-590

[93] Mitchell RT, Saunders PTK, Childs AJ, Kojima CC, Anderson RA, Wallace WHB, Kelnar CJH, Sharpe RM. Xenografting of human fetal testis tissue: A new approach to study fetal testis development and germ cell differentiation. Human Reproduction. 2010;**2510**:2405-2414

[94] Hua J, Qiu P, Zhu H, Cao H, Wang F, Li W. Multipotent mesenchymal stem cells (MSCs) from human umbilical cord: Potential differentiation of germ cells. African Journal of Biochemistry Research. 2011;**5**:113-123

[95] Zhou Q, Wang M, Yuan Y, Wang X, Fu R, Wan H, Xie M, Liu M, Guo X, Zheng Y, Feng G, Shi Q, Zhao XY, Sha J, Zhou Q. Complete meiosis from embryonic stem cell-derived germ cells *in vitro*. Cell Stem Cell. 2016;**18**:330-340

9

Ultrastructure of Spermatozoa from Infertility Patients

Elizaveta E. Bragina and Elena N. Bocharova

Abstract

Standard examination of human semen currently remains a main test for examination of male fertility disorders. Although parameters of sperm quality in fertile men are generally higher than in sterile ones, there is a substantial overlap between the two populations, indicating that other important factors affect fertility, but are not assessed in conventional assay. Currently, tests determining the functional properties of sperm have been intensively developed. This review considers an electron microscopic examination of sperm, which assesses the structure and function of the sperm nuclear, penetration and motor apparatus. The detection of sperm chromatin structure can help to understand the causes of early embryonic malformation. Genetically caused and functional disorders of the structure and function of spermatozoa are discussed. Indications for electron microscopic examination of spermatozoa in fertility disorders are given.

Keywords: sperm ultrastructure, sperm chromatin, acrosome, asthenozoospermia

1. Introduction

Standard examination of human semen currently remains a main test for male fertility disorders. The concentration (total sperm count) and motility of spermatozoa and the content of morphologically normal (typical) spermatozoa are thought to reflect the fertilization potential of the semen [1]. Although their values in fertile men are generally higher than in sterile ones, there is a substantial overlap between the two populations, indicating that other important factors affect fertility, but are not assessed in conventional assay [2]. In this regard, methods to assess the functional properties of spermatozoa and thus to evaluate their reproductive (fertilizing) potential have intensely been developed in the past years.

Light microscopy, which is employed in a conventional sperm testing, reports the numbers of sperm heads and tails, their sizes and relative arrangement, the presence and sizes of the acrosome and nuclear vacuole, and sperm movement. An ultrastructural examination makes it possible to look inside the spermatozoon and to study what is inaccessible by light microscopy, including the extent of chromatin condensation and the structures of the perinuclear theca (PT), its postacrosomal segment, the centriole, the axoneme, and periaxonemal elements of the tail.

Every function of the spermatozoon is now possible to attribute to a particular morphological structure owing to the achievements of modern molecular biology, cytology, and genetics. The morphology of spermatozoa reflects how competent they are to fertilize (enter) the oocyte and to provide for embryo development.

2. Sperm head

2.1. Chromatin structure in normal spermatozoa

The nucleus occupies a major part of the sperm head and contains condensed chromatin (**Figure 1a**), which is detected as an electron-dense homogeneous material, with small regions of lower electron density on ultrathin sections. Condensed chromatin is at least 10 times denser than ones in somatic cells [3].

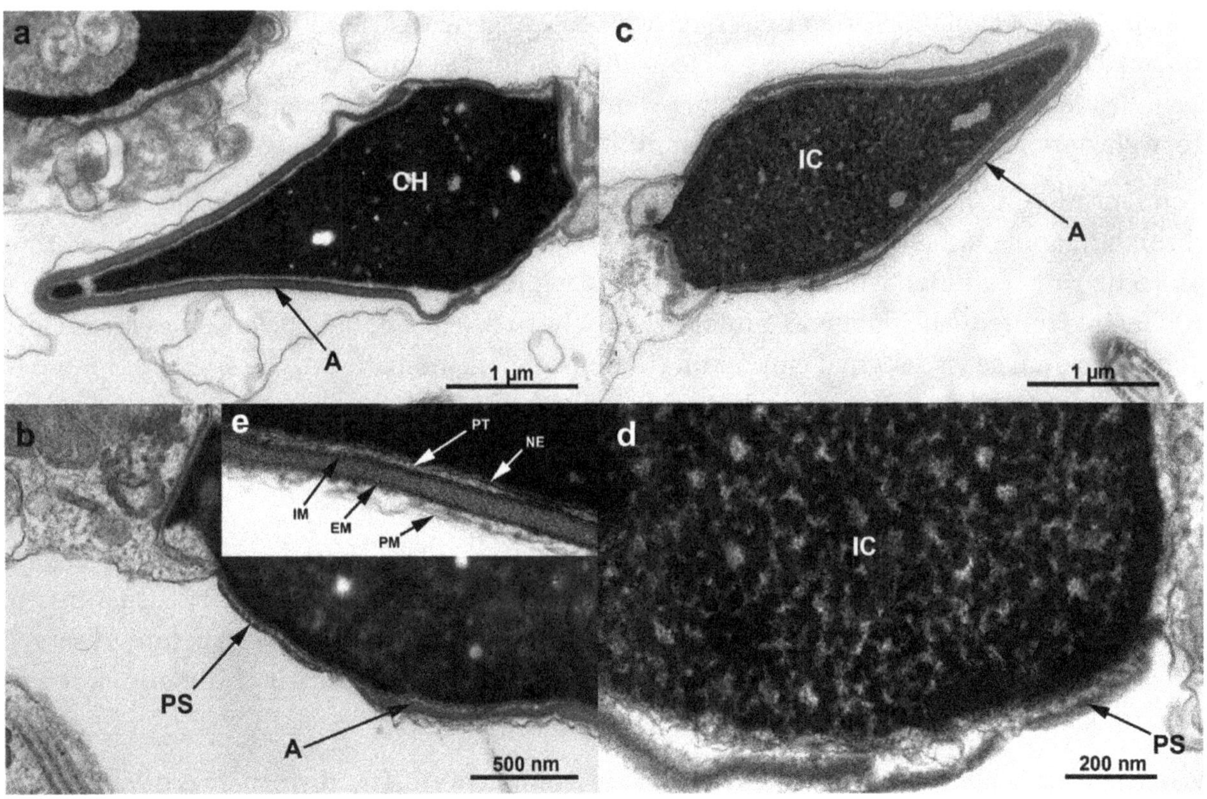

Figure 1. (a) Spermatozoon with condensed chromatin (CH) and normal acrosome (A). (b) Postacrosomal segment of perinuclear theca (PS) with characteristic intermittent striation. (c, d) Spermatozoon with immature chromatin (IC). (e) Fragment of sperm acrosome. NE, nuclear envelope; PT, perinuclear theca; IM, inner acrosome membrane; EM, extra acrosome membrane; and PM, plasma membrane.

To achieve this unique extent of compaction, sperm DNA is packaged in a specific manner, which substantially differs from chromatin packaging in somatic cells. In somatic cells, DNA is packaged to produce the so-called nucleosomes. The DNA double helix is wrapped around a specific complex of canonical histones (a histone octamer) [4].

During sperm maturation, canonical histones are replaced by testis-specific histones and then by protamines, basic proteins with lower molecular weight and high concentration of arginine and cysteine (for a review, see [5, 6]).

As spermatozoa progress through the epididymis, disulfide bridges form between cysteine residues of protamines to further stabilize the DNA-protamine complex and morphologically determine condensation of the dense nucleoprotamine complex in the sperm nucleus [7]. Sperm chromatin is decondensed and acquires a nucleosomal structure after fertilization. The organization of sperm chromatin facilitates the transfer of compacted DNA into the oocyte and ensures its reverse transformation so that genetic information becomes readily available in the developing embryo [8].

Approximately 5–10% of genomic DNA remains free of protamines and preserves a nucleosomal structure in mature human spermatozoa (for a review, see [9]). The role of the residual nucleosomes remained unclear until recently and was explained in three studies, which were published simultaneously in 2010 [10–12]. Residual nucleosomes were found to mark the genes for early embryo development factors and to perform an important function in the epigenetic regulation of embryo development. A gene distribution between protamine-associated and histone-containing (nucleosomal) regions of chromatin follows a certain pattern. Residual nucleosomes occur in the promoters of early developmental genes (e.g., *HOX* gene clusters), imprinted gene loci, and miRNA genes.

Condensation associated with histone-to-protamine replacement metabolically inactivates chromatin and, on the other hand, contributes to its mechanical and chemical stability, thus protecting the paternal genome from nucleases while spermatozoa travel through the male and female reproductive tracts and interact with the oocyte. Residual nucleosomes mark early developmental genes. Normal chromatin condensation is indicative of the sperm potential to produce a normally developing embryo.

2.2. Abnormal chromatin condensation in spermatozoa

Spermatozoa with incomplete chromatin condensation in the nucleus are almost always detectable in ejaculate samples from fertile donors. Granular and fibrillary structures of approximately 40 nm in diameter are seen in these cells. The chromatin structure observed in the spermatozoa is similar to that of elongated spermatids, and their chromatin is consequently known as immature chromatin (**Figure 1c**, **d**) [13].

What is a possible role of distorted chromatin compaction? The disturbance of chromatin condensation is a consequence of a reduced protamine content [14]. Hammoud et al. [15] have recently found that defects in histone-to-protamine exchange lead to a random distribution of nucleosomal (histone-associated and potentially active) chromatin in infertile patients, in contrast to a programmed nucleosomal chromatin distribution in fertile men. Distorted chromatin compaction in spermatozoa seems to lead to substantial post-fertilization defects. Abnormal (insufficient) chromatin condensation was shown to delay the first cell division cycle and to subsequently cause damage to the embryo [16]. Such defects can be responsible for ART failures [17] and early pregnancy losses [18].

Higher percentage of spermatozoa with immature chromatin was observed in semen of the patients with arrest of embryonic development compared with fertile men, and the difference was statistically significant. Semen samples with increased percentage of spermatozoa with immature chromatin in the men with embryo development arrest in reproductive history were 2.2 times more frequent than in the control group (44 vs. 20%) [19].

The question arises as to whether defects in chromatin condensation are associated with DNA fragmentation in spermatozoa. An early hypothesis suggested that defects in histone-to-protamine exchange and, therefore, in chromatin condensation inevitably lead to higher sperm DNA fragmentation [20].

A higher count of spermatozoa with immature, insufficiently condensed chromatin in semen provides an independent diagnostic sign and shows no association with a higher count of spermatozoa with DNA fragmentation [19, 21]. Clinically, fertility disorders are associated with both higher percentage of spermatozoa with immature chromatin and higher percentage of spermatozoa with DNA fragmentation in the ejaculate, but the disorders differ in nature between the two cases. Diagnosing the nature of damage to sperm nuclear material makes it possible to choose a treatment adequate to the observed defect [22].

2.3. Vacuoles in the sperm nucleus

Hollows, which were initially described as vacuoles varying in size and location, can be detected in chromatin of sperm nuclei [23]. Vacuoles are actually indentations in the nucleus, as is seen on ultrathin sections. Chemes and Alvarez Sedò [24] have proposed the term lacunae or lacunar defects for nuclear vacuoles. Lacunae vary in location and texture. **Figure 2a**, **b** shows a lacuna surrounded by a membrane with membrane whorls (MWs), which consist of double membranes with septal complexes [25]; the lacuna is interconnected with nuclear pockets at the base of the head (**Figure 1a**).

Invaginations of another type can also be detected in sperm nuclei. The invaginations may occur in both basal and apical parts of the nucleus, are not surrounded by a membrane, and contain granular material (**Figure 2d**, **e**). A connection (contact) between a lacuna and the subacrosomal space cannot always be seen in ultrathin sections, and the lacuna consequently appears to be a vacuole in nuclear chromatin. DNA is absent from lacunae (**Figure 2c**) [26].

Moving sperm organelle morphology examination (MSOME) using high-resolution microscopy at magnifications exceeding 5000× makes it possible to select in vivo the vacuole-free spermatozoa and to perform intracytoplasmic morphologically selected sperm injection (IMSI) [27].

There are data that IMSI of spermatozoa without vacuoles or with one small vacuole substantially increases the yield of blastocysts as compared with spermatozoa containing large vacuoles or spermatozoa with more than two small vacuoles [28].

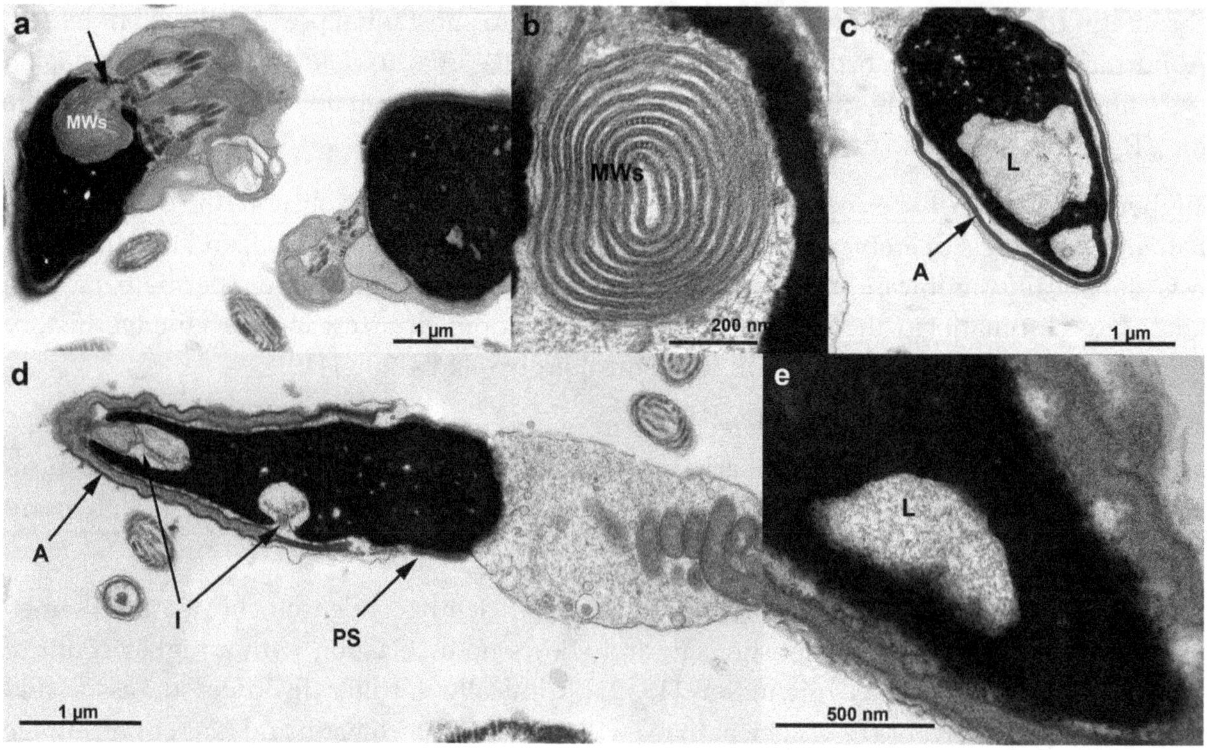

Figure 2. Vacuoles in the sperm nucleus. The lacuna surrounded by membrane with membrane whorls (MWs) (a, b). The lacuna is interconnected with nuclear pockets at the base of the head (a, arrow). Invaginations of the nucleus (I) not surrounded by membrane (d, e), and two large lacunae (L) without visible contact with the subacrosomal space (c). A, acrosome and PS, postacrosomal segment of perinuclear theca.

On the other hand, no correlation of the presence of large vacuoles in spermatozoa has been observed for spermiogram parameters, DNA damage, and live birth rate [29]. IMSI does not improve the outcome of ART after two successive IVF-ICSI failures [30].

Haraguchi et al. [31] have used immunochemistry with electron microscopy and detected proteasomes in nuclear vacuoles and clear spots of condensed chromatin. Nuclear vacuoles and nuclear pockets at the base of the nucleus were assumed to function as proteolytic centers to resorb the molecules (somatic and sperm-specific histones and transit proteins) that are released during chromatin reprogramming. A positive correlation between the presence of vacuoles and the acrosomal reaction [32], vacuoles and capacitation [33] similarly indicates that vacuoles are related to physiological properties of spermatozoa and has no effect on their fertilizing potential.

2.4. Acrosome and perinuclear theca

The acrosome is a secretory vesicle derived from the Golgi apparatus. The acrosome forms a cap on the anterior pole of the nucleus and consists of an outer membrane, inner membrane, and matrix. The outer acrosomal membrane is adjacent to the plasma membrane covering the head of the spermatozoon. A layer sandwiched between the inner acrosomal membrane and the nuclear envelope is known as the perinuclear theca (PT), which has a medium electron density and is approximately 200 nm thick (**Figure 1e**).

The acrosome covers the anterior two-thirds of the sperm head. Relative to the acrosome, the head can be divided into three regions: acrosomal, equatorial, and postacrosomal. Only the PT with its characteristic intermittent striation occurs between the nucleus and the plasma membrane in the postacrosomal region of the spermatozoon (**Figure 1b**).

Material contained in the lumen of the acrosome has a medium electron density and is known as the acrosomal matrix [34]. Zona pellucida (ZP)-binding proteins are found in the acrosomal matrix. Proacrosin is the most important of all ZP-binding proteins of the acrosome. Proacrosin was long believed to be a main lytic protein essential for sperm penetration through the ZP. However, proacrosin knockout mice were found to be fertile [35], although their spermatozoa penetrate through the ZP slower than spermatozoa of wild-type mice. Acrosin probably plays a role in maturation and packaging of other acrosomal matrix proteins. The acrosomal matrix contains several other ZP-binding proteins.

The acrosome of a capacitated spermatozoon interacts with ZP glycoprotein 1 (ZP1) of the oocyte to trigger fusion of the plasma and outer acrosomal membranes, the membrane ends fuse, and vesicles form. Then proteases are released from the acrosome and digest the ZP. The process is known as the acrosomal reaction, which consists in exocytosis and allows the spermatozoon to pass through the ZP. Acrosome-reacted spermatozoa subsequently bind with ZP2, another glycoprotein, which is responsible for sperm adhesion to the oocyte [36]. The inner acrosomal membrane remains intact.

The plasma membrane and the outer acrosomal membrane of the equatorial segment are not involved in forming vesicles during the acrosomal reaction. The equatorial segment is a region where fusion of the spermatozoon and oocyte plasma membrane is triggered. The sperm plasma membrane of the equatorial segment fuses with microvilli of the oolemma, the membranes fuse, and sperm components are thus delivered into the ooplasm. The equatorial segment protein (ESP) is found in the equatorial segment of the acrosome in human spermatozoa [37]. ESP is detectable throughout the acrosome biogenesis. It is thought that ESP plays a role in adhesion of the spermatozoon to the oocyte and their fusion at the oolemma level. Fujihara et al. [38] identified sperm equatorial segment protein 1 (SPESP1), which is specific to the equatorial segment. Spermatozoa of transgenic mice devoid of *SPESP1* (*Spesp1−/−*) fuse with eggs at a far lower rate. SPESP1 seems to be responsible for maintaining the integrity of the equatorial segment after the acrosomal reaction. Membranes of the equatorial segment are disrupted after the acrosomal reaction in Spesp1−/− mice, whereas the equatorial segment is preserved in wild-type mice.

An important role is ascribed to Izumo. The Izumo family includes four proteins, Izumo1-4. Izumo1 is a membrane immunoglobulin protein with an extracellular immunoglobulin domain of 145 residues and an N-terminal domain. The sperm protein Izumo1 on the equatorial segment of the acrosome-reacted spermatozoon recognizes its receptor, JUNO, on the oocyte surface. Human Izumo1 forms a high-affinity complex with the Juno receptor of the oocyte and changes its conformation [39].

2.5. Perinuclear theca

The PT is a cytoskeletal structure that harbors a specific oocyte-activating factor (for a review, see [40]). The PT and its postacrosomal segment remain associated with the sperm nucleus and enter the oocyte upon fertilization. In contrast to the acrosome, which rapidly responds to exogenous factors, the PT is resistant to extraction with denaturing agents and high-salt buffers.

The putative oocyte-activating factor MN13 was found in the PT [40]. MN13 is located in periodic striations, which form the postacrosomal sheath of the PT.

Phospholipase C zeta (PLCζ) is another protein found in the postacrosomal segment of the PT and is thought to act as an oocyte-activating factor [41].

Thus, PLCζ and probably other proteins of the postacrosomal sheath of the PT act as oocyte-activating factors. The postacrosomal sheath is the first to contact the oocyte, and its dissolution (disassembly) is sufficient for triggering early events of oocyte activation. The oocyte-activating factors are transmitted from the sperm PT into the oocyte cytoplasm after the incorporation and rapid dissolution of the PT. In the normal fertilization cycle, the PT dissolves in the oocyte cytoplasm simultaneously with decondensation of the sperm nucleus and initiates division of the maternal pronucleus by hydrolyzing a membrane-bound phospholipid substrate, triggering cytoplasmic Ca^{2+} oscillations [42]. In the case of ICSI, activation occurs only in the oocytes that contain a partly or completely dissolved PT. When the PT dissolves only partly, the residual PT postacrosomal sheath may persist at the apical side of the paternal pronucleus and may delay or arrest zygote development [43]. Dissolution of the subacrosomal part of the PT is essential for complete DNA decondensation in the paternal pronucleus and the start of DNA synthesis in both pronuclei.

2.6. Acrosomal abnormalities

Electron microscopic examination of the acrosome provides an experimentally grounded alternative to sperm penetration assays. The method reliably reports the integrity of the acrosome and the status of its enzymatic system and the postacrosomal segment, which is involved in sperm attachment to the oocyte. A higher percentage of spermatozoa with abnormal acrosomes in an ejaculate sample can be responsible for idiopathic infertility when the spermiogram parameters are within the normal ranges.

2.6.1. Primary lack of an acrosome

Lack of an acrosome is identified as primary when resulting from spermiogenesis defects. Globozoospermia of a presumably genetic nature provides a classical example of the primary lack of an acrosome.

Globozoospermia is an uncommon male fertility disorder. Round-headed cells may account for up to 6% of the total sperm count in the ejaculate in fertile men [44], while 100% of spermatozoa have round heads in total globozoospermia. The sperm count and motility are not affected in globozoospermia. An ultrastructural examination shows that acrosomes are completely absent from round heads or that a rudimentary acrosome occurs at the nuclear pole opposite to the tail (**Figure 3a**).

Defects of chromatin condensation in the nucleus are additionally seen in the majority of ejaculate samples. Heterogeneity is also possible; i.e., spermatozoa with normal condensed chromatin and those with decondensed chromatin may be detected in one ejaculate sample. Both

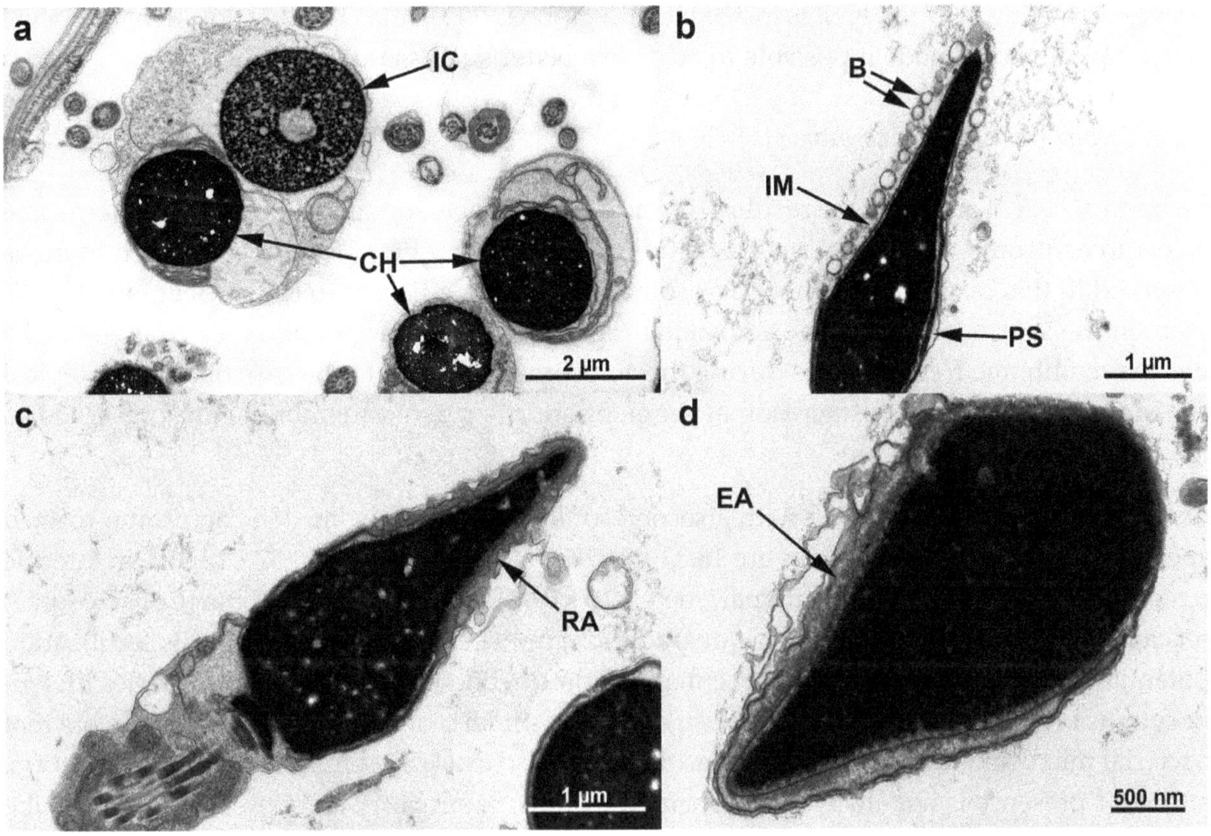

Figure 3. (a) Round acrosomeless sperm heads from globozoospermia. Some nuclei are with condensed chromatin (CH) and one nucleus with immature chromatin (IC). (b) Secondary lack of acrosome. The intact internal acrosomal membrane (IM) and postacrosomal segment (PS) are visible. The outer acrosomal membrane and the plasma membrane form bubbles (B). (c) Acrosome with irregular contours (RA); (d) "empty" acrosome (EA).

within- and between-sample heterogeneity are observed. Higher contents of spermatozoa with immature chromatin [45] were observed in globozoospermia in the majority of studies.

Kullander and Rausing [46] were the first to assume a genetic nature for globozoospermia. Cases with a family history of the disorder supported the assumption. Mutations or deletions of three genes—*SPATA16, PICK1,* and *DPY19L2*—were detected in globozoospermia in molecular genetic studies. A homozygous mutation of *SPATA16* (3q26.32) was found in three brothers with globozoospermia [47]. A mutation of *PICK1* (22q12.3-q13.2) was identified in a globozoospermia patient [48]. The protein products of the two genes occur in the Golgi apparatus and are involved in vesicular trafficking, which is necessary for acrosome biogenesis in spermatids during spermiogenesis [49]. A deletion of *DPY19L2* was observed in the majority of total globozoospermia cases; Dpy19l3 protein is essential for a nuclear flattening and the formation of the acrosome [50].

The identification of the missense mutation L967Q of the gene *VPS54* [51], gene *GM130* inactivation [52], and some others lead to phenotypic globozoospermia in mouse model. These factors are related to the function of the Golgi apparatus vesicles, and these mutations are not identified in men.

The postacrosomal sheath of the PT is absent in patients with globozoospermia. PLCζ is found in extremely small, if any, amounts in spermatozoa of mice and human patients with a *Dpy19l2* mutation and the globozoospermia phenotype [53]. Because these proteins possess oocyte-activating activity, ICSI is insufficient in globozoospermia. The development of oocyte activation methods made it possible to achieve a better success rate [54].

2.6.2. *Secondary lack of an acrosome*

Secondary lack of an acrosome results from a premature acrosomal reaction, i.e., the acrosome is lost in acrosome-reacted spermatozoa (**Figure 3b**). Disruption of the plasma membrane is observed in this case, and the inner acrosomal membrane adjacent to the nuclear envelope is seen on the sperm surface in the acrosomal region. The outer acrosomal membrane and the plasma membrane form bubbles during the acrosomal reaction. In the case of a physiological acrosomal reaction, the postacrosomal segment and its plasma membrane are preserved in the live spermatozoon.

The percentage of spermatozoa with a secondary loss of the acrosome (i.e., acrosome-reacted spermatozoa) in ejaculate samples are 18.22 ± 8.27% in fertile men and 26.37 ± 12.81% in infertile patients with normal spermiogram parameters ($p < 0.05$) [52]. A higher percentage of acrosome-reacted spermatozoa (with acrosome degradation) in the ejaculate may impair its fertilization potential. Leukocytospermia with an enhanced production of reactive oxygen species by leukocytes is one of the possible causes of an early acrosomal reaction. Our findings indicate that bacterial microcolonies present in the ejaculate may also cause a premature acrosomal reaction, and their presence is not always accompanied by an inflammatory response. We analyzed the results of electron microscopic examinations of 746 semen samples from patients with fertility disorders. Bacterial microcolonies were detected in 186 of the 746 samples (25%), and a higher (more than 20%) content of spermatozoa with a secondary loss of the acrosome was observed in 112 of the 186 samples (60%). In the absence of bacterial infection, a higher content of acrosome-reacted spermatozoa was found in 117 of the 560 samples (20%) [55].

A higher leukocyte count in the ejaculate was detected in 36 of the 186 samples with bacterial microcolonies (19%).

Electron microscopy is a gold-standard test for acrosomal reaction, although a number of other tests are now available to assess the penetrating potential of spermatozoa.

2.6.3. *Irregular acrosome*

Irregular acrosome (**Figure 3c**) and lack of acrosomal contents (**Figure 3d**) (enzymatic insufficiency of the acrosome) are found in both pronounced teratozoospermia and normospermia. Proteolytic enzymes of the acrosome dissolve the zona pellucida to allow fusion of the spermatozoon and the oolemma. When the process is disturbed as a result of acrosome loss or dysfunction, spermatozoa lose their fertilizing potential. Irregularly T-shaped acrosomes can be detected in binuclear spermatozoa (**Figure 4a**).

2.6.4. *Enlarged subacrosomal space and lack of a PT and postacrosomal segment*

Spermatozoa that have an enlarged perinuclear space and lack the postacrosomal sheath of the PT account for 2–5% of the total sperm count in semen from fertile men (**Figure 4b–d**). The abnormality is often combined with the presence of excess residual cytoplasm on the

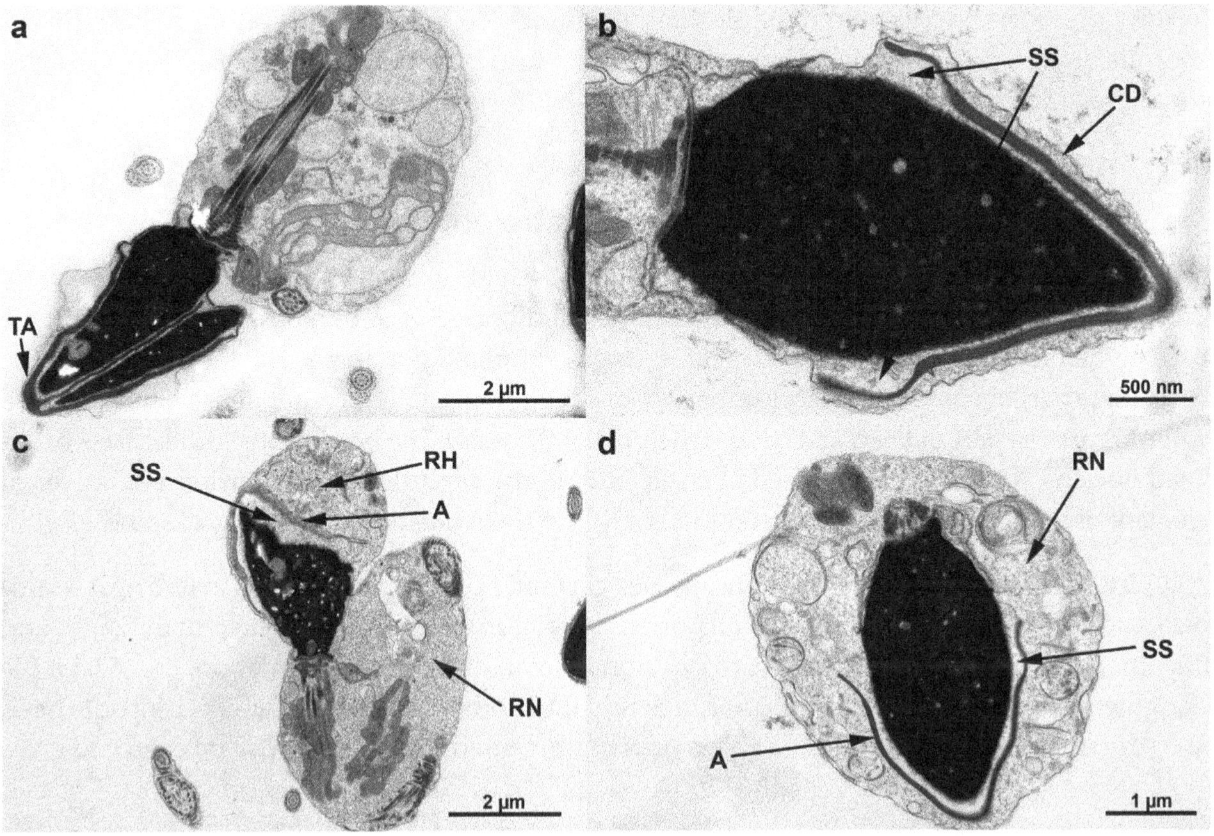

Figure 4. (a) Binuclear spermatozoa with T-shaped acrosome (TA). (b) Sperm with small cytoplasmic droplet on the head (CD) lacking the PT and its postacrosomal segment and with enlarged subacrosomal space (SS). A, irregular acrosome. (c, d) Spermatozoa with excess residual cytoplasm on the head (RH) and on the neck (RN), irregular acrosomes (A), and enlarged subacrosomal space (SS).

head (**Figure 4c, d**). The disorder is sometimes referred to as type II globozoospermia. Sperm heads appear to be spherical under a light microscope, but an ultrastructural study shows that spermatozoa have normal elongate nuclei, whereas their heads look round because of excess residual cytoplasm. This form of pathology also impairs fertility, but differs from globozoospermia [56] because lack of the PT and its postacrosomal segment suggests lack of the oocyte-activating factor.

In some cases, a small cytoplasmic droplet on the head is found in spermatozoa lacking the PT and its postacrosomal segment, so that the spermatozoa appear to be normal by light microscopy (**Figure 4b**). The pathology is detectable only by electron microscopy and may cause idiopathic infertility while the conventional spermiogram parameters are within the normal ranges. ICSI with the oocyte activation methods developed for patients with globozoospermia could solve the problem for these patients. A promising method was tested in a mouse model; i.e., recombinant PLCζ was injected to allow fertilization with spermatozoa of *PLCζ-/-I489F* mutant mice [57].

The acrosome is the most labile component of the spermatozoon. According to our data, the percentage of spermatozoa with abnormal acrosome shapes is 50.12 ± 8.70% in fertile men. Alterations of the acrosome shape or lack of the acrosomal contents are greater in men with fertility disorders. Acrosomal hypoplasia is a common component of pronounced teratozoospermia, is well detectable by electron microscopy, and is essential to diagnose because acrosomal insufficiency is possible to correct using ICSI (for a review, see [58]).

3. Connecting piece (neck) of the spermatozoon

The connecting piece connects the head with the tail (**Figure 5a**). A thin basal plate occurs at the base of the head, it has a concave shape, forming an implantation fossa. The region beneath the basal plate harbors nine striated columns, which continue caudally as outer dense fibers. Striated columns are the part of the connecting structures of the neck. The basal plate is at the base of the head nucleus. A centriole is enclosed in an electron-dense capitulum. The centriole is a universal element of animal eukaryotic cells and plays a role in the formation of the mitotic spindle.

A typical centrosome (cell center) of immature germline cells consists of two cylindrical centrioles, each consists of nine symmetrically oriented microtubule triplets, of 0.5 μm in length and 0.2 μm in diameter. Two centrioles are positioned in an orthogonal orientation, the axis of the daughter centriole being perpendicular to that of the mother centriole. A typical centriole has a 9 + 0 organization of microtubule triplets. In a mature spermatozoon, the distal centriole gives

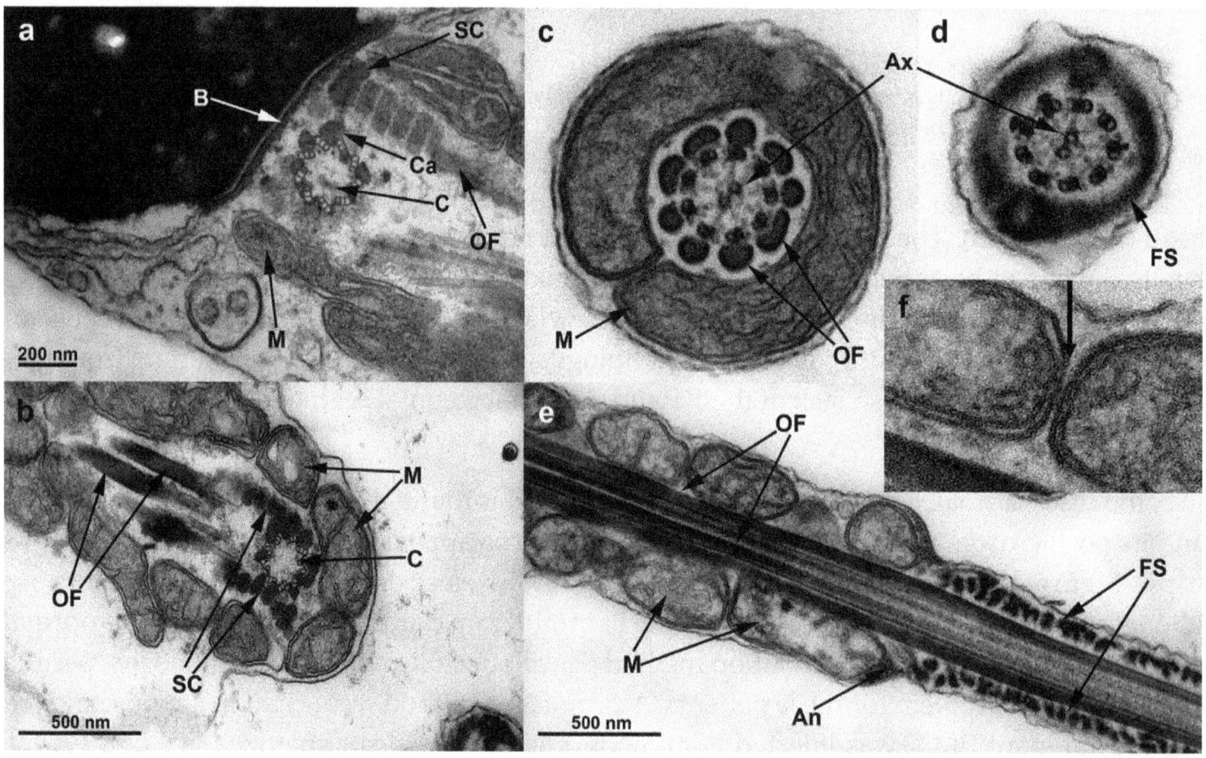

Figure 5. (a) The connecting piece of normal spermatozoon. (b) Decapitated spermatozoon. B, basal plate; C, centriole; Ca, capitulum; SC, striated column, OF, outer dense fibers; and M, mitochondria. (c) Transverse section through the mid-piece of spermatozoon tail; (d) transverse section through the principal piece of spermatozoon; (e) longitudinal section through the middle and principal piece of the tail; (f) the site of contact between mitochondria (arrow). Ax, axoneme, dynein arms of peripheral microtubule doublets are visible. M, mitochondria; FS, fibrous sheath; and An, annulus.

origin to the tail axoneme and is reduced. The proximal centriole preserves its morphology, enters the oocyte upon fertilization, and plays a role in organizing the cleavage spindle [59].

The centriole is surrounded by striated columns, which are part of the connecting structures of the neck. The basal plate is at the base of the head nucleus. The centriole is capable of functioning as an organizing center during cell division only when having a normal morphology, as was demonstrated in many somatic cell studies [60].

The role of the sperm centriole has come into focus of research relatively recently, with the development of ART methods. A paternal inheritance of the centriole was then demonstrated for humans and large mammals as opposed to rodents [61]. The centriole organizes microtubule assembly to produce the sperm aster, which forms around the paternal pronucleus 6 h after fertilization [62] and gives origin to the first mitotic spindle. The main function of the centriole is to organize a network of microtubules, which originate from the oocyte.

3.1. Centrosome abnormalities

Centrosome abnormalities were described as a cause of unsuccessful fertilization and abnormal embryo development [61, 62]. Decaudated or decapitated sperm is a rare syndrome in humans and includes the absence of the implantation fossa and the basal plate. Morphological features of the human syndrome were described comprehensively, and ultrastructural defects of spermatozoa with an abnormal fragility of the head-tail junction were studied by electron microscopy (**Figure 5b**). The proximal centriole/centrosome, which induces the formation of the basal plate and the implantation fossa, was assumed to play an essential role in attaching the flagellum to the nucleus. Dysfunction of the proximal centriole/centrosome may alter the formation of tail attachment structures, leading to decapitated sperm. Spontaneous fertilization is impossible with such spermatozoa because the tail easily detaches from the head because of the neck fragility. ICSI is the only way of fertilization in this case, but rarely is successful. Chemes et al. [63] observed lack of cleavage after ICSI. Porcu et al. [64] reported successful ICSI in two infertile couples where the men were brothers and produced acephalic spermatozoa or spermatozoa with abnormal head-tail attachments, and one birth was published by Gambera et al. [65].

A genetic origin is now commonly accepted for the syndrome. Baccetti et al. [66] assumed that recessive autosomal mutations account for the majority of sperm genetic defects. However, the genes affected by the mutations are unknown. Light microscopic signs of the syndrome vary. Multiple motile tails with single, if any, tailless heads are observed in semen in the majority of cases. Kamal et al. [67] described 16 cases with a variant of the syndrome wherein the spermiogram parameters were normal, while minimal ICSI-related manipulations caused decapitation and immobilization of spermatozoa. The head and tail usually separate at the head-neck junction; the connecting piece is preserved; the basal plate and implantation fossa are absent from the caudal pole of the nucleus.

Several variants of decapitated sperm were described. Holstein et al. [68] reported a case where the basal plate and implantation fossa were normal in morphology, while separation occurred between the proximal and distal centrioles. Baccetti et al. [66] described a patient with sperm ruptures occurring between the nucleus and centriole region, between the anterior and caudal regions of the mid-piece, and between the mid-piece and principal piece. A number of variants are most likely possible for sperm decapitation.

Cases of familial incidence of teratozoospermia with acephalic sperm suggested a genetic nature for the disorder [69]. Homo- or heterozygous mutations of the spermatid-specific SUN5 gene were found in some patients with acephalic (decapitated) sperm syndrome [70]. The protein product of the gene occurs in the immediate vicinity of the head-tail junction, and proteins of its family are known as part of the contact system that connects the inner nuclear membrane with the cytoskeleton.

4. Tail

The intact tail of a human spermatozoon is approximately 50 μm in length and consists of four regions: a connecting piece, which is attached to the head; a mid-piece, which is 3–5 μm long; a principal piece, which accounts for approximately two-thirds of the tail length; and a short end piece. In contrast to cilia, which are covered by the plasma membrane, the sperm tail has not only the axoneme but also additional structures that surround the axoneme and are known as the periaxonemal structures. A mitochondrial helix and outer dense fibers surround the axoneme in the mid-piece and a fibrous sheath in the principal piece. The axoneme has no periaxonemal structures only in the short end piece.

4.1. Axoneme

The axoneme forms a core in cilia and flagella. The sperm axoneme consists of nine pairs of microtubules (doublets) that are arranged in a ring around two central singlet microtubules (9 + 2 arrangement). The doublets are numbered clockwise, starting from the site where two doublets overlay the central pair of microtubules; the right doublet is number one (**Figure 5c**, **d**). Each peripheral doublet consists of a complete microtubule (subunit A) and an adjacent incomplete microtubule (subunit B).

Two, outer and inner, arms consisting of the protein dynein (dynein arms) with ATPase activity extend from the A subunit of each doublet towards the B subunit of the next clockwise doublet. Each dynein arm is an intricate multiprotein complex and acts as a molecular motor [71]. The microtubule doublets are connected via thin bridges of the protein nexin (nexin bridges) and project radial spokes towards the two central microtubules. This sophisticated structure sustains sliding movements of the microtubules, thus providing for undulations of the tail. The axoneme is intricate molecular machinery wherein the inner and outer dynein arms generate forces to produce bending waves and the central apparatus and radial spokes play a regulatory role [72, 73].

4.2. Periaxonemal structures of the sperm tail

4.2.1. Mid-piece of the tail

The outer dense fibers are a morphological extension of the striated columns and capitulum, which are structural elements of the connecting piece of the sperm neck [74]. The outer dense fibers surround the axoneme in the mid-piece of the tail, one fiber overlaying one peripheral microtubule doublet. ODF1 is a major protein of the outer dense fibers (**Figure 5c**, **e**).

The number of mitochondria is reduced as a large portion of the cytoplasm is eliminated with residual bodies from spermatids in the course of spermiogenesis [75]. Up to 75 mitochondria are left in a mature spermatozoon with a minor cytoplasm amount and form a helix around the outer dense fibers and axoneme. The mitochondrial helix has 11–13 turns with two mitochondria per turn. The mitochondrial helix length and the approximate number of turns are constant within a species [76].

The structure of the mitochondrial helix is stable owing to the so-called mitochondrial capsule, i.e., the outer mitochondrial membrane is coated with keratin-like molecules, which form disulfide bridges between cysteine- and proline-rich selenoprotein regions [77]. Contact zones form at the sites of contacts between mitochondria, indicating that the spermatozoon has a mitochondrial reticulum, similar to the mitochondrial network of the heart muscle rather than individual mitochondria (**Figure 5f**) [78, 79].

Active functional mitochondria were demonstrated to affect the sperm fertilizing potential in many studies. Ultrastructural defects in mitochondria are associated with lower sperm motility. The available data on the role of mtDNA mutations are discrepant. Deletions from mtDNA were considered to be responsible for sperm dysfunction and infertility [80]. However, the difference was not confirmed for several mtRNAs by rtPCR.

Metabolism of sperm mitochondria is still a matter of discussion. It is commonly accepted that ATP produced by mitochondria provides a main source of energy for the dynein motor of the axoneme. In contrast, a compartmentalization hypothesis suggests that glycolysis is a main source of energy for tail movements [81]. Because discrepant experimental data were reported from different studies, the question is still open. It is possible that mitochondria are involved in basic redox processes, which determine the fertilizing potential and lifespan of the spermatozoon, rather than in energy metabolism as a main function.

The mid-piece and principal piece of the tail are separated by a ring structure known as the annulus (**Figure 5e**), which presumably performs a barrier function to prevent molecular diffusion between the two pieces [82].

4.2.2. Principal piece of the tail

The principal piece of the tail is distal of the mid-piece and is the longest tail segment. The mitochondrial sheath is not found in the principal piece, and a fibrous sheath as another cytoskeletal element of the tail surrounds the axoneme. Two longitudinal columns of the fibrous sheath replace two opposite outer dense fibers and are connected together by numerous circumferential ribs (**Figure 5d**, **e**).

A total of 18 polypeptides were identified in the fibrous sheath. The polypeptides form a scaffold for glycolytic enzymes and act as signaling molecules upon induction of sperm motility (for a review, see [83]). A-kinase anchoring proteins 3 and 4 (AKAP3 and AKAP4) are major components of the fibrous sheath and probably form its integral cytoskeletal structure. AKAP3 and AKAP4 are associated with each other and bind to cAMP-dependent protein kinase A through its regulatory subunit. The AKAP3 and AKAP4 genes were sequenced, and the binding sites identified.

The principal piece of the tail harbors glycolytic enzymes, including sperm-specific hexokinase 1, lactate dehydrogenase, and sperm-specific glyceraldehyde 3-phosphate dehydrogenase (GAPDHs) [84].

4.3. Structural abnormalities of the tail

The complex system of tail elements with their concerted function provides the spermatozoon with the ability to move, that is, to reach and fertilize the oocyte. Any structural alteration of the system impairs sperm motility.

A functional variant of asthenozoospermia is the most common. Spermatozoa of patients display multiple heterogeneous ultrastructural changes in the axoneme and periaxonemal structures (**Figure 6a–e**), such as changes in the number and arrangement of the microtubule doublets, the shape of the outer dense fibers, or the architecture of the fibrous sheath. Quantitative changes in mitochondria and their altered localization were also associated with asthenozoospermia. The percentage of spermatozoa with ultrastructural tail defects is significantly higher in patients with asthenozoospermia. Ultrastructural defects of the tail axoneme were described in drug addicts [85]. Yet smoking and alcohol drinking were not found to affect the ultrastructural parameters of mature spermatozoa, lower sperm counts observed in alcoholics and smokers suggest testicular selection [86]. Functional asthenozoospermia can

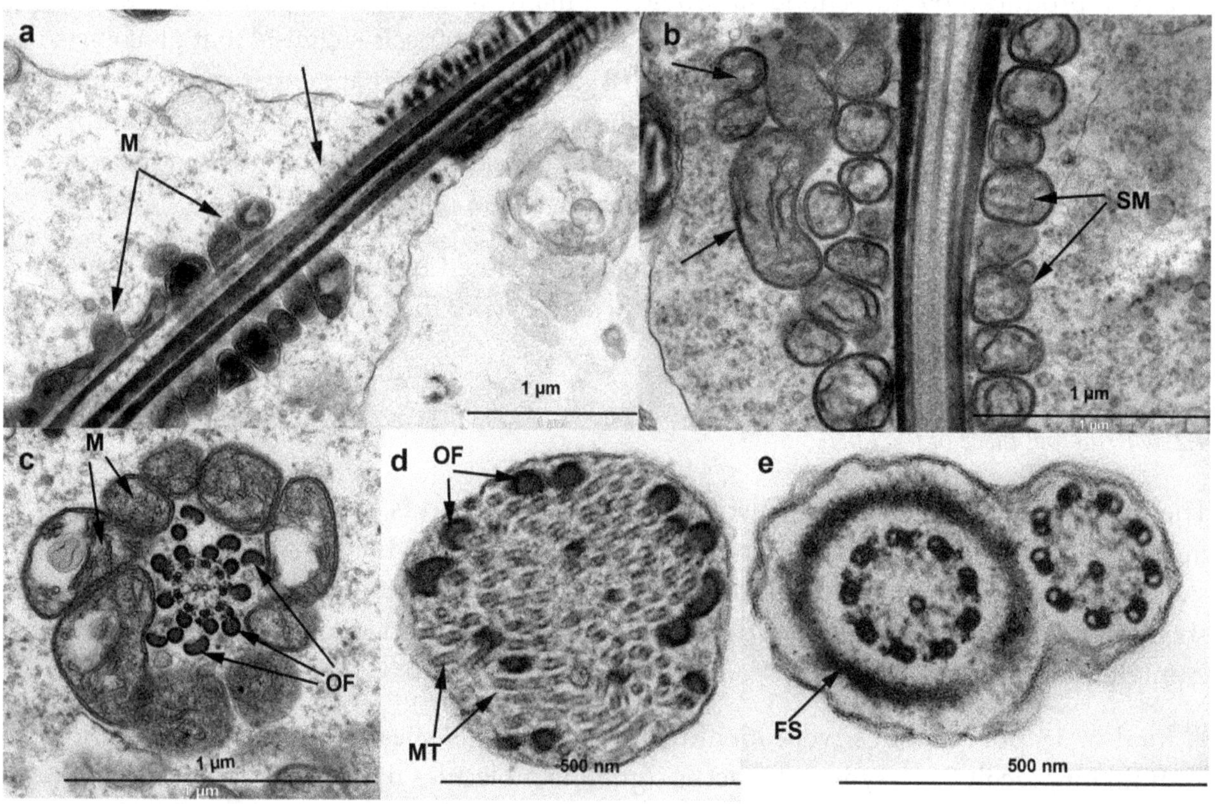

Figure 6. Longitudinal (a, b) and transverse (c–e) sections through abnormal sperm tails. (a) Lack of annulus (arrow) between the middle and principal piece of the tail; (b)swollen mitochondria (SM) and dislocation of mitochondria (arrow); (c) normal axonema structure and increased quantity of outer dense fibers (OF); (d) disorganization of axonemal microtubules (MT) and outer dense fibers (OF); (e) double tail with (9 + 1) microtubules. The absence of dynein arms in the right axoneme is revealed. FS, fibrous sheath.

be secondary to a varicocele, infections of reproductive organs, and exogenous exposures [58]. Spermiogram parameters are possible to correct with medications in men diagnosed with functional asthenozoospermia. When the treatment is ineffective, ICSI is likely to help.

4.4. Genetically determined forms of asthenozoospermia

4.4.1. Dysplasia of the fibrous sheath of the tail

Chemes et al. [87] proposed the term dysplasia of the fibrous sheath (DFS) for the disorder, which is also known as stump tail syndrome and short-tail spermatozoa. Spermatozoa have substantially reduced, if any, motility due to fibrous for DSF [88]. In spermatozoa, the location of longitudinal columns and transverse ribs of the fibrous layer has been disturbed. There are changes in the structure of the mitochondrial helix—a significant shortening and disruption of localization. Anomalies in the structure of the fibrous sheath often put together with the absence of a central pair of the axoneme microtubules (**Figure 7a–c**).

A mouse model of DFS was obtained by targeted disruption of the *Akap4* gene, and spermatozoa of mutant mice had short thick tails, which were morphologically identical to those in DFS patients [89]. However, consistent human data were reported from only one study. Baccetti et al. [90] used PCR and observed intragenic deletions of *AKAP4* and *AKAP3*, which code for major structural components of the fibrous sheath, in one DFS patient. No abnormality was detected in other samples.

We found a decrease in the activity of the glycolytic sperm-specific enzyme glyceraldehyde-3-phosphate dehydrogenase (sGAPD) and atypical localization of the enzyme. Mutations

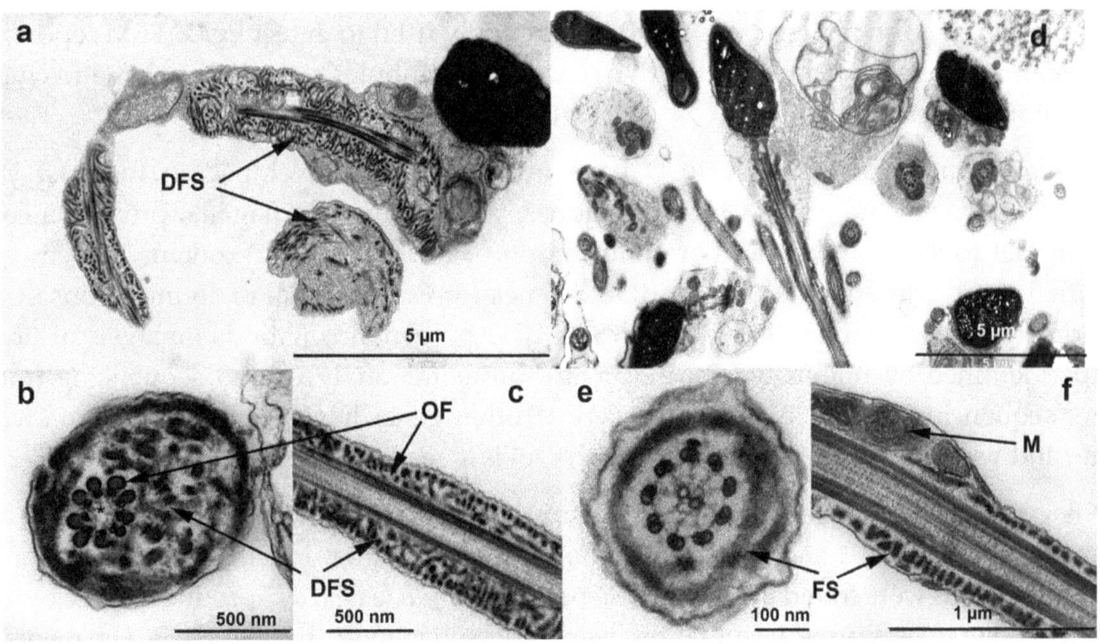

Figure 7. (a) Sperm with dysplasia of the fibrous sheath (DFS) of the tail. The lack of mitochondria is revealed (arrow). Transverse (b) and longitudinal (c) sections through the tail with DFS. The lack of the central pair of microtubules (asterisk). (d) Sperm with primary ciliary dyskinesia (PCD). Transverse (e) and longitudinal (f) sections through the tail with PCD. The absence of dynein arms is revealed on the transverse section. OF, outer dense fibers; FS, fibrous sheath; and M, mitochondria.

within human *GAPDS* gene were assayed. In all five studied semen DFS samples, a replacement of guanine by adenine was revealed in the intron region between the sixth and the seventh exons of *sGAPD* [91]. Pereira et al. [92] found heterozygous deletion in the *DNAH5* gene, but not mutations in *AKAP3* and *AKAP4* in four patients with DFS.

DSF has an autosomal recessive inheritance. The genetic risk is now impossible to estimate. A few cases of live births after ICSI with spermatozoa of DSF patients were reported in the medical literature [93].

4.4.2. Primary ciliary dyskinesia (PCD)

PCD is an autosomal recessive disorder and is highly heterogeneous genetically. PCD affects the axonemal structures (microtubules and dynein arms) of cilia and flagella (**Figure 7d–f**). Bronchial and pulmonary diseases are the main pathology in PCD because infections and bronchiectasis develop when respiratory cilia have motility defects or are immotile.

Headaches are common in PCD patients because lack of ciliary motility in the brain ventricles impairs circulation of the cerebrospinal fluid. Situs inversus is additionally observed in half of the PCD patients, possibly resulting from lack of ciliary motility in embryonic Hensen's node, which is responsible for the unidirectional fluid flow and thereby establishes left-right asymmetry [94]. The prevalence of PCD at birth is 1/10,000 to 1/20,000 [95].

Fertility is impaired in male patients because their spermatozoa are absolutely immotile or defects occur in efferent seminiferous ducts lined by ciliated epithelia. In a semen analysis, gross ejaculate parameters (volume, pH, viscosity, and color) and the concentration and count of morphologically normal spermatozoa are within the normal ranges.

Transmission electron microscopy (TEM) is commonly used to detect PCD. TEM reports lack of outer and/or inner dynein arms, the two central microtubules, or radial spokes and changes in microtubule arrangement.

Molecular methods to diagnose PCD have intensely been developed in the past years. Unicellular algae of the genus Chlamydomonas, which have two flagella, provide a convenient model to study the molecular composition of the axoneme. Axoneme protein genes identified in Chlamydomonas are candidate genes for PCD. A total of 16 mutations of PCD candidate genes were identified from 1999 to 2011 by genetic methods (analysis of linkage groups identified by homozygosity mapping), proteome analysis, and sequencing (mostly Sanger sequencing). Since 2011, mutations of 18 other genes have been described via whole-exome and whole-genome sequencing (for the review see [73, 96]).

PCD is genetically heterogeneous. Mutations of two genes, *DNAI1* and *DNAH5*, are the most common in PCD. *DNAI1* and *DNAH5* code for proteins of outer dynein arms of the axoneme. *DNAI1* mutations were found in 14% of PCD patients [97]. The *DNAH5* product is a major motor protein of outer dynein arms. Its mutations were observed in more than 25% of PCD patients [98].

Many proteins are involved in building the axoneme. Several proteins are common for epithelial cilia and sperm tails. Patients homozygous for mutations of their genes develop the total set of PCD signs, including bronchial and pulmonary diseases, changes in asymmetry of visceral organs, and immotile sperm. Other axonemal proteins are tissue specific, and mutations of their genes cause mosaic ciliopathy, such as asthenozoospermia and anosmia, or asthenozoospermia and swelling of the nasopharyngeal mucosa, which we identified in our patients.

The development of ICSI allowed men with pronounced asthenozoospermia, including forms with genetic causes, to have children. The consequences of using ICSI in PCD and DSF are poorly understood because the disorders are rare and only few live births after ICSI have been reported (20 cases according to PubMed). PCD patients with andrological symptoms naturally had no offspring before the advent of ICSI. PCD is an autosomal recessive disorder and is expressed only in homozygotes and compound heterozygotes, when both alleles of one gene are affected. This circumstance reduces PCD risk in ICSI offspring, but makes it more likely for the mutations to accumulate in the population and to occur in homozygote at a higher rate in the long term.

5. Virus infection of spermatozoa

Virus capsids morphologically identical to capsids of *Herpesviridae* family were detected in the nucleus and cytoplasmic droplet of infected spermatozoa by TEM (**Figure 8a**, **b**) (for the review see [99]). The structures shown in **Figure 8** (**8a**, **b**) are capsids of herpes simplex virus

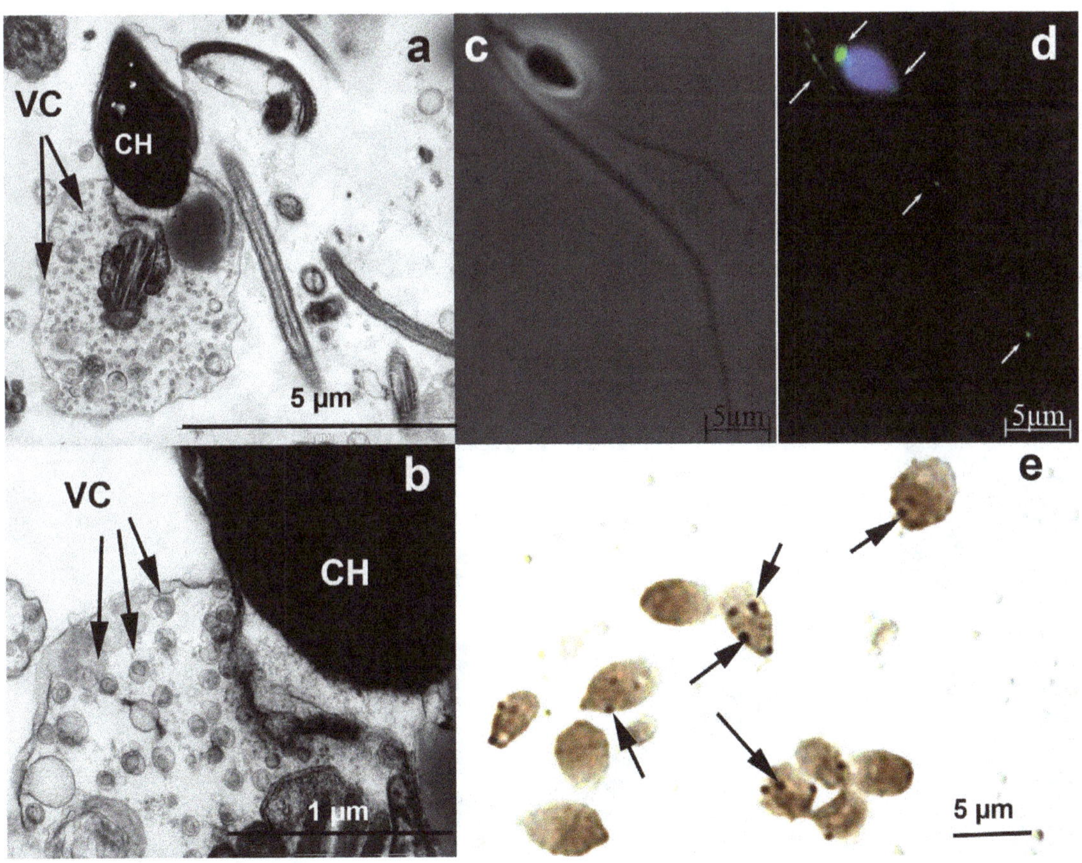

Figure 8. (a) Longitudinal section of normal sperm; (b) section through the middle piece of the tail of sperm. VC, HSV capsids; M, mitochondria; A, acrosome; CH, chromatin; and C, centriole. The hexagonal structure of some capsids is visible. Phase-contrast microscopy (c) and IF (d) of infected sperm. HSV antigen (arrows) and DAPI stain for DNA (blue); (e) FISH with probes to DNA of HSV. Localization of HSV DNA in sperm heads (arrows).

(HSV), we proved this by immunofluorescence (IF) using the monoclonal antibodies to HSV1 and HSV2 (**Figure 8c, d**) and *in situ* hybridization (ISH) with biotinylated probes for HSV (**Figure 8e**). Infection was observed in both the total sperm fraction and the isolated fraction of motile spermatozoa. The persistence of the HSV genome in motile, morphologically normal sperms indicates that the virus may be transmitted vertically to the offspring via natural fertilization or various ARTs, including IVF or ICSI.

Herpetic infection of spermatozoa was significantly more common in infertile men and men whose spouses had a history of spontaneous miscarriage or ART failure as compared with fertile men. Specific antiherpetic treatment of men diagnosed with HSV infection of spermatozoa results in a substantial, almost fivefold increase in the rates of blastocyst formation after ICSI and clinical pregnancy after ART [100].

6. Bacterial infection of the ejaculate

Bacterial colonies were detected in ejaculate samples from patients with fertility disorders. In the colonies, heteromorphic microorganisms were held together in a diffusive substance, probably of a polysaccharide nature, or covered with membranes as bacterial biofilms. The

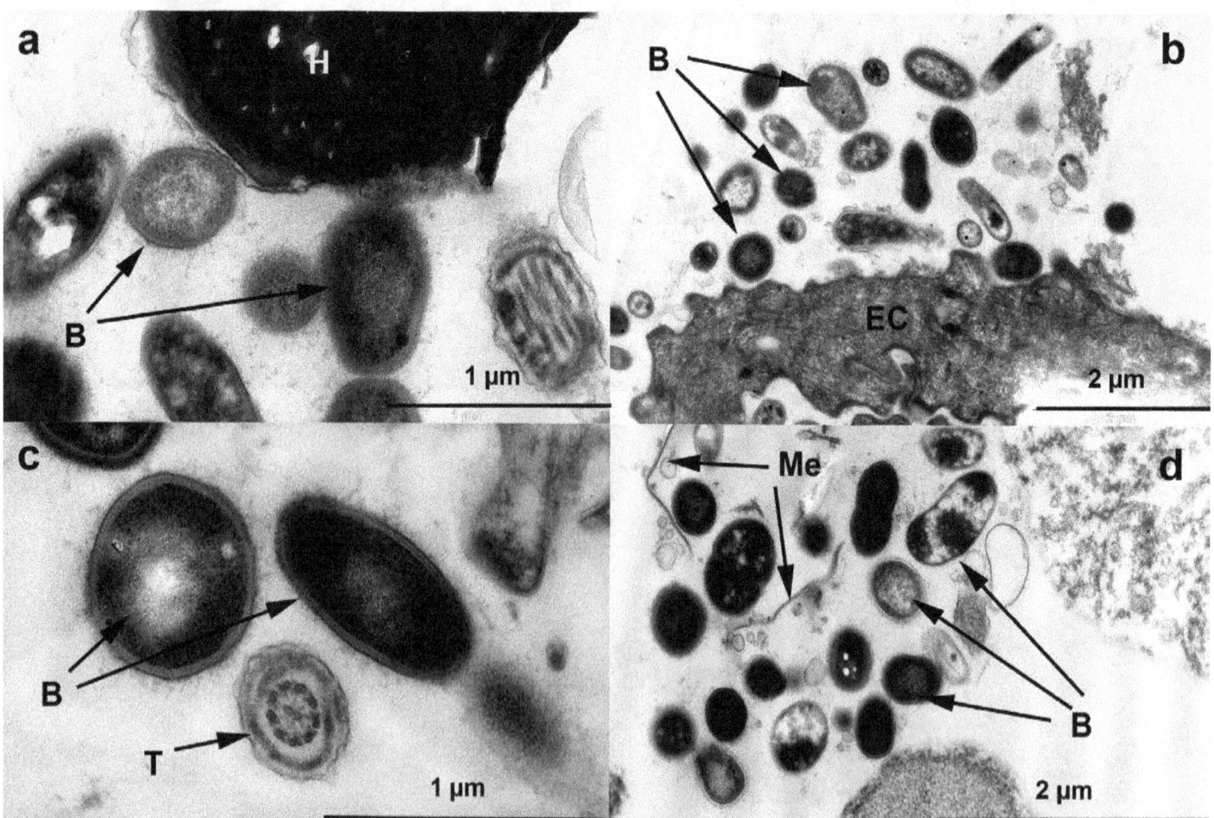

Figure 9. (a) Bacterial microcolony (B) attached to sperm head (H). (c) Bacterial microcolony (B) attached to sperm tail (T). (b, d) Bacterial microcolonies attached to the epithelial cells (EC). A diffuse substance (a–c) or membranes (Me) (d) are detected between bacterial cells.

majority of microcolonies were attached to squamous epithelial cells, whereas some were associated with sperm heads or tails (**Figure 9a–d**).

Moretti et al. [101] examined ejaculate samples from infertile patients and detected *Enteroccocus faecalis* and *Escherichia coli* most frequently and, at lower frequencies, *Streptococcus agalactiae, Ureaplasma urealyticum, Staphylococcus epidermidis, Streptococcus anginosus,* and *Morganella morganii.* With the exception of *U. urealyticum,* the microorganisms are classed with the non-specific saprophytic microflora and are not addressed in a conventional testing of infertility patients.

Bacteria may damage spermatozoa even in the absence of an overt inflammatory reaction. We observed higher contents of acrosome-reacted spermatozoa (i.e., those with a premature acrosomal reaction) in the ejaculate samples that contained bacterial microcolonies [55].

7. Conclusion

Despite the success of molecular biology, the morphological methods of research continue to play a considerable role in determining the reasons of male subfertility and infertility.

Indications for the studies using TEM are as follows:

1. Idiopathic infertility with normozoospermia or with small deviations in the semen parameters (revealing anomalies of spermatozoa that are not visible in the traditional spermiological study).
2. Examination of patients whose wives had a history of miscarriage due to abnormal embryo development, such as non-developing pregnancy or spontaneous abortion in the first trimester of natural pregnancy or ART failure.
3. Differential diagnosis of genetically determined and functional forms of asthenozoospermia and teratozoospermia.

Testing for ultrastructural sperm abnormalities makes it possible not only to identify the cause of infertility but also to choose proper clinical tactics, that is, to select treatments, to recommend ART using own spermatozoa, or to offer ART using donor sperm.

Acknowledgements

This work was supported by the Russian Science Foundation (project no. 14-50-00029) and the Russian Foundation for Basic Research (project no. 16-04-01447) and by Moscow State University Development Program PNR5.13.

Author details

Elizaveta E. Bragina[1]* and Elena N. Bocharova[2]

*Address all correspondence to: bragor@genebee.msu.ru

1 Department of Electron Microscopy, AN Belozersky Institute of Physico-Chemical Biology, MV Lomonosov Moscow State University, Moscow, Russia

2 Moscow Scientific and Practical Center of Dermatology, Moscow, Russia

References

[1] WHO Laboratory Manual for the Examination and Processing of Human Semen. 5th ed. WHO Press, World Health Organization, Geneva, Switzerland; 2010

[2] Evenson DP, Jost LK, Marshall D, Zinaman MJ, Clegg E, Purvis K, et al. Utility of the sperm chromatin structure assay as a diagnostic and prognostic tool in the human fertility clinic. Human Reproduction. 1999;**14**:1039-1049

[3] Braun RE. Packaging paternal chromosomes with protamine. Nature Genetics. 2001; **28**:10-12. DOI: 10.1038/88194

[4] Kornberg RD. Chromatin structure: A repeating unit of histones and DNA. Science. 1974;**184**:868-871

[5] Oliva R. Protamines and male infertility. Human Reproduction Update. 2006;**12**:417-435. DOI: 10.1093/humupd/dml009

[6] Castillo J, Amaral A, Oliva R. Sperm nuclear proteome and its epigenetic potential. Andrology. 2014;**2**:326-338. DOI: 10.1111/j.2047-2927.2013.00170.x

[7] Prigent Y, Muller S, Dadoune JP. Immunoelectron microscopical distribution of histones H2B and H3 and protamines during human spermiogenesis. Molecular Human Reproduction. 1996;**2**:929-935

[8] D'Occhio MJ, Hengstberger KJ, Johnston SD. Biology of sperm chromatin structure and relationship to male fertility and embryonic survival. Animal Reproduction Science. 2007;**101**:1-17. DOI: 10.1016/j.anireprosci.2007.01.005

[9] Champroux A, Torres-Carreira J, Gharagozloo P, Drevet JR, Kocer A. Mammalian sperm nuclear organization: Resiliencies and vulnerabilities. Basic and Clinical Andrology. 2016;**26**:17. DOI: 10.1186/s12610-016-0044-5

[10] Brykczynska U, Hisano M, Erkek S, Ramos L, Oakeley EJ, Roloff TC, et al. Repressive and active histone methylation mark distinct promoters in human and mouse spermatozoa. Nature Structural & Molecular Biology. 2010;**17**:679-687. DOI: 10.1038/nsmb.1821

[11] Hammoud S, Liu L, Carrell D. Protamine ratio and the level of histone retention in sperm selected from a density gradient preparation. Andrologia. 2009;**41**:88-94. DOI: 10.1111/j.1439-0272.2008.00890.x

[12] Arpanahi A, Brinkworth M, Iles D, Krawetz SA, Paradowska A, Platts AE, et al. Endonuclease-sensitive regions of human spermatozoal chromatin are highly enriched in promoter and CTCF binding sequences. Genome Research. 2009;**19**:1338-1349. DOI: 10.1101/gr.094953.109

[13] Bartoov B, Eltes F, Pansky M, Langzam J, Reichart M, Soffer Y. Improved diagnosis of male fertility potential via a combination of quantitative ultramorphology and routine semen analyses. Human Reproduction. 1994;**9**:2069-2075

[14] Arifulin EA, Bragina EE, Zamiatnina VA, Volkova EG, Sheval' EV, Golyshev SA, et al. Chromatin folding in human spermatozoa. I. Dynamics of chromatin remodelling in differentiating human spermatids. Ontogenez. 2012;**43**:143-153

[15] Hammoud SS, Nix DA, Hammoud AO, Gibson M, Cairns BR, Carrel DT. Genome-wide analysis identifies changes in histone retention and epigenetic modifications at developmental and imprinted gene loci in the sperm of infertile men. Human Reproduction. 2011;**26**:2558-2569. DOI: 10.1093/humrep/der192

[16] Ward WS. Function of sperm chromatin structural elements in fertilization and development. Molecular Human Reproduction. 2010;**16**:30-36. DOI: 10.1093/molehr/gap080

[17] Małgorzata K, Depa-Martynów M, Butowska W, Filipiak K, Pawelczyk L, Jedrzejczak P, et al. Human spermatozoa ultrastructure assessment in the infertility treatment by assisted reproduction technique. Archives of Andrology. 2007;**53**:297-302

[18] Bragina EE, Bocharova EN. Quantitative electron microscopic examination of spermatozoa in the diagnosis of male infertility. Andrology and Genital Surgery. 2014;**1**:41-50

[19] Bragina EE, Arifulin EA, Sukhomlinova MJ., Lazareva EM, Lelekova MA, Chogovadze AG et al. Lack of correlation between sperm DNA fragmentation and chromatin condensation in patients with primary infertility or embryonic development arrest. 2017; forthcoming for print

[20] Aoki VW, Emery BR, Liu L, Carrell DT. Protamine levels vary between individual sperm cells of infertile human males and correlate with viability and DNA integrity. Journal of Andrology. 2006;**27**:890-898. DOI: 10.2164/jandrol.106.000703

[21] Wyrobek AJ, Eskenazi B, Young S, Arnheim N, Tiemann-Boege I, Jabs EW, et al. Advancing age has differential effects on DNA damage, chromatin integrity, gene mutations, and aneuploidies in sperm. Proceedings of the National Academy of Sciences of the United States of America. 2006;**103**:9601-9606. DOI: 10.1073/pnas.0506468103

[22] Menezo Y, Hazout A, Panteix G, Robert F, Rollet J, Cohen-Bacrie P, et al. Antioxidants to reduce sperm DNA fragmentation: An unexpected adverse effect. Reproductive Biomedicine Online. 2007;**14**:418-421

[23] Zamboni L. Sperm structure and its relevance to infertility. An electron microscopic study. Archives of Pathology & Laboratory Medicine. 1992;**116**:325-344

[24] Chemes HE, Alvarez Sedo C. Tales of the tail and sperm headaches: Changing concepts on the prognostic significance of sperm pathologies affecting the head, neck and tail. Asian Journal of Andrology. 2012;**14**:14-23. DOI: 10.1038/aja.2011.168

[25] Fekonja N, Štrus J, Tušek Žnidarič M, Knez K, Vrtacnik Bokal E, Verdenik I, et al. Clinical and structural features of sperm head vacuoles in men included in the in vitro fertilization programme. BioMed Research International. 2014;**2014**:927841. DOI: 10.1155/2014/927841

[26] Boitrelle F, Pagnier M, Athiel Y, Swierkowski-Blanchard N, Torre A, Alter L, et al. A human morphologically normal spermatozoon may have noncondensed chromatin. Andrologia. 2015;**47**:879-886. DOI: 10.1111/and.12341

[27] Bartoov B, Berkovitz A, Eltes F. Selection of spermatozoa with normal nuclei to improve the pregnancy rate with intracytoplasmic sperm injection. The New England Journal of Medicine. 2001;**345**:1067-1068. DOI: 10.1056/NEJM200110043451416

[28] Vanderzwalmen P, Hiemer A, Rubner P, Bach M, Neyer A, Stecher A, et al. Blastocyst development after sperm selection at high magnification is associated with size and number of nuclear vacuoles. Reproductive Biomedicine Online. 2008;**17**:617-627

[29] Fortunato A, Boni R, Leo R, Nacchia G, Liguori F, Casale S, et al. Vacuoles in sperm head are not associated with head morphology, DNA damage and reproductive success. Reproductive Biomedicine Online. 2016;**32**:154-161. DOI: 10.1016/j.rbmo.2015.10.009

[30] Gatimel N, Parinaud J, Leandri RD. Intracytoplasmic morphologically selected sperm injection (IMSI) does not improve outcome in patients with two successive IVF-ICSI failures. Journal of Assisted Reproduction and Genetics. 2016;**33**:349-355. DOI: 10.1007/s10815-015-0645-5

[31] Haraguchi CM, Mabuchi T, Hirata S, Shoda T, Tokumoto T, Hoshi K, et al. Possible function of caudal nuclear pocket: degradation of nucleoproteins by ubiquitin-proteasome system in rat spermatids and human sperm. The Journal of Histochemistry and Cytochemistry. 2007;**55**:585-595. DOI: 10.1369/jhc.6A7136.2007

[32] Kacem O, Sifer C, Barraud-Lange V, Ducot B, De Ziegler D, Poirot C, et al. Sperm nuclear vacuoles, as assessed by motile sperm organellar morphological examination, are mostly of acrosomal origin. Reproductive Biomedicine Online. 2010;**20**:132-137

[33] Montjean D, Belloc S, Benkhalifa M, Dalleac A, Ménézo Y. Sperm vacuoles are linked to capacitation and acrosomal status. Human Reproduction. 2012;**27**:2927-2932. DOI: 10.1093/humrep/des266

[34] Kim KS, Cha MC, Gerton GL. Mouse sperm protein sp56 is a component of the acrosomal matrix. Biology of Reproduction. 2001;**64**:36-43

[35] Baba T, Niida Y, Michikawa Y, Kashiwabara S, Kodaira K, Takenaka M, et al. An acrosomal protein, sp32, in mammalian sperm is a binding protein specific for two proacrosins and an acrosin intermediate. The Journal of Biological Chemistry. 1994;**269**:10133-10140

[36] Okabe M. The acrosome reaction: A historical perspective. Advances in Anatomy, Embryology, and Cell Biology. 2016;**220**:1-14. DOI: 10.1007/978-3-319-30567-7_1

[37] Wolkowicz MJ, Shetty J, Westbrook A, Klotz K, Jayes F, Mandal A, et al. Equatorial segment protein defines a discrete acrosomal subcompartment persisting throughout acrosomal biogenesis. Biology of Reproduction. 2003;**69**:735-745. DOI: 10.1095/biolreprod.103.016675

[38] Fujihara Y, Murakami M, Inoue N, Satouh Y, Kaseda K, Ikawa M, et al. Sperm equatorial segment protein 1, SPESP1, is required for fully fertile sperm in mouse. Journal of Cell Science. 2010;**123**:1531-1536. DOI: 10.1242/jcs.067363

[39] Aydin H, Sultana A, Li S, Thavalingam A, Lee JE. Molecular architecture of the human sperm IZUMO1 and egg JUNO fertilization complex. Nature. 2016;**534**:562-565. DOI: 10.1038/nature18595

[40] Manandhar G, Toshimori K. Fate of postacrosomal perinuclear theca recognized by monoclonal antibody MN13 after sperm head microinjection and its role in oocyte activation in mice. Biology of Reproduction. 2003;**68**:655-663

[41] Amdani SN, Jones C, Coward K. Phospholipase C zeta (PLCζ): oocyte activation and clinical links to male factor infertility. Advances in Biological Regulation. 2013;**53**:292-308. DOI: 10.1016/j.jbior.2013.07.005

[42] Nomikos M, Sanders JR, Kashir J, Sanusi R, Buntwal L, Love D, et al. Functional disparity between human PAWP and PLCζ in the generation of Ca^{2+} oscillations for oocyte activation. Molecular Human Reproduction. 2015;**21**:702-710. DOI: 10.1093/molehr/gav034

[43] Sutovsky P, Manandhar G, Wu A, Oko R. Interactions of sperm perinuclear theca with the oocyte: Implications for oocyte activation, anti-polyspermy defense, and assisted reproduction. Microscopy Research and Technique. 2003;**61**:362-378. DOI: 10.1002/jemt.10350

[44] Florke-Gerloff S, Topfer-Petersen E, Muller-Esterl W, Mansouri A, Schatz R, Schirren C, et al. Biochemical and genetic investigation of round-headed spermatozoa in infertile men including two brothers and their father. Andrologia. 1984;**16**:187-202

[45] Talebi AR, Ghasemzadeh J, Khalili MA, Halvaei I, Fesahat F. Sperm chromatin quality and DNA integrity in partial versus total globozoospermia. Andrologia. 2017. DOI: 10.1111/and.12823

[46] Kullander S, Rausing A. On round-headed human spermatozoa. International Journal of Fertility. 1975;**20**:33-40

[47] Dam AH, Koscinski I, Kremer JA, Moutou C, Jaeger AS, Oudakker AR, Tournaye H, Charlet N, Lagier-Tourenne C, van Bokhoven H, et al . Homozygous mutation in

SPATA16 is associated with male infertility in human globozoospermia. American Journal of Human Genetics 2007;**81**:813-820. DOI: 10.1086/521314

[48] Liu G, Shi QW, Lu GX. A newly discovered mutation in PICK1 in a human with globozoospermia. Asian Journal of Andrology. 2010;**12**:556-560. DOI: 10.1038/aja.2010.47

[49] Xiao N, Kam C, Shen C, Jin W, Wang J, Lee KM, et al. PICK1 deficiency causes male infertility in mice by disrupting acrosome formation. The Journal of Clinical Investigation. 2009;**119**:802-812. DOI: 10.1172/JCI36230

[50] Pierre V, Martinez G, Coutton C, Delaroche J, Yassine S, Novella C, et al. Absence of Dpy19l2, a new inner nuclear membrane protein, causes globozoospermia in mice by preventing the anchoring of the acrosome to the nucleus. Development. 2012;**139**:2955-2965. DOI: 10.1242/dev.077982

[51] Jockusch H, Holland A, Staunton L, Schmitt-John T, Heimann P, Dowling P, Ohlendieck K. Pathoproteomics of testicular tissue deficient in the GARP component VPS54: The wobbler mouse model of globozoospermia. Proteomics. 2014;**14**:839-852. DOI: 10.1002/pmic.201300189

[52] Han F, Liu C, Zhang L, Chen M, Zhou Y, Qin Y, et al. Globozoospermia and lack of acrosome formation in GM130-deficient mice. Cell Death and Disease. 2017 May;**8**(1):e2532. DOI: 10.1038/cddis.2016.414

[53] Escoffier J, Yassine S, Lee HC, Martinez G, Delaroche J, Coutton C, et al. Subcellular localization of phospholipase Cζ in human sperm and its absence in DPY19L2-deficient sperm are consistent with its role in oocyte activation. Molecular Human Reproduction. 2015;**21**:157-168. DOI: 10.1093/molehr/gau098

[54] Karaca N, Akpak YK, Oral S, Durmus T, Yilmaz RA. successful healthy childbirth in a case of total globozoospermia with oocyte activation by calcium ionophore. Journal of Reproduction & Infertility. 2015;**16**:116-120

[55] Bragina EE, Aniskova BY, Gigalenko AR, Bocharova EN. Semen infection. In: Proceedings of the XXI International Conference of the Russian Association of Human Reproduction. The text of this abstract is Russian. We can pun square brackets [Semen infection]; Sep 8-10, 2011; St. Petersburg. 2011. p. 116

[56] Dam AH, Ramos L, Dijkman H, Woestenenk R, Robben H, van den Hoven L, et al. Morphology of partial globozoospermia. Journal of Andrology 2011;**32**:199-206. DOI: 10.2164/jandrol.109.009530

[57] Nomikos M, Stamatiadis P, Sanders JR, Beck K, Calver BL, Buntwal L, et al. Male infertility-linked point mutation reveals a vital binding role for the C2 domain of sperm PLCζ. The Biochemical Journal. 2017;**474**:1003-1016. DOI: 10.1042/BCJ20161057

[58] Chemes HE, Rawe VY. Sperm pathology: A step beyond descriptive morphology. Origin, characterization and fertility potential of abnormal sperm phenotypes in infertile men. Human Reproduction Update. 2003;**9**:405-428

[59] Manandhar G, Schatten H, Sutovsky P. Centrosome reduction during gametogenesis and its significance. Biology of Reproduction. 2005;**72**:2-13. DOI: 10.1095/biolreprod.104.031245

[60] Schatten H, Sun Q-Y. The role of centrosomes in mammalian fertilization and its significance for ICSI. Molecular Human Reprod. 2009;**15**:531-538. DOI: 10.1093/molehr/gap049

[61] Sathananthan AH, Kola I, Osborne J, Trounson A, Ng SC, Bongso A, Ratnam SS. Centrioles in the beginning of human development. Proceedings of the National Academy of Sciences of the United States of America. 1991;**88**:4806-4810

[62] Nakamura S, Terada Y, Horiuchi T, Emuta C, Murakami T, Yaegashi N, et al. Human sperm aster formation and pronuclear decondensation in bovine eggs following intracytoplasmic sperm injection using a Piezo-driven pipette: A novel assay for human sperm centrosomal function. Biology of Reproduction. 2001;**65**:1359-1363

[63] Chemes HE, Puigdomenech ET, Carizza C, Olmedo SB, Zanchetti F, Hermes R. Acephalic spermatozoa and abnormal development of the head-neck attachment: A human syndrome of genetic origin. Human Reproduction. 1999;**14**:1811-1818

[64] Porcu G, Mercier G, Boyer P, Achard V, Banet J, Vasserot M, et al. Pregnancies after ICSI using sperm with abnormal head-tail junction from two brothers: Case report. Human Reproduction. 2003;**18**:62-67

[65] Gambera L, Falcone P, Mencaglia L, Collodel G, Serafini F, de Leo V, et al. Intracytoplasmic sperm injection and pregnancy with decapitated sperm. Fertility and Sterility 2010;**93**:1347.e7-1347.e12. DOI: 10.1016/j.fertnstert.2008.12.087

[66] Baccetti B, Capitani S, Collodel G, Di Cairano G, Gambera L, Moretti E, Piomboni P. Genetic sperm defects and consanguinity. Human Reproduction. 2001;**16**:1365-1371

[67] Kamal A, Mansour R, Fahmy I, Serour G, Rhodes C, Aboulghar M. Easily decapitated spermatozoa defect: A possible cause of unexplained infertility. Human Reproduction. 1999;**14**:2791-2795

[68] Holstein AF, Schill WB, Breucker H. Dissociated centriole development as a cause of spermatid malformation in man. Journal of Reproduction and Fertility. 1986;**78**:719-725

[69] Baccetti B, Burrini AG, Collodel G, Magnano AR, Piomboni P, Renieri T, et al. Morphogenesis of the decapitated and decaudated sperm defect in two brothers. Gamete Research. 1989;**23**(2):181-188

[70] Zhu F, Wang F, Yang X, Zhang J, Wu H, Zhang Z, et al. Biallelic SUN5 mutations cause autosomal-recessive acephalic spermatozoa syndrome. American Journal of Human Genetics. 2016;**99**:942-949. DOI: 10.1016/j.ajhg.2016.08.004

[71] Schmidt H, Gleave E, Carter A. Insights into dynein motor domain function from a 3.3-Å crystal structure. Nature Structural & Molecular Biology. 2012;**19**:492-497. DOI: 10.1038/nsmb.2272

[72] Inaba K. Sperm flagella: Comparative and phylogenetic perspectives of protein components. Molecular Human Reproduction. 2011;**17**:524-538. DOI: 10.1093/molehr/gar034

[73] Pereira R, Sá R, Barros A, Sousa M. Major regulatory mechanisms involved in sperm motility. Asian Journal of Andrology 2017;**19**:5-14. doi: 10.4103/1008-682X.167716

[74] Fawcett DW. The mammalian spermatozoon. Developmental Biology. 1975;**44**:394-436

[75] Kerr JB. Ultrastructure of the seminiferous epithelium and intertubular tissue of the human testis. Journal of Electron Microscopy Technique. 1991;**19**:215-240. DOI: 10.1002/jemt.1060190208

[76] Olson GE, Winfrey VP. Structural organization of surface domains of sperm mitochondria. Molecular Reproduction and Development. 1992;**33**:89-98. DOI: 10.1002/mrd.1080330113

[77] Ursini F, Heim S, Kiess M, Maiorino M, Roveri A, Wissing J, et al. Dual function of the selenoprotein PHGPx during sperm maturation. Science. 1999;**285**:1393-1396

[78] Bakeeva LE, YS T. The mitochondrial reticulum: The structure and some functional properties. [Itogi nauki i tehniki]. Actual Problems of Biology. 1989;**9**:104-114

[79] Huang X, Sun L, Ji S, Zhao T, Zhang W, Xu J, et al. Kissing and nanotunneling mediate intermitochondrial communication in the heart. Proceedings of the National Academy of Sciences of the United States of America. 2013;**110**:2846-2851. DOI: 10.1073/pnas.1300741110

[80] StJohn JC, Jokhi RP, Barratt CL. The impact of mitochondrial genetics on male infertility. International Journal of Andrology. 2005;**28**:65-73. DOI: 10.1111/j.1365-2605.2005.00515.x

[81] Miki K, Qu W, Goulding EH, Willis WD, Bunch DO, Strader LF, et al. Glyceraldehyde 3-phosphate dehydrogenase-S, a sperm-specific glycolytic enzyme, is required for sperm motility and male fertility. Proceedings of the National Academy of Sciences of the United States of America. 2004;**101**:16501-16506. DOI: 10.1073/pnas.0407708101

[82] Kwitny S, Klaus AV, Hunnicutt GR. The annulus of the mouse sperm tail is required to establish a membrane diffusion barrier that is engaged during the late steps of spermiogenesis. Biology of Reproduction. 2010;**82**:669-678. DOI: 10.1095/biolreprod.109.079566

[83] Eddy EM, Toshimori K, O'Brien DA. Fibrous sheath of mammalian spermatozoa. Microscopy Research and Technique. 2003;**61**:103-115. DOI: 10.1002/jemt.10320

[84] Kim YH, Haidl G, Schaefer M, Egner U, Mandal A, Herr JC. Compartmentalization of a unique ADP/ATP carrier protein SFEC (Sperm Flagellar Energy Carrier, AAC4) with glycolytic enzymes in the fibrous sheath of the human sperm flagellar principal piece. Developmental Biology. 2007;**302**:463-476. DOI: 10.1016/j.ydbio.2006.10.004

[85] El_Shoura SM, Abdel_Aziz M, Ali ME, El_Said MM, Ali KZM, Kemeir MA, et al. Deleterious effects of khat addiction on semen parameters and sperm ultrastructure. Human Reproduction. 1995;**10**:2295-2300

[86] Joo KJ, Kwon YW, Myung SC, Kim TH. The effects of smoking and alcohol intake on sperm quality: Light and transmission electron microscopy finding. The Journal of International Medical Research. 2012;**40**:2327-2335. DOI: 10.1177/030006051204000631

[87] Chemes HE, Olmedo SB, Carrere C, Oses R, Carizza C, Leisner M, et al. Ultrastructural pathology of the sperm flagellum: association between flagellar pathology and fertility prognosis in severely asthenozoospermic men. Human Reproduction. 1998;**13**:2521-2526

[88] Moretti E, Collodel G. Three cases of genetic defects affecting sperm tail: A FISH study. Journal of Submicroscopic Cytology and Pathology. 2006;**38**:137-141

[89] Miki K, Willis WD, Brown PR, Goulding EH, Fulcher KD, Eddy EM. Targeted disruption of the Akap4 gene causes defects in sperm flagellum and motility. Developmental Biology. 2002;**248**:331-342

[90] Baccetti B, Collodel G, Estenoz M, Manca D, Moretti E, Piomboni P. Gene deletions in an infertile man with sperm fibrous sheath dysplasia. Human Reproduction. 2005;**20**:2790-2794. DOI: 10.1093/humrep/dei126

[91] Elkina YL, Kuravsky ML, Bragina EE, Kurilo LF, Khayat SS, Sukhomlinova MY, et al. Detection of a mutation in the intron of sperm-specific glyceraldehyde-3-phosphate dehydrogenase gene in patients with fibrous sheath dysplasia of the sperm flagellum. Andrologi. 2017;**49**:1-8. DOI: 10.1111/and.12606

[92] Pereira R, Oliveira J, Ferraz L, Barros A, Santos R, Sousa M. Mutation analysis in patients with total sperm immotility. Journal of Assisted Reproduction and Genetics. 2015 Jun;**32**(6):893-902. DOI: 10.1007/s10815-015-0474-6

[93] Olmedo SB, Rawe VY, Nodar FN, Galaverna GD, Acosta AA, Chemes HE. Pregnancies established through intracytoplasmic sperm injection (ICSI) using spermatozoa with dysplasia of fibrous sheath. Asian Journal of Andrology. 2000;**2**:125-130

[94] Basu B, Brueckner M. Cilia multifunctional organelles at the center of vertebrate left-right asymmetry. Current Topics in Developmental Biology. 2008;**85**:151-174. DOI: 10.1016/S0070-2153(08)00806-5

[95] Kuehni CE, Frischer T, Strippoli MP, Maurer E, Bush A, Nielsen KG, et al. Factors influencing age at diagnosis of primary ciliary dyskinesia in European children. The European Respiratory Journal. 2010;**36**:1248-1258. DOI: 10.1183/09031936.00001010

[96] Bragina EE, Arifulin EF, Senchenkov EP. Genetically determined and functional human sperm motility decrease. Russian Journal of Developmental Biology. 2016;**47**:239-253

[97] Zariwala MA, Leigh MW, Ceppa F, Kennedy MP, Noone PG, Carson JL, et al. Mutations of DNAI1 in primary ciliary dyskinesia: Evidence of founder effect in a common mutation. American Journal of Respiratory and Critical Care Medicine. 2006;**174**:858-866. DOI: 10.1164/rccm.200603-370OC

[98] Hornef N, Olbrich H, Horvath J, Zariwala M, Fliegauf M, Loges NT, et al. DNAH5 mutations are a common cause of primary ciliary dyskinesia with outer dynein arm defects. American Journal of Respiratory and Critical Care Medicine. 2006;**174**:120-126. DOI: 10.1164/rccm.200601-084OC

[99] Bragina EE, Bocharova EN, Azova MA. Spermatozoon as a vehicle for viruses. International Journal of Cell Science and Molecular Biology. 2017;**2**(4):555593. DOI: 10.19080/IJCSMB.2017.02.555593

[100] Bragina EE, Vinogradov IV, Suhomlinova MJ, Kurilo LF, Gablija MJ. The improving ICSI outcome from patients with intragamete herpesvirus infection. Andrology and Genital Surgery. 2011;**1**:65-69

[101] Moretti E, Capitani S, Figura N, Pammolli A, Federico MG, Giannerini V, et al. The presence of bacteria species in semen and sperm quality. Journal of Assisted Reproduction and Genetics. 2009;**26**:47-56. DOI: 10.1007/s10815-008-9283-5

10

The Role of Human Semen as an Early and Reliable Tool of Environmental Impact Assessment on Human Health

Luigi Montano, Paolo Bergamo,
Maria Grazia Andreassi and Stefano Lorenzetti

Abstract

Several studies have shown a dramatic reduction of semen quality in many industrialized countries and infertility is becoming a public health top priority, whose incidence is associated to late-onset adult diseases, especially cancer, shorter life expectancy and trans-generational effects. The male reproductive system is particularly sensitive to a broad variety of reproductive and developmental toxicants, including many environmental pollutants and recent studies suggest that human semen is an early and sensitive environmental and health marker. A set of semen biomarkers is described for reproductive health effects in relation to environmental exposure, where human semen seems to be an early and sensitive source of biomarkers than blood to monitor high environmental pressure on human health. Environmental health should consider reproductive health and development, from intrauterine life to childhood and puberty: these are both vulnerable targets and high-value protection goals, inasmuch as they represent the future of our societies. Hence, biomarkers of reproductive health should be exploited as early signals of environmental pressure and increased risk of adverse chronic health effects so that the use of "*human seminal model*" might be the main objective to be considered in the agenda of public prevention policies for early detection and innovative programs of health surveillance in environmental risk areas.

Keywords: semen quality, pollution, DNA sperm damage, environmental marker, health marker, endocrine disruptors, sperm telomere, redox status, epigenetic, aneuploidies, reproductive health, environmental health

1. Introduction

Since the early 1950s, in several demographic surveys a steady decline of birth rates in all European countries has been observed [1]. In particular semen quality was highly decreased in many industrialized countries [2–4] and in many European, Japanese and American young people poor semen quality was associated with subfertility or even infertility [5, 6]. The risk is that semen quality of a significant proportion of young men in developed countries will impair the fecundity potential causing on a short-term basis just a longer waiting time to pregnancy without to considerably family sizes of modern couples [7, 8], but on a middle-, long-term basis, strongly contributing (along with socio-economic factors) to the already observed European decrease in the birth rate. While there was a considerable variability in trends in sperm counts over the past 20 years, several recent studies have reported that 20–30% of young men today have sperm concentration below 40×10^6/ml, which is associated with reduced fecundity [9–11]. Among life-style changes that contribute to a reduced birth rate, affecting semen parameters and/or semen quality, there are: increased age at conception of both parents (although as a consequence of socio-economic factors), the increase in obesity, physical inactivity and the exposure to environmental and dietary environmental and chemical contaminants, including drugs. Exposure to man-made chemicals, in particular in the workplace, is recognized as major risk factors for male infertility in both epidemiological and experimental studies [12–16]. Individuals exposed for professional reasons to environmental contaminants show a reduction of concentration, motility, morphology and/or sperm DNA damage. In addition, toxicological studies in animal models are reporting DNA damages or epigenetic alterations within the germline: exposure to environmental xenobiotics during the fetal development and in early post-natal life, caused congenital malformations or reproductive tissue alterations or reduced fertility or signs of reproductive syndromes, such as the testicular dysgenesis syndrome, in particular when multiple *in utero* exposure to chemicals are tested. Furthermore, gene expression of genes mediating hormone (e.g. sex steroid hormones) actions is affected by epigenetic alterations even after some generation from the exposure to chemicals showing that the adverse effects can be eventually recorded only in next generations. A milestone in understanding the pathogenesis of testicular tumor has been the discovery of the fact that its onset in adults results from cancer cells *in situ*, which are transformed germ cells of the gonocyte type, which have failed to differentiate into spermatogonia during the fetal period [17, 18]. More strikingly, especially in industrialized countries, the reduction of semen quality and/or semen count present differences in areas within the same country or even in the same region supporting the idea that environmental factors, present in some areas but not in others, may be responsible for the decline in semen quality and sperm count [19–27]. Furthermore, different studies have reported that in high environmental pressure areas there is both an increase of infertility, urogenital malformation and chronic disease (cancer, diabetes, etc.) [28–32]. These epidemiological data are important to understand the shared biological mechanisms mediated by contaminants. In fact, infertility is becoming a public health top priority because, in addition to psychological distress and high economic costs, there are more and more evidences of diseases associated with poor semen quality [33] including cross-generational effects [34, 35], shorter life expectancy [36], testicular cancer [37–41] and overall other types of cancer [42, 43]. However, the first systematic study regarding environmental pollution and human reproduction has been conducted in the Czech Republic within the research program "Teplice" [44]. In particular, with regard to the impact on the semen quality, it has been proved a positive correlation between the increased concentration of polycyclic aromatic hydrocarbons (PAHs) in atmospheric pollution as well as of airborne particulate matter (PM), with an aerodynamic diameter smaller than 10 μm (PM10), mainly in winter, and an increase in fragmentation of sperm chromatin, DNA-PAHs adducts, abnormal sperm shapes and in the rate of sperm aneuploidies [45]. Other human biomonitoring studies have documented widespread human exposure to chemicals [46, 47] and actually the European Commission has financed the Human Biomonitoring Initiative (HBM) (https://ec.europa.eu/research/conferences/2016/hbm4eu/index.cfm) to promote the generation of current HBM data throughout Europe as well as the development of new biomarkers of exposure for chemicals. However, knowing the environmental pollutant concentrations in the environment and their seasonal variability, is essential to consider each source of exposure related to individual lifestyle (including living places, dietary habits, use of cosmetics, plastic bottles, personal computers, wireless internet and much more), and the plausibility of the cause-to-effect relationship among the real life mixture of dietary and environmental contaminants, the tissue/biological fluid levels at which chemicals (or their metabolites) are present in the human body and human disorders and/or pathologies. From this stage onwards, how much chemical values are measurable in fluids or tissues (biomarkers of exposure) and to which extent they are associated with a biological effect (biomarkers of effect) depending on specific, individual response (markers of genetic susceptibility, polymorphisms, etc.) will define a complete risk assessment founded on a reliable Adverse Outcome Pathway (AOP) in which each sequential step is linked to the other. Furthermore, in order to adopt an effective primary prevention strategy, it will be important to identify not only the source and extent of the exposure but also the tissue or organ most sensitive to such exposure and, simultaneously, the biological tool more sensitive and reliable to predict future alterations and to detect the earliest clinical risk indices. Dietary and environmental chemicals exposure may influence human endocrine and metabolic homeostasis and, especially, the reproductive system. Among the reproductive system targets, the male reproductive system could be considered a general health check detector since it is particularly and uniquely sensitive to a broad variety of reproductive and developmental toxicants, including many environmental pollutants, throughout the lifespan. Indeed, spermatogenesis and secretory fluids of the differentiated accessory glands of the male reproductive system are continuously renovated starting from newly differentiating staminal cells, thus making them a feasible target to study both short- and long-term effects of chemical exposure. The male germline accumulates mutations faster than the female one [48, 49]. For instance, it is thought that sperm cells are more susceptible than eggs to the effects of oxidative damage [50] and recent studies have demonstrated the association between semen quality and state of health, correlating the semen quality with either chronic degenerative diseases, comorbidities and even mortality [51–53]. Thus, spermatogenesis is a cycle extremely complex and vulnerable to endogenous and exogenous stress and that human semen can become an important "environmental and health marker". In this way, the qualitative assessment of human semen might be envisaged as a potential focus for future development of public prevention policies. Therefore, the use of reproductive biomarkers as environmental health risks was proposed as a promising/ innovative strategy for the early detection and prevention of environmental health [54].

2. Main

With the release of the Silent Spring in 1962 [55] the issues related to chemical pollution have begun to become a topic of political and scientific debate by laying the basis of environmental chemistry and ecotoxicology as we know them. Environmental toxicology concerns the way in which toxic substances reach the organism and affect human health. At present many chemicals [56] have been detected in tissues and biological fluids of human body (**Figures 1** and **2**).

2.1. Organic pollutants and reproduction

Persistent organic pollutants (POPs) are very durable toxic chemicals which include polychlorinated dibenzodioxins polychlorinated dibenzofurans polychlorinated biphenyls (PCBs), chlorinated organic pesticides, PAHs, hexachlorobenzene and many other substances that we find in daily life such as polybrominated diphenyl ethers (PBDEs), perfluorooctane sulfonate, Perfluorottanoic acid ammonium salt, brominated flame retardants, food additives such as bisphenols and phthalates (plasticizers) and parabens (preservatives), according to recent experimental acquisitions, are known as endocrine disruptors (Endocrine Disrupting Chemicals). They are able to interfere with the production, release, transport, metabolism, binding, action or elimination of natural hormones of the body responsible for maintaining the homeostasis and the setting of endocrine reproductive processes [57–59]. They can also alter the cellular oxido-reductive homeostasis (redox status), resulting in a condition known as biochemical oxidative stress [60–62] a genotoxic action featuring a genetic and epigenetic damage transmissible through the germ line to the offspring (transgenerational effect). This last aspect is definitely very disturbing to future generations' public health and justifies the growing interest of the scientific community in the study of the reproductive system in recent years [63–65]. These substances, very stable and soluble in fats, are found in semen that has a considerable lipid amount [66, 67].

2.2. Inorganic pollutants and reproduction

Metals toxicity depends on several factors, including their ability to bonds to reactive groups of enzymes and proteins (e.g. thiol groups) thus altering their structure and/or function. They may also interfere with the bioaccumulation of essential metals (e.g. iron, calcium and zinc) thus negatively affect those physiological mechanisms depending upon their bioavailability. Heavy metals accumulation in living organisms, in particular lead, cadmium, arsenic, mercury, depend upon the exposure to contaminated environment and may trigger acute and chronic degenerative diseases: In particular, genotoxic elements (Arsenic, Cadmium and Nickel) may damage the DNA structure either directly (through the production of oxygen radicals) or indirectly (via the alteration of enzymes responsible for DNA repair) and they may interfere in the activities of regulators of proliferation, apoptosis, differentiation and cell transformation [68–71]. Metals also include "trace metals," such as zinc, copper, iron, manganese, present in humans under physiological conditions, which are toxic at high concentrations. The risk assessment of the exposure to metals is achieved through human biomonitoring studies and their quantification in human biological fluids such as blood, serum and urine,

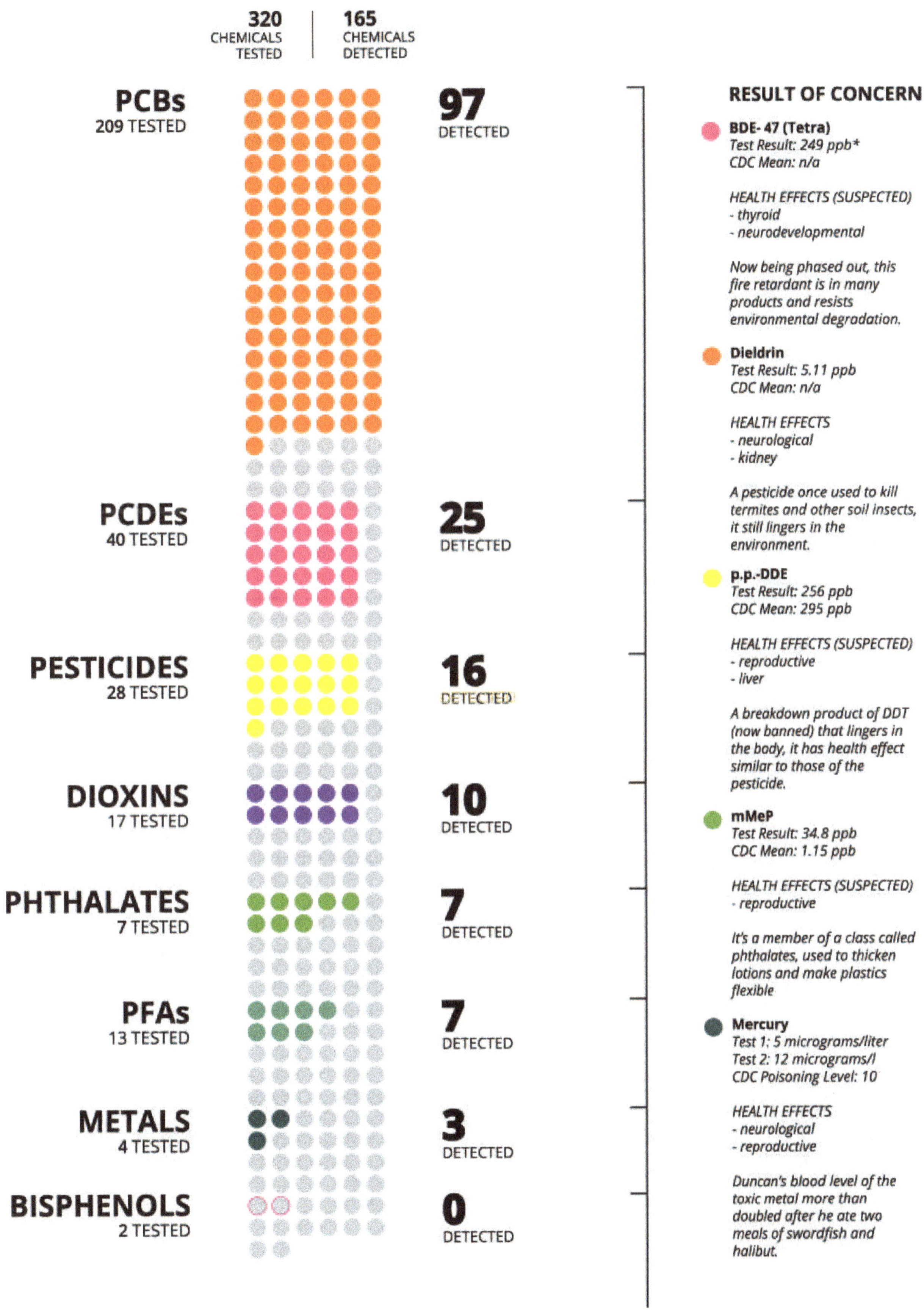

Figure 1. List of some of the chemicals tested and detected.

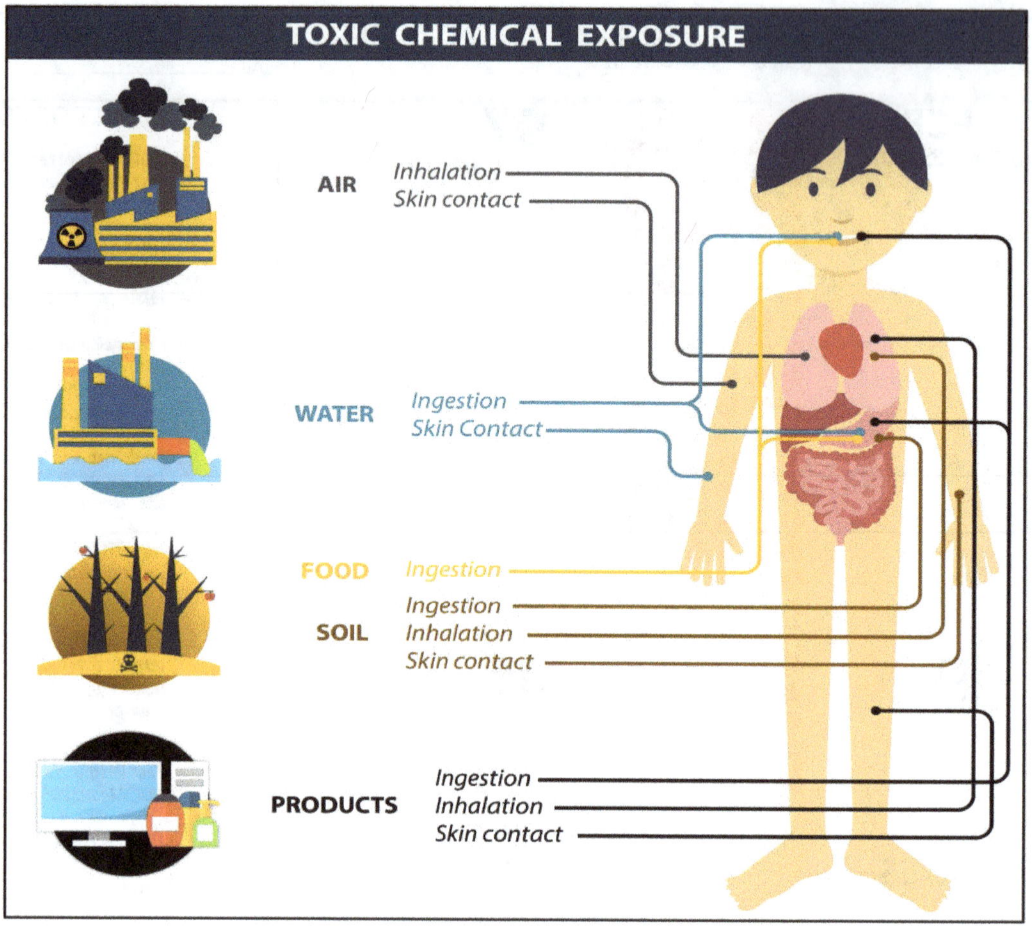

Figure 2. The entry routes of the contaminants into the body.

being an indispensable tool to evaluate the possible influence of environmental determinants on human health. The level of metals in human fluids reflects the amount entering the body *via* all exposure routes (ingestion, inhalation and dermal absorption). Moving into the bloodstream, they are compartmentalized in organs or tissues, where they carry out their harmful effects according to the concentration and to their inherent toxicity. Even though several papers have covered the report of qualitative parameters of the seminal fluid with the occupational exposure to metals [72, 73], environmental impact studies in urban areas are still unsatisfactory [74]. An Italian study [68] has compared, through statistical methods, the sperm counts with the geochemistry distribution of heavy metals in soils of the metropolitan area of Naples, observing a strong correlation in the case of lead, whereas a lesser correlation has been found in the case of mercury and zinc. In addition, data have been reported regarding the effects of changes in concentration of zinc, magnesium and calcium on semen quality parameters and infertility [75].

2.3. Mechanisms involved in male reproductive dysfunction

2.3.1. Oxidative stress

Oxidative stress plays an important role in the etiology of male infertility by impairing negatively the quality and the function of the sperm [76] although the relationship between the bioaccumulation of environmental pollutants and the alteration of the seminal redox status has not been elucidated yet, and neither the possible mechanism of action. The imbalance of antioxidant defenses and detoxification processes provides a logical explanation to the onset of diseases caused by oxidative stress in men [77] and increases the organism susceptibility to pollutants toxicity [78]. After all, the balance between oxidation and anti-oxidation is critically important in maintaining healthy any biological system.

The fact remains however, that pro-oxidant activity of PM [79] PAHs [60] on human health has been demonstrated in clinical data, whereas the harmful effects caused by toxic heavy metals or pesticides organophosphates [80] have been proved in animal studies. Reactive oxygen species (ROS), at low physiological levels, play an important role in sperm maturation and function [81]. On the contrary, excessive amounts of ROS produced by leukocytes and immature spermatozoa can damage mature sperm and DNA integrity [82–84]. The mechanism of DNA damage by ROS is mainly due to the high susceptibility of spermatozoa to ROS for their high content of polyunsaturated fatty acids, major components of cellular and intracellular membranes (**Figure 3**). An increase in oxidative stress has been found in 80% of infertile men clinically tested, and it seems that exposure to environmental toxicants contributes to this increment [60, 78–80]. In addition, a positive correlation between ROS and sperm DNA fragmentation has been reported in studies [85]. However, the Nuclear factor (erythroid-derived 2)-like 2 (Nrf2), plays a key role in the modulation of antioxidant response, which basically modulates both synthesis and the recycling of the main cellular antioxidant, that is the reduced glutathione. The reduced activity of glutathione reductase, has been associated with oxidative stress-related diseases [77], just like an increased susceptibility to adverse effects induced by pollutants [78] has also been associated with increased expression of p53 [86] (**Figure 4**).

Notably, detoxifying/antioxidant defenses can be modulated by diet. However, it is known that improper eating habits (*i.e.*, increased intake of carbohydrates, high protein and total fat) have been linked to poor sperm quality [87], although the protective effects of a proper diet towards pro-oxidants effects caused by bioaccumulation of environmental pollutants have not yet been demonstrated. In summary, although supplementation with antioxidants may improve pregnancy and birth rates for infertile couples [88] the efficacy of dietary supplements in improving the quality of male sperm is still controversial [89] and the link among bioaccumulation of environmental pollutants, diet and semen quality remains to be demonstrated.

2.3.2. Genetic alterations

Endocrine Disrupting Chemicals affect spermatogenesis both through alterations in the hypothalamic–pituitary axis, and direct damage to spermatozoa [90–92]. In recent decades, several studies have shown disorders of spermatogenesis due to genetic causes (15–30% of infertile males) [93, 94] and chromosomal aberrations, either numerical or structural, can profoundly affect fertility. It is estimated that the frequency of chromosomal aberrations in the general population is about 0.6% [95], and 2–14% in infertility male [96]. In particular, chromosomal aberrations increase with the increasing severity of infertility. Moreover, some genetic polymorphisms involved in the metabolism and detoxification activities as well as in DNA repair capacity influence individual susceptibility to environmental exposure leading to changes in

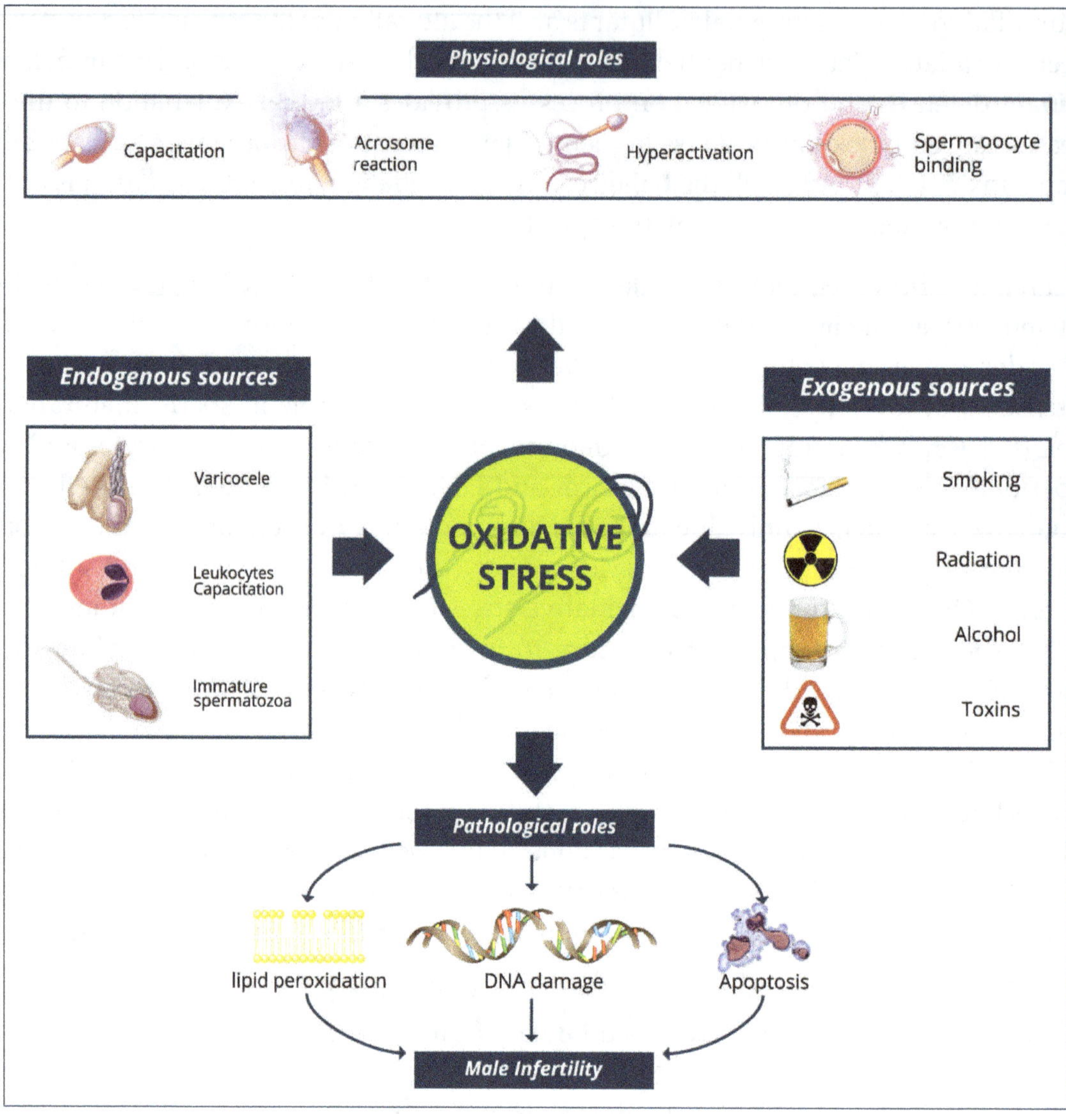

Figure 3. The positive and negative effects on spermatogenesis and steroidogenesis of controlled or uncontrolled oxidative stress.

sperm quality [60]. The main alteration responsible for male infertility is represented by DNA and chromatin alterations, highly sensitive to exogenous contaminants [97]. Some studies have suggested that environmental toxins affect sperm DNA's integrity and it has been observed that exposure to air pollutants such as PM, is capable of producing disomy of sexual chromosome in nemasperm DNA [98]. In fact, most chromosomal abnormalities are lethal and so they either manifest as a sperm's inability or as miscarriage [99].

In particular, aneuploidy defined as structural and numerical aberrations of chromosomes [100], is an informative effect biomarker, for male reproductive toxicants and a hallmark of cancer [101–104]. There are some substances known that induce sperm aneuploidy and can be carcinogenic [105, 106] and for this reason sperm aneuploidy is associated with both increased risk of cancer and reproductive toxicity. Fortunately, sperm aneuploidy assessment has become very easy and this opens up to a growing use of health risk assessment from chemical hazard [107] so that, it could be integrated with current aneuploidy and chromosome imbalance

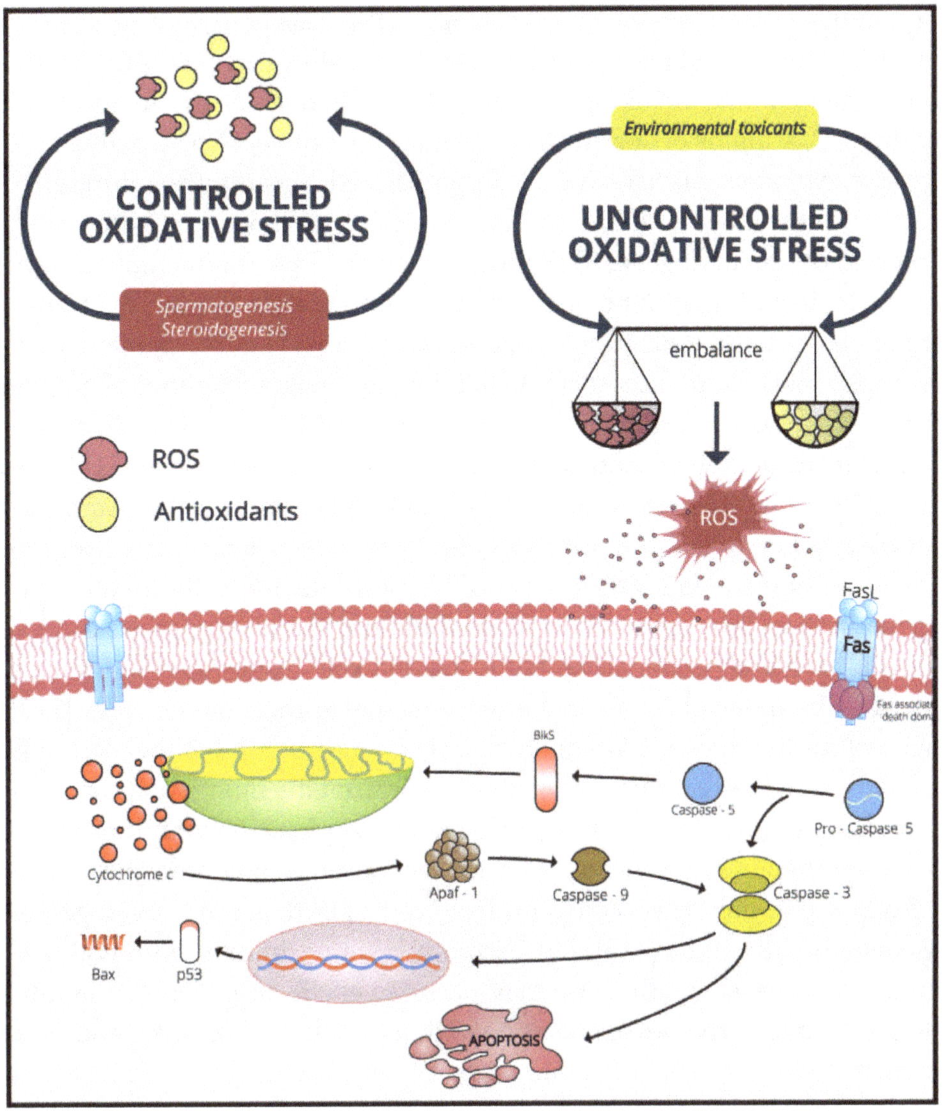

Figure 4. Exogenous and endogenous factors inducing oxidative stress: Pathological and physiological roles on sperm function.

assessments in place for somatic cells [108]. In conclusion, sperm aneuploidy evaluation is informative well beyond the standard sperm parameters (number, motility, morphology) useful for comprehensive evaluation of carcinogenicity and reproductive toxicity.

With regard to sperm DNA's integrity, it is a great indicator of male fertility, since men with normal sperm parameters may also have a high degree of DNA fragmentation, leading cause of undiagnosed /inexplicable infertility. In fact, the damage to sperm DNA contributes not only to infertility, but also on the frequency of miscarriages and birth defects in the offspring. The data supporting this are primarily derived from animal toxicology studies, which unequivocally demonstrate that the genetic integrity of the male germ line play an important role in determining the normal embryonic development [109].

The results of studies by toxicologists using several compounds in increasing doses prove adverse effects on the development of the embryo, on animal behavior, postnatal growth, longevity of progeny, as well as increased susceptibility to cancer. These toxicology animal-data support the hypothesis that toxic substances can act on the male germ line by interfering with the development of human pregnancies and the health of the unborn. To support this, there are associations between paternal smoking, oxidative DNA damage of sperm and the incidence of cancer in children. The origins of sperm DNA damage are not yet clearly defined, but in light of recent discoveries, six main mechanisms are hypothesized: (1) apoptosis during the process of spermatogenesis; (2) breakage of DNA strands created from the sperm chromatin remodeling during the process of spermatogenesis; (3) post-testicular DNA fragmentation induced mainly by oxygen radicals, including nitric oxide and hydroxyl radicals, during the transport of spermatozoa through the seminiferous tubules and epididymis; (4) DNA fragmentation induced by endogenous caspase and endonuclease; (5) DNA damage induced by radiotherapy and chemotherapy; (6) DNA damage induced by environmental toxins [110]. The damage in testicular sperm DNA is statistically lower than what is found in ejaculated sperm [111]. Sperm nuclear DNA fragmentation is the last phase of apoptosis, a highly controlled programmed cell death program that plays a key role in different biological processes such as embryonic development and maintenance of homeostasis. High cell proliferation rate and cell differentiation processes occur during maturation from stem cell to haploid mature sperm. Apoptosis is needed to avoid the excess of cell proliferation and it seems to have a role in germ cells differentiation. This process might also be induced by several environmental stimuli or damages [112]. In case of DNA damage within the male germ line, the adverse outcome(s) will depend either from the type of damage or from the genomic region affected or from the timing of the damage itself and, as an overall consequence, from the ability of the embryo repair system to properly counteract any damage earlier than the first mitotic division will occur. In any case, the embryo could not always effectively repair damages carried on from male germ as it occurs in genetic dominant diseases, such as achondroplasia [113]. Furthermore, healthy children born with assisted reproduction from DNA-damaged sperm [114] may possess genetic or epigenetic alterations generating a phenotypic change in the next generation(s) due to double recessive gene expression or in the birth of a male upon chromosome X mutations. Finally, it is also possible that DNA-damaged sperm can cause offspring defects not recognized at birth. The recent discovery that DNA damage in sperm of males due to aging is associated with the onset of epilepsy, schizophrenia, autism, and bipolar illness [115, 116].

Strikingly, an increased risk of sperm DNA fragmentation was associated to high levels of air pollution, in fact seems that the classical sperm parameters -motility, concentration, morphology- do not change related to high smog levels, while sperm DNA fragmentation appeared to be much more sensible [98]. In this direction, also in Campania Region (Southern Italy), preliminary data of EcoFoodFertility initiative [54], indicated an increased sperm DNA damage associated to environmental pressure, measured with two techniques. In fact, healthy, no-smoking, no-drinker, no professionally exposed to environmental stresses males (n = 175, mean age 30 $\pm$ 4) were enrolled in areas of High or Low environmental impact. According to their stable residence in "Land of Fires", a wide area between the towns of Naples and Caserta (High Environmental Impact Area—HIP; n = 70) or in Alto-Medio Sele in Salerno province (Low Environmental Impact Area – LIP; n = 105), data of the enrolled men were compared by their DNA Fragmentation Index (DFI). DFI was evaluated by using the sperm DNA fragmentation Kit (Halosperm®, Halotech DNA SL). Furthermore, the spermatic p53 levels were also assessed by using the DuoSet® ELISA (R&D) [117]. The results obtained so far support the effectiveness of the considered markers in the quantification of DNA damages as well as the relationship between the extent of the observed sperm DNA damage and the environmental characteristics of the area of residence (HIP versus LIP areas). In conclusion, these data showed sperm DNA damage measured as DFI by SCD and p53 overexpression to be an early and sensitive marker of environmental pollution [118].

In recent years, an increasing interest has been directed on other biomarkers of DNA integrity in male germinal cells: telomere. Telomeres are noncoding double-stranded DNA repeats (in humans, TTAGGG sequences extended 10–15 kbIn dividing cells, the synthesis of new telomeric DNA repeats requires the activity of telomerase, a protein complex composed of the TERT enzyme and of the telomere-associated proteins, able to recognize the 150–200 nt 3′-single stranded (G-strand) overhang. During aging in most adult somatic cells, a progressive telomere shortening occurs and, in turn, telomerase activity decrease or completely disappear. In contrast to such adult somatic cells, germ cells maintain high telomerase activity, long telomeres and high proliferative potential [119, 120]. In particular, the sperm telomere length (STL) seems to be of fundament importance for fertilization and early embryo development [121]. To date, the relationship between telomere function and aspects of semen quality is an area of great attention. Indeed, it has been reported that sperm TL is lower in oligozoospermic than in normozoospermic men [122]. Furthermore, spermatozoa from elderly males have significantly longer telomeres than those from younger males, but the biological implications of this paradoxical effect are unknown [123]. Additionally, telomere dysfunction is a relevant mechanism driving cancers in humans [124]. Indeed, critical telomere attrition results in chromosomal aberration which in the absence of normal cellular DNA repair and apoptosis can lead to genetic instability. On the other hand, long telomeres may permit cells to escape growth arrest and increase the chance of acquiring mutations, especially in the presence of an external exposure, i.e. smoking and sun exposure. In fact, longer telomeres have been associated with some types of cancers, especially melanoma and lung cancer [125]. Recently, a Mendelian randomization study reported that longer telomeres were associated with increased risk of several cancers but reduced risk of some non-neoplastic diseases [126].

Interestingly, accumulating evidence indicates that leukocyte telomeric DNA may be one important target of environmental [127–132]. Accordingly, a very recent study has shown a possible association between high environmental pressure in polluted area and the STL [133]. In particular, a preliminary study was carried out evaluate the influence of environmental exposure to the telomere length (TL) of leukocytes (LTL) and of STL. This pilot study was conducted on young healthy men living in HEI or in LEI area and the data obtained showed that STL was significantly greater in subjects while no significant difference was observed between LTL and HEI in the LEI group and no correlation between STL and sperm parameters was found [134]. These findings support the view that STL is a more sensible marker than LTL to environmental pollution and it is a further evidence that the genetic structure of spermatozoa is particularly sensitive to environmental insults.

2.3.3. Epigenetic alterations

In recent years, interest has grown on new acquisitions that regulate gene expression and epigenetic mechanisms. In fact, if the interaction between genes and environment in determining human phenotypes has been known for many years, the real innovation provided by epigenetic studies concerns specific gene expression changes without any change in their sequence. Therefore, as genetic variants make the organism vulnerable to certain environmental insults, epigenetic alterations induced by the environment may have the same effect and especially could be transmitted to the offspring. Thus, birth defects, greater susceptibility to diseases in adulthood, may be the result of a gene/environment interaction that occurred in one of the parents, not the subject itself. Studying the sperm epigenome represents a new frontier in the field of human reproduction, and numerous studies have shown the importance of epigenetic mechanisms as potential biomarkers in hazard identification and risk assessment attributable to environmental exposures. Epigenetic mechanisms responsible for these alterations are represented by DNA methylation, histone modifications and noncoding microRNAs [135]. The association between sperm DNA methylation and idiopathic male infertility is already documented with studies [136–139]. Other studies have shown that DNA hypermethylation of gene promoters (like *MTHFR, PAX8, NTF3, SFN* and others) plays a crucial role in determining male infertility. On the contrary, hypomethylation of other genes, including the check zone *IGF2/H19 1* (ICR1), is found in patients with lower sperm concentration and motility compared to controls with normal sperm kinetics [140–145]. Nuclear condensation in the spermatozoon represents the most delicate and sensitive stress related event, inducing genetic and epigenetic alterations. During this phase, in fact, about 85% of histones (rich in lysine) bound to DNA, are replaced with proteins of transition and arginine-rich proteins: the protamine [146, 147]. In contrast to histones, which form a ring-like association with DNA (nucleosomes), protamines are linked to DNA helix grooves, wrapping themselves tightly around the DNA strands (about 50 kb of DNA and protamines), to form tight loops highly organized. The spermatozoon's nuclear condensation is obtained by the intramolecular disulfide bonds between cysteine-rich protamines resulting in the reduction of about 10% of the size of the nucleus. The bromodomain testis-specific protein is the key factor mediating the chromatin compaction promoting nuclear remodeling ensuring the transition between a histone chromatin organization, which is somatic, and the protamine one typical of the mature sperm. The sperm genome is protected from physiological and environmental stresses by this peculiar nuclear compaction, but also from genetic mutations and chromosomal abnormalities that can interfere with the mechanisms of spermatogenesis [148]. These alterations may result in an abnormal chromatin structure, a feature incompatible with fertility. The resulting genomic material defects that are found in mature sperm may be packing defects (defective replacements of histones-protamines), defects in the maturation of the nucleus, DNA fragmentation defects (that is, single or double strand breaks), sperm DNA integrity defects or chromosomal aneuploidy and changes in gene expression (epigenetic modifications). In fact, an increasing amount of data now supports the hypothesis that in the mature spermatozoon of mammals the DNA is actually not homogeneously rich of protamine [149]. Defects in the action of protamine affect the transcription of genes. For example, in mice, the deregulation of the protamine action process results in premature chromatin condensation, interruption of the transcription, and failure of spermatogenesis [150]. The human sperm's nucleus preserves 10–15% of its original histone content, which is distributed heterogeneously in the genome [142]. An analysis of the entire genome of seven infertile patients has clearly demonstrated that five out of seven infertile men had a random process of protamine action in comparison with normal fertile men where the preservation of histone quota was programmatic [143]. Specific errors in the epigenetic control, damaging male fertility and embryonic development, can occur at each stage of spermatogenesis [144]. At the mitotic level, epigenetic alterations can affect the expression of specific genes involved in the early stages of spermatogenesis, decreasing the overall differentiation process. At the meiotic level, epigenetic alterations can trigger double strand breaks or chromosomal nondisjunction and, during the spermiogenesis, protamine replacement errors may induce, in turn, epigenetic alterations due to defects in the above described histone-protamine transition [144]. Taken together, these facts suggest that the different characteristics of male infertility, including alterations in sperm count or morphology, DNA fragmentation chromosomal, aneuploidy, alterations in the chromatin density, could all be related to epigenetic mechanisms that occur at different stages of spermatogenesis. Great attention is then lately directed to the role of microRNA (miRNA) and so to the posttranscriptional regulation. Increasing evidence has shown that miRNAs play a critical role in mitosis and meiosis as well as in spermatogenesis [151–153]. MiRNAs are expressed specifically during spermatogenesis and participate in the control of every phase of the male germ cell differentiation. Genetically altered rat models have shown the importance of miRNA's pathway for the development of a normal spermatogenesis and functional studies have been conducted to establish the roles of specific miRNAs [154]. Finally, clinical studies have shown that spermatozoa from patients with sperm alterations present an altered miRNA profile [155, 156]. Hence, a strong emphasis on the crucial role of miRNA in spermatogenesis: indeed, the miRNA profile expression can be also seen as a new reliable and non-invasive diagnostic biomarker for the study of male fertility. Recently, a pool of sperm samples obtained from fertile and infertile men was examined and shown that alterations in miRNA profiles both in azoospermia and asthenozoospermia conditions can be found [157]. In particular, the level of seven miRNAs was significantly lower in patients with azoospermia and higher in the asthenozoospermia, compared to fertile subjects considered as case–control, leading to the hypothesis that these seven miRNAs may have confirmatory molecular diagnostic value for male infertility. Furthermore, miR-I9B and let-7 bis expression pattern was analyzed in patients affected by idiopathic infertility, azoospermia or non-obstructive oligozoospermia: it was showed that both miRNAs were expressed at higher levels in infertile patients compared to fertile individuals [158]. Therefore, it was concluded that miR-I9B and let-7 bis may be considered good diagnostic molecular markers for non-obstructive azoospermia cases with primary infertility or oligozoospermia. Similarly, it was recently identified miR-155 serum level as a potential biomarker of male fertility [159]. Interestingly, the miR-155 serum has been associated with male subfertility regardless of the systemic inflammation grade or androgenic alteration. Ultimately, the damage assessment to the spermiogenesis caused by pollution, of genotoxic, genetic and epigenetic type, are a major concern not only for the susceptibility to chronic diseases in adulthood, but also and especially for the vulnerability to diseases of future generations (transgenerational effects). (**Figures 5** and **6**).

2.4. The semen as an early marker of environmental exposure (environmental sentinel)

Semen qualitative and quantitative changes observed by several epidemiological studies, by Carlsen and latest ones [2–5], show how these changes are induced by individual lifestyle and

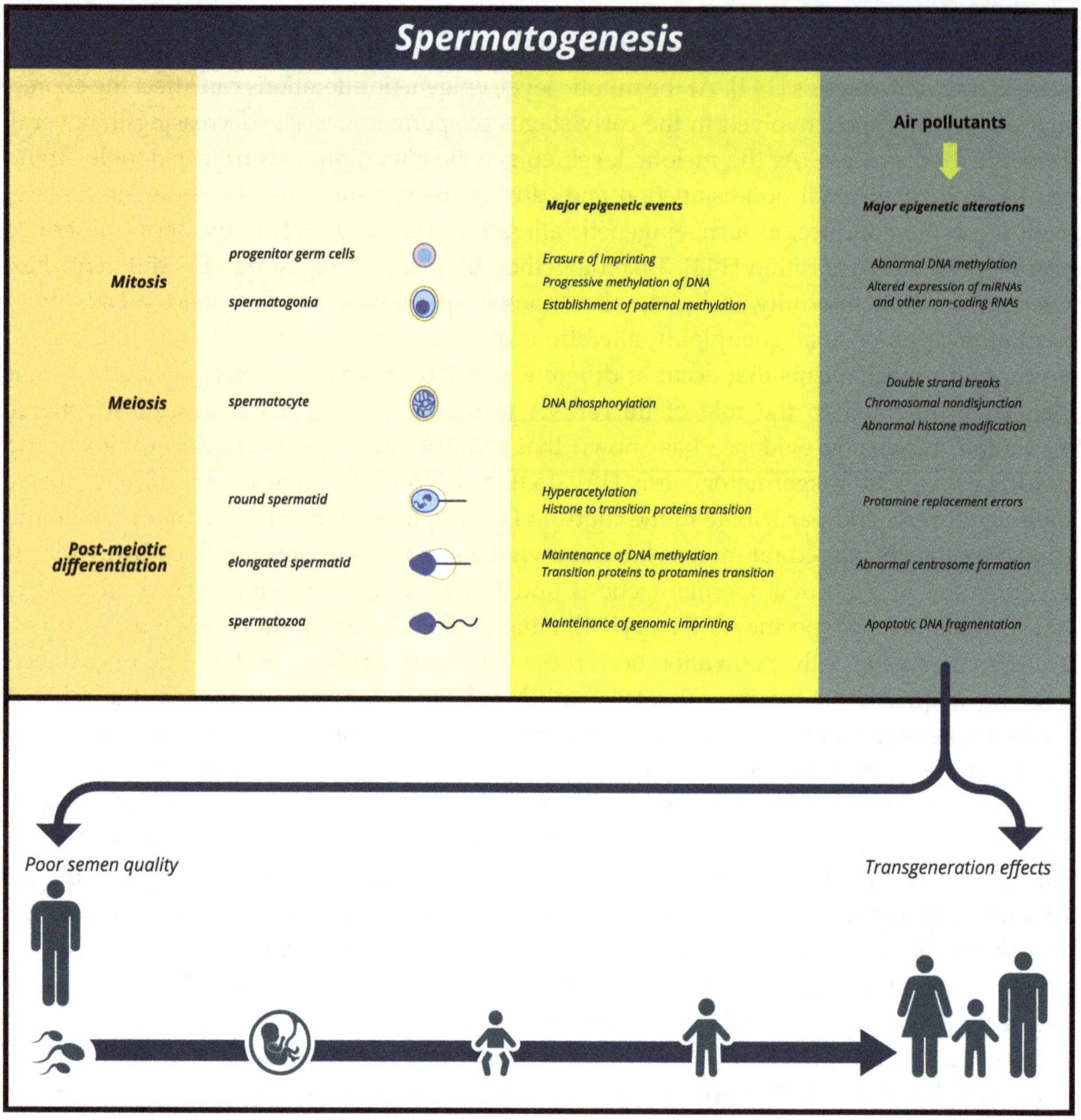

Figure 5. Epigenetic alterations by environmental factors affects sperm quality and when fertilization occurs, transgenerational epigenetic effects may compromise embryo development, favoring congenital diseases at birth and diseases in adulthood.

from the environment. Epidemiological studies on individuals exposed for professional reasons or living in contaminated areas and nearby settlements, demonstrate significant alterations of the semen: reduction of the motility, concentration, of sperm's morphology, sperm DNA damage, sperm aneuploidies, alteration of sperm epigenome that result in increased cases of infertility, recurrent miscarriage, congenital malformations. Toxicological studies conducted on mice, show how some of the major environmental organic and inorganic contaminants reduce seminal quality. Significant changes of semen quality are noticed in different environments [22–27]. Exposure to air pollution has been associated with abnormalities in sperm parameters. In recent studies the negative effect on sperm motility was estimated, in

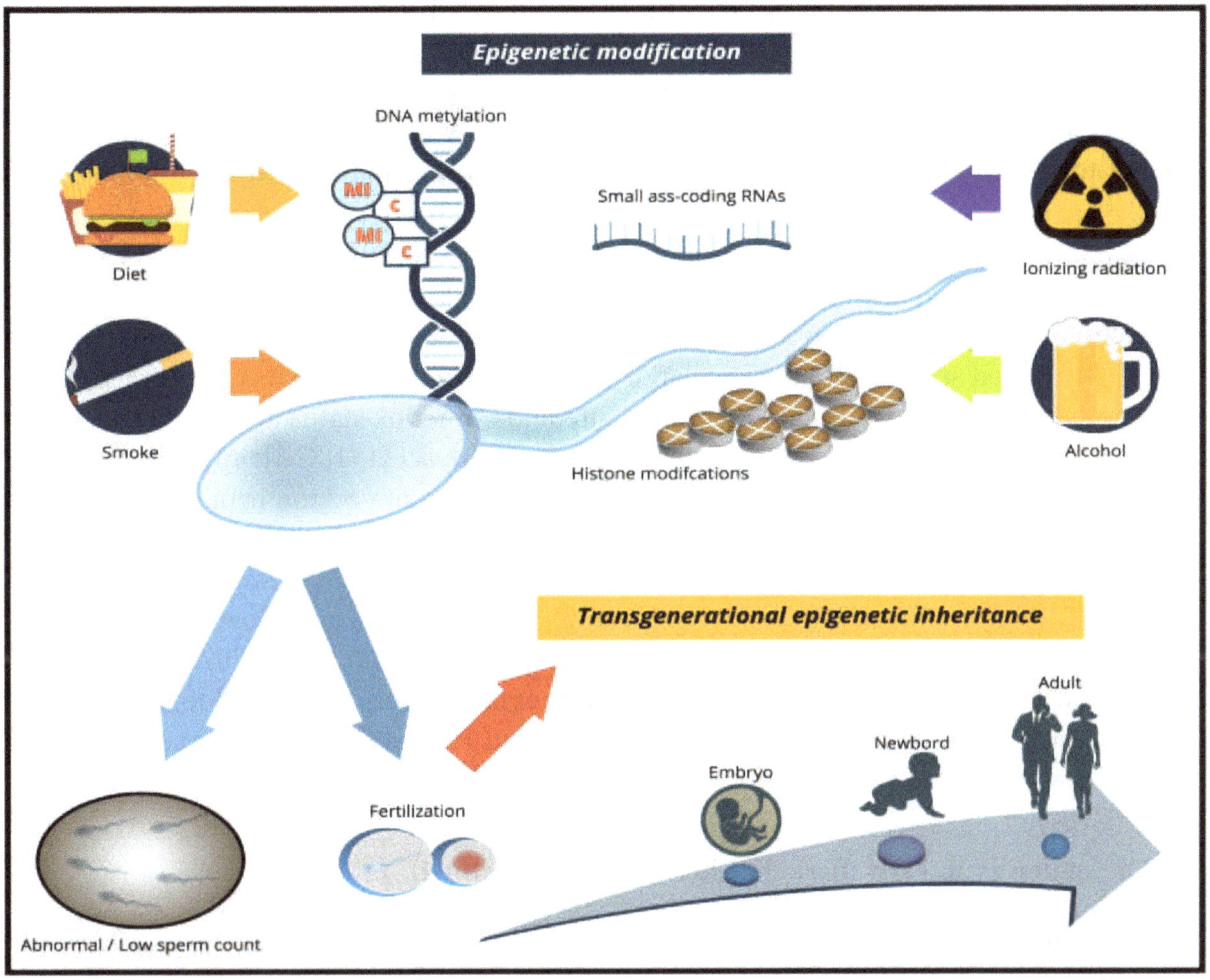

Figure 6. Environmental, life style and diet factors causing with different epigenetic mechanisms (histone modifications, DNA methylation, small ass-coding RNAs) alterations of the sperm epigenome and subsequent transgenerational effects.

particular on sperm DNA's integrity from carbon monoxide, nitrogen dioxide, sulfur dioxide, ozone, lead and PM 2.5, the latter being of particular interest, because it contains several trace elements and PAHs, powerful endocrine disruptors [160].

Spermatogenesis unlike oogenesis from puberty onward is continuously and therefore more easily exposed to insults in his stages of continuous replication. Moreover, biologically a 20-year-old's sperm has undergone about 160 rounds of chromosome replication, a 40-year-old's has undergone 610 and many male germline mutations fall into the "replicative" category or the "non-replicative," such as those caused by environmental exposure, so male germline accumulates mutations faster than female one [48, 49]. For instance, it is thought that sperm cells are more susceptible than eggs to the effects of oxidative damage as a consequence of: (i) the limited cytoplasmic space where to host the enzymes involved in the antioxidant protection, and (ii) the higher amount of polyunsaturated fatty acids within the sperm membranes rendering them more susceptible to oxidative stress, such as lipid peroxidation [50]. Furthermore, in semen it is possible to measure simultaneously environmental contaminants and *in vivo* effects on sperm cells, which are readily available, with features sensitive to environmental pollutants such as motility, morphology and the integrity of the DNA strand.

In 2010, Rubes while assessing seasonal differences of exposure of police officers who worked in the Centre of Prague (Czech Republic), found that sperm DNA fragmentation was significantly higher in winter (high exposure) rather than in spring (low exposure) in samples of all men, including non-smokers [161]. Also in the metropolitan area of Naples studies support the relationship between low sperm motility and high environmental exposure to emissions of traffic or heavy metals [162]. In addition, significantly higher level of sperm DNA damage, measured by means two different techniques, was found in healthy male volunteers living in HIP area as compared with that measured in volunteers living in LIP [118]. Human semen sensitivity to pollution-induced alteration of semen redox status was recently confirmed in a recently published study [26]. In particular, it was demonstrated that semen is more susceptible than blood plasma to pollution-associated alteration of redox status and that STL, but not LTS, was significantly influenced by the environmental impact [134] Certainly, the possibility for measuring simultaneously in human semen the presence of environmental contaminants and checking *in vivo* effects on sperm cells, readily available, with sensitive features to environmental pollutants such as motility, morphology, integrity of DNA strand, semen redox status, sperm aneuploidies, STL, make it an ideal way to assess the adverse effects of environmental exposure for measuring the environmental impact on human health. In conclusion, human semen seems an earlier and sensitive source of biomarkers than blood to monitor high environmental pressure on human health, hence useful for innovative prevention programs and health surveillance, especially in risk areas.

2.5. The semen as an early marker of health (health sentinel)

The spermatogenesis cycle is extremely complex and vulnerable to endogenous and exogenous stress, so it is not surprising that it can be an important indicator of the state of well-being of the organism. Recent studies have demonstrated the association between semen quality and state of health, correlating the semen quality with either chronic degenerative diseases, comorbidities and even mortality [36, 42, 43, 51–53].

In a first study of Eisenberg [53] a group of 9387 men was examined, average age 38 years, which had been evaluated for infertility issues between 1994 and 2011. Within the group, 44% had at least one medical diagnosis not related to infertility. Using the Charlson Comorbidity Index, researchers have shown that men with a higher index of chronic conditions had a lower count of sperm volume and motility, of total number of sperms and of normal shape. Sperm abnormalities rates were significantly higher among men with endocrine-metabolic, circulatory or genitourinary disorders and skin diseases, compared to other men without these conditions. Vascular hypertension, cerebrovascular disease and ischemic heart disease were associated with higher rates of sperm abnormalities. On the other hand, about 15% of all human genes are directly involved in reproduction and the majority of these genes may also play an important role in other parts of the body.

In a second study of Eisenberg [42] 2238 men recruited in an infertility clinic of Texas were analyzed: 451 of which with azoospermia and 1787. It was compared the incidence of cancer on with that on the general population of Texas. At the first evaluation of infertility, the average age was 35.7 years. After a 6–7 years follow-up, it was shown that 29 of the infertile men developed a cancer, 10 (2.2%) among those ones with azoospermia and 19 (1.1%) among those ones without it. In comparison to the overall population of Texas, this subset of infertile men had a significantly higher risk of overall cancers and such a was significantly higher in men with azoospermia than in those without azoospermia.

The same Eisenberg linked semen quality with mortality rates [53] and found that men with damaged seminal parameters, including low sperm volume, concentration, sperm motility, had higher death rates than men with normal sperm parameters. Men with at least two abnormal sperm parameters had a 2.3-fold higher death risk (95% CI 1.12–4.65) than men with normal sperm. This further study of association, shows that men with poor semen parameters have an increased mortality rate in subsequent years and suggests that the fertility assessment may be an indicator of overall health.

3. Conclusion

A certain number of regions in all the world experience a higher incidence of health disorders (reproductive, pediatric, cancer, etc.) due to environmental pollution: the societal costs associated with poor health and the interventions to reduce pollution are stirring debates and concerns. It is important a science-based guidance for preventing/reducing health risks in many high environmental pressure areas.

Information about levels of exposure to contaminants (chemical, physical) is critical to evaluate and to manage environmental and professional risks and, as a result, as much as possible, to measure the biological risk expressed in terms of probability of reaching potential harm through the exposure to certain chemical and/or physical stress. There are new analytical tools today that first identify and measure biomarkers, quantitative end-point and intermediate pathways of biological tissue/fluid fluids to identify early signs of functional or structural modification before clinical damage. Therefore, in order to have greater preventive efficacy and raise the level of attention and protection especially to populations living in areas with greater environmental exposure, it is important consider to organofunctional "*sentinel*" systems more susceptible to endogenous and exogenous modifications, those that suffer effects before others. For this reason and in relation to the new primary prevention approaches, the endocrine-metabolic system, and in particular the male reproductive, considering "*double function*" of human semen (Health and Environmental marker), represent an ideal tool for investigating and promoting health surveillance. Human semen seems to be a time-effective, sensitive and informative source of biomarkers, providing information about the presence of biologically active exposures, useful for innovative prevention programs and health surveillance, especially in environmental risk areas. Furthermore, maintaining a good semen quality and fertility is a prevention coverage. Bad lifestyles and environmental contaminants can impair reproductive health and overall health, encouraging the development of chronic degenerative diseases affecting the adult and, through the sperm epigenome changes, future generations. Environmental health should consider reproductive health and development, from intrauterine life to childhood and puberty: these are both vulnerable targets and high-value protection goals, inasmuch as they represent the future of our societies, in particular, biomarkers of reproductive health should be exploited as early signals of environmental pressure and increased risk of adverse chronic health effects. Hence, the use of reproductive biomarkers for early detection and prevention of environmental health risks represents a useful initiative for public health. Thus, identifying risk factors to improve the management of human wellness and health throughout standardized analysis, which correlates the toxic bioaccumulation of the seminal fluid with the multiple semen parameters, might be the main objective to be considered in the agenda of public prevention policies.

Acknowledgements

The authors would like to thank EcoFoodFertility research group and Silvia Letizia Piscopo for the English revision.

Author details

Luigi Montano[1]*, Paolo Bergamo[2], Maria Grazia Andreassi[3] and Stefano Lorenzetti[4]

*Address all correspondence to: luigimontano@gmail.com

1 Andrology Unit of the "San Francesco d'Assisi" Hospital, ASL Salerno, Oliveto Citra, Salerno, Italy

2 National Research Council (CNR), Institute of Food Sciences, Avellino, Italy

3 National Research Council (CNR), Institute of Clinical Physiology, Pisa, Italy

4 Department of Food Safety, Nutrition and Veterinary Public Health, Istituto Superiore di Sanità (ISS), Rome, Italy

References

[1] Lutz W, O'Neill BC, Scherbov S. Demographics. Europe's population at a turning point. Science. 2003;**299**(5615):1991-1992

[2] Carlsen E, Giwercman A, Keiding N, Skakkebæk NE. Evidence for decreasing quality of semen during past 50 years. British Medical Journal. 1992;**305**:609-613

[3] Rolland M, Le MJ, Wagner V, Royere D, De MJ. Decline in semen concentration and morphology in a sample of 26,609 men close to general population between 1989 and 2005 in France. Human Reproduction. 2013;**28**:462-470

[4] Andersen AG. Semen quality and reproductive hormones in normal young men and in partners of pregnant women [PhD thesis]. Copenhagen: Univ. of Copenhagen; 2001

[5] Sengupta P, Borges EJ, Dutta S, Krajewska-Kulak E. Decline in sperm count in European men during the past 50 years. Human & Experimental Toxicology 2017. DOI: 10.1177/0960327117703690 [Epub ahead of print]

[6] Kollin C, Karpe B, Hesser U, Granholm T, Ritzen EM. Surgical treatment of unilaterally undescended testes: Testicular growth after randomization to orchiopexy at age 9 months or 3 years. The Journal of Urology. 2007;**178**:1589-1593

[7] Andersson AM, Jørgensen N, Main KM, Toppari J, Rajpert-De Meyts E, Leffers H, Juul A, Jensen TK, Skakkebæk NE. Adverse trends in male reproductive health: We may have reached a crucial "tipping point". International Journal of Andrology. 2008;**31**: 74-80

[8] Slama R, Kold-Jensen T, Scheike T, Ducot B, Spira A, Keiding N. How would a decline in sperm concentration over time influence the probability of pregnancy? Epidemiology. 2004;**15**:458-465

[9] Bonde JP, Ernst E, Jensen TK, Hjollund NH, Kolstad H, Henriksen TB, et al. Relation between semen quality and fertility: A population-based study of 430 first-pregnancy planners. Lancet. 1998;**352**:1172-1177

[10] Guzick DS, Overstreet JW, Factor-Litvak P, Brazil CK, Nakajima ST, Coutifaris C, et al., National Cooperative Reproductive Medicine Network. Sperm morphology, motility, and concentration in fertile and infertile men. The New England Journal of Medicine. 2001;**345**: 1388-1393

[11] Slama R, Eustache F, Ducot B, Jensen TK, Jørgensen N, Horte A, et al. Time to pregnancy and semen parameters: A cross-sectional study among fertile couples from four European cities. Human Reproduction. 2002;**17**:503-515

[12] Selevan SG, Borkovec L, Slott VL, Zudova Z, Rubes J, Evenson DP, et al. Semen quality and reproductive health of young Czech men exposed to seasonal air pollution. Environmental Health Perspectives. 2000;**108**:887-894

[13] Rubes J, Selevan SG, Evenson DP, Zudova D, Vozdova M, Zudova Z, et al. Episodic air pollution is associated with increased DNA fragmentation in human sperm without other changes in semen quality. Human Reproduction. 2005;**20**:2776-2783

[14] Guven A, Kayikci A, Cam K, Arbak P, Balbay O, Cam M. Alterations in semen parameters of toll collectors working at motorways: Does diesel exposure induce detrimental effects on semen? Andrologia. 2008;**40**:346-351

[15] Hammoud A, Carrell DT, Gibson M, Sanderson M, Parker-Jones K, Peterson CM. Decreased sperm motility is associated with air pollution in Salt Lake City. Fertility and Sterility. 2010;**93**:1875-1879

[16] Deng Z, Chen F, Zhang M, Lan L, Qiao Z, Cui Y, et al., Association between air pollution and sperm quality: A systematic review and meta-analysis. Environmental Pollution. 2016;**208**:663-669

[17] Sonne SB, Kristensen DM, Novotny GW, Olesen IA, Nielsen JE, et al. Testicular dysgenesis syndrome and the origin of carcinoma in situ testis. International Journal of Andrology. 2008;**31**:275-287

[18] Skakkebaek NE. Carcinoma in situ of the testis: possible origin from gonocitys and precursor of all types of germ cell tumours except spermatocytoma. International Journal of Andrology. 1987;**26**:2-15

[19] Auger J, Kunstmann JM, Czyglik F, Jouannet P. Decline in semen quality among fertile men in Paris during the past 20 years. New England Journal of Medicine. 1995;**332**:281-285 (9)

[20] Mendiola J, Jorgensen N, Andersson AM, Stahlhut RW, Liu F, Swan SH. Reproductive parameters in young men living in Rochester, New York. Fertility and Sterility. 2014;**101**: 1064-1071

[21] Le Moal J, Rolland M, Goria S, Wagner V, De Crouy-Chanel P, Rigou A, et al. Semen quality trends in French regions are consistent with a global change in environmental exposure. Reproduction. 2014;**147**:567-567

[22] Hauser R, Sokol R. Science linking environmental contaminant exposures with fertility and reproductive health impacts in the adult male. Fertility and Sterility. 2008;**89**:e59-e65

[23] Akre O, Cnattingius S, Bergstrom R, Kvist U, Trichopoulos D, Ekbom A. Human fertility does not decline: Evidence from Sweden. Fertility and Sterility. 1999;**71**:1066-1069

[24] Menchini-Fabris F, Rossi P, Palego P, Simi S, Turchi P. Declining sperm counts in Italy during the past 20 years. Andrologia. 1996;**28**:304-332

[25] Nordkap L, Joensen UN, Blomberg Jensen M, Jørgensen N. Regional differences and temporal trends in male reproductive health disorders: Semen quality may be a sensitive marker of environmental exposures. Molecular and Cellular Endocrinology. 2012;**355**(2): 221-230

[26] Bergamo P, Volpe MG, Lorenzetti S, Mantovani A, Notari T, Cocca E, et al. Human semen as an early, sensitive biomarker of highly polluted living environment in healthy men: A pilot biomonitoring study on trace elements in blood and semen and their relationship with sperm quality and RedOx status. Reproductive Toxicology. 2016;**66**:1-9

[27] Zhou N, Cui Z, Yang S, Han X, Chen G, Zhou Z, et al. Air pollution and decreased semen quality: A comparative study of Chongqing urban and rural areas. Environmental Pollution. 2014;**187**:145-152

[28] Pirastu R, Comba P, Conti S, Iavarone I, Fazzo L, Pasetto R, Zona A, Crocetti E, Ricci P. Sentieri-Epidemilogical Study of residents in National Priority Contaminated Sites: Mortality, cancer incidence and hospital discharges. Epidemiologia e Prevenzione. 2014;**38**:25-33

[29] Jagai JS, Messer LC, Rappazzo KM, Gray CL, Grabich SC, Lobdell DT. County-level cumulative environmental quality associated with cancer incidence. Cancer. Aug 1, 2017;**123**(15):2901-2908. DOI: 10.1002/cncr.30709 [Epub May 8, 2017]. PMID: 28480506

[30] Tagliabue G, Borgini A, Tittarelli A, van Donkelaar A, Martin RV, Bertoldi M, Fabiano S, Maghini A, Codazzi T, Scaburri A, Favia I, Cau A, Barigelletti G, Tessandori R, Contiero P. Atmospheric fine particulate matter and breast cancer mortality: A population-based cohort study. BMJ Open 2016 Nov 14;**6**(11):e012580. doi: 10.1136/bmjopen-2016-012580. PMID: 28076275

[31] Martuzzi M, Mitis F, Bianchi F, Minichilli F, Comba P, Fazzo L. Cancer mortality and congenital anomalies in a region of Italy with intense environmental pressure due to waste. Occupational and Environmental Medicine. 2009;**66**:725-732. DOI: 10.1136/oem.2008.044115

[32] Pasetto R, Zengarini N, Caranci N, De Santis M, Minichilli F, Santoro M, Pirastu R, Comba P. Environmental justice in the epidemiological surveillance system of residents in Italian National Priority Contaminated Sites (SENTIERI project). Epidemiologia e Prevenzione Jan–Feb 2017;**41**(2):134-139

[33] Asklund C, Jorgensen N, Skakkebaek NE, Jensen TK. Increased frequency of reproductive health problems among fathers of boys with hypospadias. Human Reproduction. 2007;**22**:2639-2646

[34] Barazani Y, Katz BF, Nagler HM, Stember DS. Lifestyle, environment, and male reproductive health. The Urologic Clinics of North America. 2014;**41**:55-66

[35] Guerrero-Bosagna C, Skinner MK. Environmentally induced epigenetic transgenerational inheritance of male infertility. Current Opinion in Genetics & Development. 2014;**26**: 79-88

[36] Jensen K, Jacobsen R, Christensen K, Nielsen NC, Bostofte E. Good semen quality and life expectancy: A cohort study of 43,277 men. American Journal of Epidemiology. 2009; **170**:559-565

[37] Baker JA, Buck GM, Vena JE, Moysich KB. Fertility patterns prior to testicular cancer diagnosis. Cancer Causes & Control. 2005;**16**:295-299

[38] Jorgensen N, Vierula M, Jacobsen R, Pukkala E, Perheentupa A, Virtanen HE, et al., Recent adverse trends in semen quality and testis cancer incidence among Finnish men. International Journal of Andrology. 2011;**34**:e37-e4811-12

[39] Raman JD, Nobert CF, Goldstein M. Increased incidence of testicular cancer in men presenting with infertility and abnormal semen analysis. The Journal of Urology. 2005; **174**:1819-1822

[40] Ostrowski KA, Walsh TJ. Infertility with testicular cancer The Urologic Clinics of North America. 2015;**42**:409-420

[41] Hanson HA, Anderson RE, Aston KI, Carrell DT, Smith KR, Hotaling JM. Subfertility increases risk of testicular cancer: Evidence from population-based semen samples. Fertility and Sterility. 2016;**105**:322-328

[42] Eisenberg ML, Li S, Brooks JD, Cullen MR, Baker LC. Increased risk of cancer in infertile men: Analysis of U.S. claims data. The Journal of Urology. 2015;**193**:1596-1601

[43] Rogers MJ, Walsh TJ. Male infertility and risk of cancer. Seminars in Reproductive Medicine. 2017;**35**:298-303

[44] Srám RJ, Benes I, Binková B, Dejmek J, Horstman D, Kotěsovec F, et al. Teplice program: The impact of air pollution on human health. Environmental Health Perspectives. 1996; **104**(Suppl 4):699-714

[45] Srám RJ, Binková B, Rössner P, Rubes J, Topinka J, Dejmek J. Adverse reproductive outcomes from exposure to environmental mutagens. Mutation Research. 1999;**428**:203-215

[46] Frederiksen H, Jensen TK, Jorgensen N, Kyhl HB, Husby S. Skakkebaek NE, Main KM, Juul A, Anderson AM. Human urinary excretion of non-persistent environmental chemicals: An overview of Danish data collected between 2006 and 2012.Reproduction. 2014;**147**:555-565

[47] CDC Report. Fourth national Report on Human Exposure to Environmental Chemicals, Updates Tables. Atlanta, USA: Ceners for Disease Control and Prevention, National Center for Enviornmetal Health; February 2015. pp. 1-1095

[48] Ségurel L, Wyman MJ, Przeworski M. Determinants of mutation rate variation in the human germline. Annual Review of Genomics and Human Genetics. 2014;**15**:47-70 (5)

[49] Blumenstiel JP. Sperm competition can drive a male-biased mutation rate. Journal of Theoretical Biology. Dec 7, 2007;**249**(3):624-632

[50] Aitken RJ, Gibb Z, Baker MA, Drevet J, Gharagozloo P. Causes and consequences of oxidative stress in spermatozoa. Reproduction, Fertility, and Development. 2016;**28**(1–2): 1-10. DOI: 10.1071/RD15325

[51] Eisenberg ML, Li S, Behr B, Pera RR, Cullen MR. Relationship between semen production and medical comorbidity. Fertility and Sterility. 2015;**103**:66-71

[52] Latif T, Kold Jensen T, Mehlsen J, Holmboe SA, Brinth L, Pors K, et al. Semen quality is a predictor of subsequent morbidity. A Danish cohort study of 4,712 men with long-term follow-up. American Journal of Epidemiology. May 11, 2017. DOI: 10.1093/aje/kwx067 [Epub ahead of print]

[53] Eisenberg ML, Li S, Behr B, Cullen MR, Galusha D, Lamb DJ, Lipshultz LI. Semen quality, infertility and mortality in the USA. Human Reproduction. 2014;**29**:1567-1574

[54] Montano L, Iannuzzi L, Rubes J, Avolio C, Pistos C, Gatti A, Raimondo S, Notari N. EcoFoodFertility – Environmental and food impact assessment on male reproductive function. Andrology. 2014;**2**(Suppl 2):69 http://dx.doi.org/10.1111/andr.267

[55] Carson R. Silent Spring. Boston: Houghton Mifflin; 1962

[56] ECHA. European Chemicals Agency, List of Registered Substances. 2016. Available from: https://echa.europa.eu/information-on-chemicals/registered substances. [Accessed: Nov 20, 2016]

[57] Kavlock RJ, Daston GP, DeRosa C, Fenner-Crisp P, Gray LE, Kaattari S, et al. Research needs for the risk assessment of health and environmental effects of endocrine disruptors:

A report of the U.S. EPA-sponsored workshop. Environmental Health Perspectives. 1996; (Suppl 4):715-740

[58] Den Hond E, Tournaye H, De Sutter P, Ombelet W, Baeyens W. Covaci A, et al. Human exposure to endocrine disrupting chemicals and fertility: A case-control study in male subfertility patients. Environment International. 2015;**84**:154-160

[59] Marques-Pinto A, Carvalho D. Human infertility: Are endocrine disruptors to blame? Endocrine Connections. 2013;**17**:R15-R29

[60] Singh R, Sram RJ, Binkova B, Kalina I, Popov TA, Georgieva T, et al. The relationship between biomarkers of oxidative DNA damage, polycyclic aromatic hydrocarbon DNA adducts, antioxidant status and genetic susceptibility following exposure to environmental air pollution in humans. Mutation Research. 2007;**620**:83-92

[61] Singh R, Kaur B, Kalina I, Popov TA, Georgieva T, Garte S, et al. Effects of environmental air pollution on endogenous oxidative DNA damage in humans. Mutation Research. 2007;**620**:71-82

[62] Wright C, Milne S, Leeson H. Sperm DNA damage caused by oxidative stress: Modifiable clinical, lifestyle and nutritional factors in male infertility. Reproductive Biomedicine Online. 2014;**28**:684-703

[63] Guerrero-Bosagna CM, Skinner MK. Epigenetic transgenerational effects of endocrine disruptors on male reproduction. Seminars in Reproductive Medicine. 2009;**27**(5):403-408

[64] Xin F, Susiarjo M, Bartolomei MS. Multigenerational and transgenerational effects of endocrine disrupting chemicals: A role for altered epigenetic regulation? Seminars in Cell & Developmental Biology. 2015;**43**:66-75

[65] Walker DM, Gore AC. Transgenerational neuroendocrine disruption of reproduction. Nature Reviews Endocrinology. 2007;**7**(4):197-207

[66] Kamarianos A, Karamanlis X, Theodosiadou E, Goulas P, Smokovitis A. The presence of environmental pollutants in the semen of farm animals (bull, ram, goat, and boar). Reproductive Toxicology. 2003;**17**(4):439-445

[67] Jurewicz J, Hanke W, Radwan M, Bonde JP. Environmental factors and semen quality. International Journal of Occupational Medicine and Environmental Health. 2009;**22**(4): 305-329

[68] Giaccio L, Cicchella D, De Vivo B, Lombardi G, De Rosa M. Does heavy metals pollution affects semen quality in men? A case of study in the metropolitan area of Naples (Italy). Journal of Geochemical Exploration. 2012;**112**:218-225

[69] Mínguez-Alarcón L, Mendiola J, Roca M, López-Espín JJ, Guillén JJ, Moreno JM, et al. Correlations between different heavy metals in diverse body fluids: Studies of human semen quality. Advances in Urology. 2012;**2012**:420893

[70] Srikanth K, Pereira E, Duarte AC, Ahmad I. Glutathione and its dependent enzymes' modulatory responses to toxic metals and metalloids in fish – A review. Environmental Science and Pollution Research International 2013;**20**:2133-2149

[71] Li P, Zhong Y, Jiang X, Wang C, Zuo Z, Sha A. Seminal plasma metals concentration with respect to semen quality. Biological Trace Element Research. 2012;**148**:1-6

[72] Danadevi K, Rozati R, Reddy PP, Grover P. Semen quality of Indian welders occupationally exposed to nickel and chromium. Reproductive Toxicology. 2003;**17**:451-456

[73] Mendiola J, Torres-Cantero AM, Moreno-Grau JM, Ten J, Roca M, Moreno-Grau S, et al. Exposure to environmental toxins in males seeking infertility treatment: A case-controlled study. Reproductive Biomedicine Online. 2008;**16**:842-850

[74] Altomare M, Vicari LO, Fiore M, Ferrante M, Fallico R, Condorelli RA, et al. Relationships between occupational exposure and heavy metal levels in men living in an eastern sicily industrial area. In: ISEE Conference - August 26–30, 2012 - Columbia, South Caroline. In Epidemiology. 2012. Vol. 23(5S). Philadelphia: Editore Lippincot Willuiams & Wilkins; Sep 2012

[75] Marzec-Wróblewska U, Kamiński P, Łakota P, Szymański M, Wasilow K, Ludwikowski GM, et al. Zinc and iron concentration and SOD activity in human semen and seminal plasma. Biological Trace Element Research. 2011;**143**:167-177

[76] Tremellen K. Oxidative stress and male infertility: a clinical perspective. In: Agarwal A, et al. editors. Applied Basic Research and Clinical Practice. Humana Press; 2012. p. 325-353

[77] Hybertson BM, Gao B, Bose SK, McCord JM. Oxidative stress in health and disease: The therapeutic potential of Nrf2 activation. Molecular Aspects of Medicine. 2011;**32**:234-246

[78] Williams MA, Rangasamy T, Bauer SM, Killedar S, Karp M, Kensler TW, et al. Disruption of the transcription factor Nrf2 promotes pro-oxidative dendritic cells that stimulate Th2-like immuno responsiveness upon activation by ambient particulate matter. Journal of Immunology. 2008;**181**:4545-4559

[79] Risom L, Møller P, Loft S. Oxidative stress-induced DNA damage by particulate air pollution. Mutation Research. 2005;**592**:119-137

[80] Ojha A, Srivastava N. Redox imbalance in rat tissues exposed with organophosphate pesticides and therapeutic potential of antioxidant vitamins. Ecotoxicology and Environmental Safety. 2012;**32**:234-246

[81] De Lamirande E, Jiang H, Zini A. Reactive oxygen species and sperm physiology. Reviews of Reproduction. 1997;**2**:48-54

[82] Said TM, Agarwal A, Sharma RK. Human sperm superoxide anion in generation and correlation with semen quality in patients with male infertility. Fertility and Sterility. 2004;**82**:871-877

[83] Gil-Guzman E, Ollero M, Lopez MC. Differential production of reactive oxygen species by subsets of human spermatozoa at different stages of maturation. Human Reproduction. 2001;**16**:1922-1930

[84] Sharma RK, Pasqualotto AE, Nelson DR. Relationship between seminal white blood cell counts and oxidative stress in men treated at an infertility clinic. Journal of Andrology. 2001;**22**:575-583

[85] Metelev AY, Bogdanov AB, Ivkinl EV, Mitrokhin AA, Vodneva MM, Veliev EI. Hyperbaric oxygen therapy in the treatment of male infertility associated with increased sperm DNA fragmentation and reactive oxygen species in semen. Urologia. 2015;**5**:74-76

[86] Faraonio R, Vergara P, Di Marzo D, Pierantoni MG, Napolitano M, Russo T, et al. p53 suppresses the Nrf2-dependent transcription of antioxidant response genes. The Journal of Biological Chemistry. 2006;**281**:39776-39784

[87] Attaman JA, Toth TL, Furtado J, Campos H, Hauser R, Chavarro JE. Dietary fat and semen quality among men attending a fertility clinic. Human Reproduction. 2012;**27**:1466-1474

[88] Showell MG, Mackenzie-Proctor R, Brown J, Yazdani A, Stankiewicz MT, Hart RJ. Antioxidants for male subfertility.Cochrane Database of Systematic Reviews. 2014;**12**: CD007411

[89] Yao DF, Mills JN. Male infertility: Lifestyle factors and holistic, complementary, and alternative therapies. Asian Journal of Andrology. 2016;**18**:410-418

[90] Sharma R, Biedenharn KR, Fedor JM, Agarwal A. Lifestyle factors and reproductive health: Taking control of your fertility. Reproductive Biology and Endocrinology. 2013;**16**(11):66

[91] Anawalt BD. The silent spermatozoon: Are man-made endocrine disruptors killing male fertility? Asian Journal of Andrology. 2013;**15**:165-168

[92] Veras MM, Caldini EG, Dolhnikoff M, Saldiva PH. Air pollution and effects on reproductive-system functions globally with particular emphasis on the Brazilian population. Journal of Toxicology and Environmental Health. Part B, Critical Reviews 2010; **13**:1-15

[93] Ferlin A, Raicu F, Gatta V, Zuccarello D, Palka G, Foresta C. Male infertility: Role of genetic background. Reproductive Biomedicine Online. 2007;**14**:734-745

[94] Esteves SC. A clinical appraisal of the genetic basis in unexplained male infertility. Journal of Human Reproductive Sciences. 2013;**6**:176-182

[95] Berger R. The incidence of constitutional chromosome aberrations. Journal de Génétique Humaine. 1975;**23**:42-49

[96] Shi Q, Martin RH. Aneuploidy in human sperm: A review of the frequency and distribution of aneuploidy, effects of donor age and lifestyle factors. Cytogenetics and Cell Genetics. 2000;**90**:219-226

[97] McAuliffe ME, Williams PL, Korrick SA, Altshul LM, Perry MJ. Environmental exposure to polychlorinated biphenyls and p,p′-DDE and sperm sex-chromosome disomy. Environmental Health Perspectives 2012;**120**:535-540

[98] Rubes J, Selevan SG, Evenson DP, Zudova D, Vozdova M, Zudova Z, Robbins WA, Perreault SD. Episodic air pollution is associated with increased DNA fragmentation in human sperm without other changes in semen quality. Human Reproduction. Oct 2005; **20**(10):2776-2783. [Epub Jun 24, 2005]

[99] Aitken RJ, De Iuliis GN, McLachlan RI. Biological and clinical significance of DNA damage in male germ line. International Journal of Andrology. 2009;**32**:46-56

[100] Dyer A, Jong K, Ratter J. Aneuploidy: A redefinition. Notes from the Royal Botanic Garden Edinburgh. 1970;**30**:177-182

[101] Albertini RJ, Anderson D, Douglas GR, Hagmar L, Hemminki K, Merlo F, et al. IPCS guidelines for the monitoring of genotoxic effects of carcinogens in humans. International Programme on Chemical Safety. Mutation Research. 2000;**46**:111-172

[102] Norppa H. Cytogenetic biomarkers. IARC Scientific Publications. 2004;**157**:179-205

[103] Gordon DJ, Resio B, Pellman D. Causes and consequences of aneuploidy in cancer. Nature Reviews. Genetics. 2012;**13**:189-203

[104] Torres EM, Williams BR, Amon A. Aneuploidy: Cells losing their balance. Genetics. 2008;**179**(2):737-746

[105] Schrader SM, Marlow KL. Assessing the reproductive health of men with occupational exposures. Asian Journal of Andrology. 2014;**16**(1):23-30

[106] NTP. Report on Carcinogens. 12th ed. Collingdale, Pennsylvania, USA: DIANE Publishing Company; 2011

[107] Martinez G, Gillois P, Le Mitouard M, Borye R, Esquerre-Lamare C, Satre V, et al. FISH and tips: A large scale analysis of automated versus manual scoring for sperm aneuploidy detection. Basic and Clinical Andrology. 2013;**23**:13

[108] Fenech M, Kirsch-Volders M, Rossnerova A, Sram R, Romm H, Bolognesi C, et al. HUMN project initiative and review of validation, quality control and prospects for further development of automated micronucleus assays using image cytometry systems. International Journal of Hygiene and Environmental Health. 2013;**216**:541-545

[109] Adler ID. 2000. Spermatogenesis and mutagenicity of environmental hazards: Extrapolation of genetic risk from mouse to man. Andrologia. 2000;**32**:233-237

[110] Sakkas D, Alvarez JG. Sperm DNA fragmentation: Mechanisms and origin, impact on reproductive outcame, and analysis. Fertility and Sterility. 2010;**934**:1027-1036

[111] Moskovtsev SI, Jarvi K, Brendan J, Mullen M, Cadesky KI, Hannam T, et al. Testicular spermatozoa have statistically significantly lower DNA damage compared with ejaculated spermatozoa in patients with unsuccessful oral antioxidant treatment. Fertility and Sterility. 2010;**93**:1142-1146

[112] Slama R, Darrow L, Parker J, Woodruff TJ, Strickland M, Nieuwenhuijsen M, et al. Meeting report: Atmospheric pollution and human reproduction. Environmental Health Perspectives. 2008;**116**(6):791

[113] Crow JF. The origins, patterns and implication of human spontaneous mutation. Nature Reviews. Genetics. 2000;**1**:40-47

[114] Gandini L, Lombardo F, Paoli D, Caruso F, Eleuteri P, Leter G, et al. Full-term pregnancies achieved with ICSI despite high levels of sperm chromatin damage. Human Reproduction. 2004;**19**:1409-1417

[115] Sipos A, Rasmussen F, Harrison G, Tynelius P, Lewis G, Leon DA, Gunnell D. Paternal age and schizophrenia: A population based cohort study. British Medical Journal. 2004; **329**:1070

[116] Frans EM, Sandin S, Reichenberg A, Lichtenstein P, Langstrom N, Hultman CM. Advancing paternal age and bipolar disorder. Archives of General Psychiatry. 2008;**65**: 1034-1040

[117] Raimondo S, Gentile T, Cuomo F, De Filippo S, Aprea GE, Guida J. Quantitative evaluation of p53 as a new indicator of DNA damage in human spermatozoa. Journal of Human Reproductive Sciences. Jul 2014;**7**(3):212-217. DOI: 10.4103/0974-1208.142490

[118] Montano L, Notari T, Raimondo S, Bergamo P, Rossi M, Luongo D, et al. Campania region group research EcoFoodFertility . Evaluation of environmental impact on sperm DNA integrity by sperm chromatin dispersion test and p53 ELISA. Preliminary data (ECOFOODFERTILITY project). Reproductive Toxicology. 2015;**56**:20

[119] Červenák F, Juríková K, Sepšiová R, Neboháčová M, Nosek J, Tomáška L. Double-stranded telomeric DNA binding proteins: Diversity matters. Cell Cycle. 2017;**16**:1568-1577. DOI: 10.1080/15384101.2017.1356511

[120] Thilagavathi J, Venkatesh S, Dada R. Telomere length in reproduction. Andrologia. 2013; **45**:289-304

[121] Zalenskaya IA, Bradbury EM, Zalensky AO. Chromatin structure of telomere domain in human sperm. Biochemical and Biophysical Research Communications. 2000;**279**:213-218

[122] Yang Q, Zhao F, Dai S, Zhang N, Zhao W, Bai R, et al. Sperm telomere length is positively associated with the quality of early embryonic development. Human Reproduction. 2015;**30**:1876-1881

[123] Aston KI, Hunt SC, Susser E, Kimura M, Factor-Litvak P, et al. Divergence of sperm and leukocyte age-dependent telomere dynamics: Implications for male-driven evolution of telomere length in humans. Molecular Human Reproduction. 2012;**18**:517-522

[124] Hou L, Zhang X, Gawron AJ, Liu J. Surrogate tissue telomere length and cancer risk: Shorter or longer? Cancer Letters. 2012;**319**:130-135

[125] Rode L, Nordestgaard BG, Bojesen SE. Long telomeres and cancer risk among 95,568 individuals from the general population. International Journal of Epidemiology. 2016;**45**: 1634-1643

[126] Haycock PC, Burgess S, Nounu A, Zheng J, Okoli GN, Bowden J, et al., Telomeres Mendelian Randomization Collaboration. Association between telomere length and risk

of cancer and non-neoplastic diseases: A Mendelian Randomization Study. JAMA Oncology. 2017;**3**:636-651

[127] Hoxha M, Dioni L, Bonzini M, Pesatori AC, Fustinoni S, Cavallo D, et al. Association between leukocyte telomere shortening and exposure to traffic pollution: A cross-sectional study on traffic officers and indoor office workers. Environmental Health. 2009;**8**:41

[128] Shin JY, Choi YY, Jeon HS, Hwang JH, Kim SA, Kang JH, et al. Low-dose persistent organic pollutants increased telomere length in peripheral leukocytes of healthy Koreans. Mutagenesis. 2010;**25**:511-516

[129] Hou L, Wang S, Dou C, Zhang X, Yu Y, Zheng Y, et al. Air pollution exposure and telomere length in highly exposed subjects in Beijing, China: A repeated-measure study. Environment International. 2012;**48**:71-77

[130] Dioni L, Hoxha M, Nordio F, Bonzini M, Tarantini L, Albetti B, et al. Effects of short-term exposure to inhalable particulate matter on telomere length, telomerase expression, and telomerase methylation in steel workers. Environmental Health Perspectives. 2011;**119**: 622-627

[131] Li H, Engström K, Vahter M, Broberg K. Arsenic exposure through drinking water is associated with longer telomeres in peripheral blood. Chemical Research in Toxicology. 2012;**25**:2333-2339

[132] Gao J, Roy S, Tong L, Argos M, Jasmine F, Rahaman R, et al. Arsenic exposure, telomere length, and expression of telomere-related genes among Bangladeshi individuals. Environmental Research. 2015;**136**:462-469. DOI: 10.1016/j.envres.2014.09.040

[133] Ling X, Zhang G, Chen Q, Yang H, Sun L, Zhou N, et al. Shorter sperm telomere length in association with exposure to polycyclic aromatic hydrocarbons: Results from the MARHCS cohort study in Chongqing, China and in vivo animal experiments. Environment International. 2016;**95**:79-85. DOI: 10.1016/j.envint.2016.08.001

[134] Vecoli C, Montano L, Borghini A, Notari T, Guglielmino A, Mercuri A, et al. Effects of highly polluted environment on sperm telomere length: A pilot study. International Journal of Molecular Sciences. 2017;**18**:1703. DOI: 10.3390/ijms18081703

[135] Feng S, Jacobsen SE, Reik W. Epigenetic reprogramming in plant and animal development. Science. 2010;**330**:622-627

[136] Houshdaran S, Cortessis VK, Siegmund K, Yang A, Laird PW, Sokol RZ. Widespread epigenetic abnormalities suggest a broad DNA methylation erasure defect in abnormal human sperm. PLoS One. 2007;**2**:e1289

[137] Urdinguio RG, Bayón GF, Dmitrijeva M, Toraño EG, Bravo C, Fraga M, et al. Aberrant DNA methylation patterns of spermatozoa in men with unexplained infertility. Human Reproduction. 2015;**30**:1014-1028

[138] Du Y, Li M, Chen J, Duan Y, Wang X, Qiu Y, et al. Promoter targeted bisulfite sequencing reveals DNA methylation profiles associated with low sperm motility in asthenozoospermia. Human Reproduction. 2016;**31**:24-33

[139] Laurentino SS, Borgmann J, Gromoll J. On the origin of sperm epigenetic heterogeneity. Reproduction. 2016;**151**:R71-R78 (16)

[140] Hammoud SS, Purwar J, Pflueger C, Cairns BR, Carrell DT. Alterations in sperm DNA methylation patterns at imprinted loci in two classes of infertility. Fertility and Sterility. 2010;**94**:1728-1733

[141] Kobayashi H, Sato A, Otsu E, Hiura H, Tomatsu C, Utsunomiya T, Sasaki H, Yaegashi N, Arima T. Aberrant DNA methylation of imprinted loci in sperm from oligospermic patients. Human Molecular Genetics. 2007;**16**:2542-2551

[142] Marques CJ, Costa P, Vaz B, Carvalho F, Fernandes S, Barros A, Sousa M. Abnormal methylation of imprinted genes in human sperm is associated with oligozoospermia. Molecular Human Reproduction. 2008;**14**:67-74

[143] Khazamipour N, Noruzinia M, Fatehmanesh P, Keyhanee M, Pujol P. MTHFR promoter hypermethylation in testicular biopsies of patients with non-obstructive azoospermia: The role of epigenetics in male infertility. Human Reproduction. 2009;**24**:2361-2364

[144] Wu W, Shen O, Qin Y, Niu X, Lu C, Xia Y, et al. Idiopathic male infertility is strongly associated with aberrant promoter methylation of methylenetetrahydrofolate reductase (MTHFR). PLoS One. 2010;**5**:e13884

[145] Rajender S, Avery K, Agarwal A. Epigenetics, spermatogenesis and male infertility. Mutation Research. 2011;**727**:62-71

[146] Hammoud SS, Nix DA, Hammoud AO, Gibson M, Cairns BR, Carrell DT. Genome-wide analysis identifies changes in histone retention and epigenetic modifications at developmental and imprinted gene loci in the sperm of infertile men. Human Reproduction. 2011;**26**:2558-2569

[147] Paradowska AS, Miller D, Spiess AN, Vieweg M, Cerna M, Dvorakova-Hortova K, et al. Genome wide identification of promoter binding sites for H4K12ac in human sperm and its relevance for early embryonic development. Epigenetics. 2012;**7**:1057-1070

[148] Dada R, Kumar M, Jesudasan R, Fernández JL, Gosálvez J, Agarwal A. Epigenetics and its role in male infertility. Journal of Assisted Reproduction and Genetics. 2012;**29**:213-223

[149] Rousseaux S, Caron C, Govin J, Lestrat C, Faure AK, Khochbin S. Establishment of male-specific epigenetic information. Gene. 2005;**345**:139-153

[150] Weber M, Hellmann I, Stadler M.B, Ramos L, Paabo S, Rebhan M, Schubeler D. Distribution, silencing potential and evolutionary impact of promoter DNA methylation in the human genome. Nature Genetics. 2007;**39**:457-466

[151] Hayashi K, Chuva de Sousa Lopes SM, Kaneda M, Tang F, Hajkova P, Lao K, et al. MicroRNA, biogenesis is required for mouse primordial germ cell development and spermatogenesis. PLoS One. 2008;**3**:e1738

[152] Maatouk DM, Loveland KL, McManus MT, Moore K, Harfe BD. Dicer1 is required for differentiation of the mouse male germline. Biology of Reproduction. 2008;**79**:696-703

[153] Huszar JM, Payne CJ. MicroRNA 146 (Mir146) modulates spermatogonial differentiation by retinoic acid in mice. Biology of Reproduction. 2013;**88**:15

[154] Kotaja N. MicroRNAs and spermatogenesis. Fertility and Sterility. 2014;**101**:1552-1562

[155] Khazaie Y, Nasr Esfahani MH. MicroRNA and male infertility: A potential for diagnosis. International Journal of Fertility & Sterility. 2014;**8**:113-118

[156] Salas-Huetos A, Blanco J, Vidal F, Godo A, Grossmann M, Pons MC, et al. Spermatozoa from patients with seminal alterations exhibit a differential micro-ribonucleic acid profile. Fertility and Sterility. 2015;**104**:591-601

[157] Wang C, Yang C, Chen X, Yao B, Yang C, Zhu C, et al. Altered profile of seminal plasma microRNAs in the molecular diagnosis of male infertility. Clinical Chemistry. 2012;**57**: 1722-1731

[158] Wu W, Hu Z, Qin Y, Dong J, Dai J, Lu C, et al. Seminal plasma microRNAs: Potential biomarkers for spermatogenesis status. Molecular Human Reproduction. 2012;**18**:489-497

[159] Tsatsanis C, Bobjer J, Rastkhani H, Dermitzaki E, Katrinaki M, Margioris AN, et al. Serum miR-155 as a potential biomarker of male fertility. Human Reproduction. 2015; **30**:853-860

[160] Radwan M, Jurewicz J, Polańska K, Sobala W, Radwan P, Bochenek M, et al. Exposure to ambient air pollution. Does it affect semen quality and the level of reproductive hormones? Annals of Human Biology. 2016;**43**:50-56

[161] Rubes J, Rybar R, Prinosilova P, Veznik Z, Chvatalova I, Solansky I, Sram RJ. Genetic polymorphisms influence the susceptibility of men to sperm DNA damage associated with exposure to air pollution. Mutation Research. Jan 5, 2010;**683**(1–2):9-15

[162] De Rosa M, Zarrilli S, Paesano L, Carbone U, Boggia B, Petretta M, Maisto A, Cimmino F, Puca G, Colao A., Lombardi G. Traffic pollutants affect fertility in men. Human Reproduction. 2003;**18**:1055-1061

11

Physiological and Pathological Roles of Free Radicals in Male Reproduction

Eva Tvrdá, Peter Massanyi and Norbert Lukáč

Abstract

Oxidative stress (OS) is a condition caused by an imbalance between reactive oxygen species (ROS) overgeneration and decreased antioxidant defense mechanisms in the cell. OS has become a prominent factor in male reproductive dysfunction as ROS cause damage to sperm DNA, lipids and proteins, alterations to critical sperm structures and signaling pathways, leading to a decreased sperm activity and fertilizing capacity. At the same time, small amounts of ROS play vital roles in events leading to sperm maturation and acquisition of functional activity, which is why a proper oxidative balance is of paramount importance for a proper male fertility. Understanding the physiological and pathological roles of ROS in male reproduction has become an essential pillar of modern andrology; however, numerous questions related to the controversial behavior of ROS in male reproductive cells and tissues still remain unanswered. This chapter aims to summarize current evidence available on the relationships between free radicals, antioxidants and male reproduction and to trigger more scientific interest, particularly with respect to the design of efficient strategies to diagnose or treat male sub- or infertility associated with OS.

Keywords: free radicals, reactive oxygen species, oxidative stress, antioxidants, spermatozoa, male infertility

1. Introduction

Aerobic life inherently depends on oxygen, which is essential for a controlled oxidation of molecules containing carbon, subsequently leading to the release of energy. Nevertheless, aerobic cells, including spermatozoa, are persistently counteracting the so-called Oxygen Paradox: while oxygen is crucial to sustain aerobic life, it is simultaneously toxic to the cell survival [1]. Normal aerobic metabolism leads to the generation of by-products called free radicals (FR) [2, 3], which, under physiological conditions, are necessary for a normal cell function [4]. On the other hand, if FR concentrations become too high, either because of their overgeneration or due to low levels of antioxidant defense mechanisms, oxidative stress (OS) emerges with unpredictable consequences on the cell behavior and survival [5].

Oxidative stress has been implicated in the pathogenesis of a variety of human diseases such as atherosclerosis, cancer, diabetes, liver damage, AIDS, Parkinson's disease and health complications associated with premature birth [6]. In the meantime, seminal OS is believed to be one of the main factors in the pathogenesis of sperm dysfunction in male sub- or infertility [7–9]. Several intrinsic and extrinsic factors have the ability to promote reactive oxygen species (ROS) generation in the testicular as well as post-testicular (e.g. epididymal) environment, resulting in defective spermatogenesis and altered sperm function [9]. As expected, approximately 25% of infertile patients exhibit higher ROS levels in semen as opposed to fertile men [7, 10–12].

Although the origin of ROS generation in semen and their roles in male reproduction have only recently been uncovered, numerous questions still remain unanswered, thus offering multiple strategies for future research. As such, the role of free radicals and oxidative stress in fertility and subfertility is an area requiring continuous scientific attention.

2. Free radicals: general characteristics

A free radical (FR) is defined as any atom, molecule or a fragment of atoms and molecules with one or more unpaired electrons, capable of short independent existence. The abstraction or gain of one electron by a nonradical molecule may (or may not) convert it to a radical species [13]. Free radicals may have a positive, negative or a neutral charge [14]:

$A \rightarrow$ minus one electron $\rightarrow A^{+\bullet}$.

$B \rightarrow$ plus one electron $\rightarrow B^{-\bullet}$.

It is precisely the presence of an unpaired electron that results in certain common properties shared by most radicals. Free radicals are generally unstable and highly reactive. They can either donate an electron to or accept an electron from other molecules, thus behaving as oxidants or reductants [13].

In cells, one-electron modification of molecules can yield sulfur-, oxygen-, carbon- and nitrogen-derived free radicals [14]. Furthermore, ions of transition metals have a radical nature [13].

The most common and important free radicals related to biological systems are oxygen-derived radicals called reactive oxygen species (ROS) and nitrogen-derived molecules, defined as reactive nitrogen species (RNS) [15]. ROS represent a broad category of molecules including radical and non-radical oxygen derivatives [16]. Reactive nitrogen species are nitrogen-free radicals and commonly accepted as a subclass of ROS [13, 15]. A summary of the most common oxygen- and nitrogen-derived free radicals is provided in **Table 1**.

Radicals		Non-radicals	
Reactive oxygen species (ROS)			
Superoxide	$O_2^{\bullet -}$	Hydrogen peroxide	H_2O_2
Hydroxyl radical	$OH^{\bullet}$	Hypochlorous acid	HOCl
Peroxyl radical	$ROO^{\bullet}$	Hypobromous acid	HOBr
Alkoxyl radical	$RO^{\bullet}$	Ozone	O_3
Hydroperoxyl radical	$HO_2^{\bullet}$	Singlet oxygen	$^1\Delta_g$
Lipid peroxyl radical	$LOO^{\bullet}$	Lipid peroxide	LOOH
Reactive nitrogen species (RNS)			
Nitric oxide	$NO^{\bullet}$	Nitrous acid	HNO_2
Nitrogen dioxide	$NO_2^{\bullet}$	Nitrosyl cation	NO^+
		Nitroxyl anion	NO^-
		Dinitrogen tetroxide	N_2O_4
		Dinitrogen trioxide	N_2O_3
		Peroxynitrite	$ONOO^-$
		Peroxynitrous acid	ONOOH
		Nitronium (nitryl) cation	NO_2^+
		Nitryl chloride	NO_2Cl
		Alkyl peroxynitrite	ROONO

Table 1. Overview of reactive oxygen and nitrogen species.

3. Sources of ROS in semen

Virtually every ejaculate may contain potential sources of ROS. Leukocytes activated by multiple factors, especially inflammation and infection, are among significant ROS producers in semen [17]. Subpopulations of leukocytes, which may be found in semen, mainly consist of polymorphonuclear (PMN) leukocytes (50–60%) and macrophages (20–30%) [18]. PMN leukocytes represent an important source of ROS due to their abundant presence in semen. Furthermore, external stimuli induce the activation of macrophages, leading to an oxidative burst and ROS overgeneration. Under normal circumstances, these monocytes are of paramount importance in defending male reproductive structures against nearby cells and pathogens [19].

The Endz test based on myeloperoxidase staining is an efficient technique to quantify seminal leukocytes during semen quality assessment [20]. According to the World Health Organization (WHO), if the leukocyte concentration in the ejaculate exceeds 1×10^6/mL, leukocytospermia is present [21].

Numerous reports have studied possible relationships between seminal leukocytes and male reproductive dysfunction, resulting in two different directions. On the one hand, some studies failed to reveal any correlation between leukocytospermia and sperm damage [22], whereas inversely, other studies emphasized on a strong link between the presence of seminal leukocytes and abnormal sperm quality [23]. In particular, Sharma et al. [24] observed that even small numbers of white blood cells may be responsible for seminal OS, and hence subthreshold levels of leukocytes, as seen in ejaculates collected from otherwise healthy subjects, may not be considered safe as previously believed. Moreover, activated leukocytes may be responsible for a 100-fold increase in ROS production in comparison to non-activated white blood cells [25].

Leukocytospermia has been furthermore associated with increased ROS production by spermatozoa, most likely triggered by a direct cell-to-cell contact of the leukocyte with the sperm cell or by the release of soluble products acting on the spermatozoon [23, 24].

Spermatozoa have also been reported to generate ROS independently of leukocytes, and this ability primarily depends on the maturation level of the sperm cell. During the epididymal transit, the main morphological change that takes place in the spermatozoon is the migration of the cytoplasmic droplet, a remnant of the cytoplasm associated with testicular sperm. The droplet migrates from the proximal to the distal position during maturation and is normally shed from spermatozoa during or shortly after ejaculation [26]. Failure to extrude excess cytoplasm during sperm differentiation and maturation traps a number of enzymes, including glucose-6-phosphate dehydrogenase (G6PD) and ß-nicotinamide adenine dinucleotide phosphate (NADPH) oxidase, which have been associated with ROS generation through the formation of the NADPH intermediate [27]. As such, immature and functionally defective spermatozoa with abnormal head morphology and cytoplasmic retention are another important source of ROS in semen [12]. According to Gil-Guzman et al. [28] there is a strong positive correlation between immature spermatozoa and ROS production, which in turn is negatively correlated with semen quality. The study revealed that after a density gradient separation of human ejaculates, the layer of immature spermatozoa produced the highest levels of ROS. Furthermore, elevated concentrations of immature spermatozoa were accompanied by increased amounts of mature spermatozoa with damaged DNA [28].

Sertoli cells have also been revealed to have the ability to generate ROS, which may be inhibited by the addition of scavestrogens (J811 and J861). Scavestrogens are derivates of 17alpha-estradiol and serve as effective FR-quenching molecules that able to inhibit iron-catalyzed cell damage *in vitro*. As such, Sertoli cells may play a vital role in ROS-mediated spermatogenesis. Due to currently limited evidence, there is a need to further understand the function of Sertoli cells in the process of ROS generation [29, 30].

Varicocele is defined as the excessive dilation of the *pampiniform venous plexus* around the spermatic cord and this endogenous condition is highly linked to testicular and seminal OS. While its role in male infertility is well researched, recent studies have linked higher grades of varicocele with higher ROS levels [29]. In addition, research has shown that spermatozoa from varicocele patients tend to have high levels of oxidative DNA damage [31]. The most common management option is varicocelectomy, which has been effective in the reduction of ROS levels in affected patients [29, 31].

3.1. Endogenous ROS production by sperm

Superoxide ($O_2^{\bullet-}$) is considered to be the primary ROS produced by respiring cells, including spermatozoa [32]. It is a regular by-product of oxidative phosphorylation, created between complex I and III of the electron transport chain as a result of a monovalent reduction of oxygen and the addition of a single electron [33].

In the male gamete, $O_2^{\bullet-}$ is predominantly generated through two reduced forms of ß-nicotinamide adenine dinucleotide phosphate (NADPH) oxidases that are similar to those found in phagocytic leukocytes: the NADH-dependent oxidoreductase located in the inner mitochondrial membrane and the NAD(P)H-oxidase found in the plasma membrane [34]. The hypothesis that these enzymes are primarily responsible for low-level generation of $O_2^{\bullet-}$ important in cell signaling events in spermatozoa is based essentially on two observations. Firstly, adding pharmacological doses of NADPH to purified sperm suspensions has led to an increase in $O_2^{\bullet-}$ production, subsequently leading to a decline in the sperm function [34, 35]. Secondly, such increased $O_2^{\bullet-}$ production could be inhibited by superoxide dismutase (SOD), which protects male reproductive cells against the toxic effects of NADPH [34]. Additionally, the cytoplasmic enzyme G6PD controls the rate of glucose flux and intracellular availability of NADPH through the hexose monophosphate shunt. This in turn serves as a source of electrons by spermatozoa to fuel $O_2^{\bullet-}$ generation through the NADPH oxidase [35, 36]. Lastly, another relevant source of $O_2^{\bullet-}$ in spermatozoa is electron leakage from the mitochondrial electron transport [34].

Although $O_2^{\bullet-}$ is relatively unreactive, in the presence of hydrogen (H^+) it undergoes either a spontaneous or SOD-catalyzed dismutation into hydrogen peroxide (H_2O_2)—a membrane permeable molecule [15], which is considered to be the major initiator of peroxidative damage in the plasma membrane of spermatozoa [27]. H_2O_2 can be either scavenged by glutathione peroxidase (GPx) or catalase, catalyzing its dismutation into water and oxygen.

Moreover, $O_2^{\bullet-}$ as well as H_2O_2 can undergo a series of cellular transformations to generate the highly reactive hydroxyl radical ($OH^\bullet$) through the Fenton and Haber-Weiss reactions, comprising a reduction of ferric (Fe^{3+}) to ferrous ion (Fe^{2+}) in the presence of $O_2^{\bullet-}$, followed by the H_2O_2 conversion to $OH^\bullet$. Furthermore, $O_2^{\bullet-}$ has the ability to interact with nitric oxide ($NO^\bullet$) to generate peroxynitrite ($ONOO^-$), subsequent reactions of which may lead to either apoptosis or necrosis [30].

3.2. Endogenous RNS production by sperm

The primary RNS species produced by male gametes is nitric oxide ($NO^\bullet$). Its production is catalyzed by nitric oxide synthase (NOS) in a redox reaction between L-arginine and oxygen, initiated by NADPH, and with L-citrulline as a byproduct. $NO^\bullet$ interacts with $O_2^{\bullet-}$ to create peroxynitrite ($ONOO^-$), a highly toxic-free radical [13]. Interestingly, both high and low concentrations of $NO^\bullet$ may result in significant alterations of the sperm function as a result of the production of $ONOO^-$ [30].

Inversely, physiological $NO^\bullet$ levels are reported to have beneficial effects, acting in signal transduction pathways involved in spermatozoa motility, capacitation and acrosome reaction [37].

3.3. External sources of ROS

ROS generation can be exacerbated by a multitude of environmental, infectious and lifestyle-related etiologies.

A wide range of industrial by-products and waste chemicals (e.g. polychlorinated biphenyls, nonylphenol or dioxins) have been associated with several adverse health effects, many of which are related to male infertility. These chemicals have been shown to increase the production of reactive species such as $O_2^{\bullet-}$ and H_2O_2 in the testes, damage sperm DNA and impair spermatogenesis [38]. Persistent environmental contaminants, such as heavy metals and pesticides, may also lead to OS, particularly among workers exposed to such pollutants. These individuals often present with a decreased semen volume and density, accompanied by increased oxidative damage to the sperm lipids, proteins and DNA [39].

Radiation is a natural source of energy with significant effects on living organisms. Mobile devices are becoming more accessible to the general population, particularly to adolescent males and men of reproductive age. Cell phones release radiofrequency electromagnetic radiation, exposure to which has shown to increase the risk of oligo-, astheno- or teratozoospermia. Furthermore, *in vitro* studies have demonstrated that EMR induces ROS generation and DNA fragmentation in human spermatozoa, alongside a decreased sperm concentration, motility and vitality depending on the duration of exposure to radiation [40].

Various components of cigarette smoke have been associated with OS exacerbation. Cigarettes contain a broad array of free radical-inducing agents such as nicotine, cotinine, hydroxycotinine, alkaloids and nitrosamines [41, 42]. The prime component of tobacco is nicotine, which is a well-known ROS producer in spermatozoa with detrimental effects on the sperm count, motility and morphology. Moreover, smokers exhibited a lower hypo-osmotic swelling test percentage, indicating a weaker plasma membrane integrity when compared to non-smokers [41]. Smoking increases ROS production by causing leukocytospermia as shown by Saleh et al. [42], who also demonstrated that in smokers, the seminal ROS and total antioxidant capacity score was increased—a direct indication of oxidative imbalance in affected ejaculates. A different study showed that levels of seminal plasma antioxidants were diminished in smokers. This was furthermore confirmed by the presence of increased levels of 8-hydroxy-2′-deoxyguanosine [43].

By directly affecting the liver, alcohol intake increases ROS production while simultaneously decreasing the antioxidant capacity of the body. Although alcohol consumption has been repeatedly associated with systemic OS, its effect on semen parameters has not been explored to a larger extent. In a study comprising 8344 subjects, moderate alcohol consumption did not negatively affect semen parameters [44]. Nevertheless, it was revealed that chronic drinkers had reduced levels of testosterone, possibly due to an impaired hypothalamic-pituitary axis and damage to the Leydig cells [45]. Increased alcohol levels block gonadotropin-releasing hormone, leading to reduced luteinizing hormone and testosterone levels. Furthermore, alcohol has been shown to increase ROS generation when consumed by malnourished individuals [44].

Lastly, diet may affect semen parameters. In a Danish study, men with the highest saturated fat intake presented with a significantly lower total sperm count and concentration in comparison to those with the lowest saturated fat intake [46]. These observations were supported by a later report focused on studying the link between dairy food intake and male fertility and revealing that a low-fat dairy diet may lead to a higher spermatogenesis [47]. On the other hand, omega-3 fatty acids and omega-6 fatty acids were shown to improve sperm count, motility and morphology [48]. With regard to obesity and its relation to semen parameters, currently available data are conflicting. In a study on Iranian men, it was found that overweight men tend to have lower sperm counts [49]. Inversely, a different study reported that underweight subjects had lower sperm counts than normal and overweight men [48]. Moreover, a study comprising Tunisian men revealed that sperm concentration, motility and morphology did not vary across different BMI values [50].

4. Physiological roles of ROS

Aerobic metabolism utilizing oxygen is essential for energy requirements of reproductive cells, and free radicals do play a significant role in physiological processes occurring within the male reproductive tract. Spermatozoa themselves produce small amounts of ROS that are essential for a variety of physiological processes such as capacitation, hyperactivation, acrosome reaction and sperm-oocyte fusion [30].

4.1. Sperm maturation

During transit and storage in the epididymis, spermatozoa undergo membrane, nuclear and enzymatic remodeling, involving the release, attachment and rearrangement of surface proteins [6, 30, 51]. Such changes are based on the assembly of several signal transduction pathways necessary for the subsequent ability of spermatozoa to undergo hyperactivation and capacitation.

ROS are essential for a proper chromatin packing during the maturation of mammalian spermatozoa, leading to a characteristic chromatin stability. This unique chromatin architecture results from an extensive inter- and intra-molecular disulfide bond stabilization between the cysteine residues of protamines—small nuclear proteins that replace histones during spermatogenesis. Oxidation of the thiol groups in protamines takes place during the transport of spermatozoa from the caput to the cauda epididymis [52]. As demonstrated by Aitken et al. [53], a spontaneous luminol peroxidase signal indicating the presence of ROS was exclusive to mature spermatozoa collected from the cauda region. ROS may act as oxidizing agents in this process, hence facilitating the formation of disulfide bonds, increasing chromatin stability and protecting DNA from possible damage [30, 52]. As spermatozoa possess minimal to none repair mechanisms [9], chromatin condensation is a crucial protective mechanism, in which ROS actually protect male gametes against future oxidative insults.

Likewise, peroxides have been associated with formation of the mitochondrial capsule—a coat surrounding sperm mitochondria providing protection against possible proteolytic degradation [54]. It is suggested that during spermatogenesis peroxides may oxidize the active form of phospholipid hydroperoxide glutathione peroxidase (PHGPx), creating an intermediate that subsequently interacts with thiol groups to form a seleno-disulfide bond. The resulting mitochondrial capsule is made out of a complex protein network rich in disulfide bonds. Mitochondria require such protection as their proper function is crucial for metabolism, cell cycle control and oxidative balance [51, 53, 54].

Although several studies have reported improved sperm DNA integrity and reduced ROS production as a result of daily antioxidant consumption [55], an unusual decondensation of sperm DNA has been revealed as well [56]. Hence it may be hypothesized that high antioxidant levels may alter the oxidative conditions necessary for a proper formation of the inter- and intra-molecular disulfide bonds, leading to a lower DNA compaction.

4.2. Capacitation

Capacitation is a prominent process of final maturation that spermatozoa undergo in the female reproductive tract, during which sperm motility changes from a progressive state to a highly energetic one. It is hypothesized that capacitation occurs exclusively in mature spermatozoa in order to reach the oocyte taking advantage of hyperactive motility and an increased responsiveness to chemotactic agents. Numerous receptors on the sperm head become activated, providing energy to the sperm to penetrate the zona pellucida. As such, capacitation sets up the path necessary for subsequent hyperactivation and acrosome reaction [57]. Most prominent molecular processes associated with capacitation include Ca^{2+} and HCO_3^- influx, cholesterol efflux, increased cAMP activity, ROS generation, pH, protein phosphorylation and membrane hyperpolarization [32, 58].

Numerous of studies on both human and animal spermatozoa indicate that H_2O_2 is the primary ROS responsible for capacitation to occur. This process is associated with an increase in tyrosine phosphorylation, and it has been shown that the amount and banding pattern of tyrosine phosphorylation by adding exogenous H_2O_2 was similar to that observed during endogenous ROS production, providing evidence that H_2O_2 may be responsible for the enhancement of capacitation [32, 57, 58]. This hypothesis was further confirmed by Rivlin et al. [59] who showed that catalase decreased, while H_2O_2 increased the tyrosine phosphorylation in a dose-dependent manner, thereby solidifying the involvement of H_2O_2 in the process of capacitation.

At the same time, de Lamirande and Gagnon [58] indicated that $O_2^{\bullet-}$ may be also involved in this process. Of note is also the role of $NO^{\bullet}$, which is present in the female genital tract. $NO^{\bullet}$ may initiate the acrosome reaction, the effects of which are likely achieved through a complex mechanism involving H_2O_2 [59, 60].

Finally, a combination of $O_2^{\bullet-}$ and $NO^{\bullet}$ forms $ONOO^-$, which allows oxysterol to be produced. Oxysterol, which removes cholesterol from the lipid bilayer, inhibits tyrosine phosphate and promotes cyclic adenosine 3′,5′-monophosphate (cAMP) production [60]. This process is vital as cAMP must increase in concentration for capacitation to occur. cAMP and its subsequent pathways involve protein kinase A, which phosphorylates MEK (extracellular signal-regulated kinase)-like proteins as well as tyrosine present in fibrous sheath proteins [57, 58].

The results of the above studies show that ROS can positively enhance sperm capacitation, but diverge over the specific ROS involved. Both $O_2^{\bullet-}$ and H_2O_2 may stimulate different molecules in the biochemical pathways, and depending on the *in vitro* method used to induce capacitation, specific ROS involved may therefore differ. Several studies have confirmed the lack of molecular specificity in the activation of capacitation and tyrosine phosphorylation, as both SOD and catalase have been shown to negate the positive effect exogenously induced capacitation and hyperactivation [59].

Although physiological ROS levels are necessary for capacitation, their overgeneration may trigger apoptosis. When the levels of oxysterols and lipid aldehydes increase, cell-mediated suicide may occur accompanied by an enhanced mitochondrial $O_2^{\bullet-}$ production, lipid peroxidation (LPO), cytochrome c release and subsequent caspase activation [53, 61].

4.3. Motility and hyperactivation

Hyperactivation is an incompletely understood process to be observed in the final maturation stage of spermatozoa and is considered a subcategory of capacitation. Normally spermatozoa exhibit a low amplitude flagellar movement accompanied by low, linear velocity. In the hyperactivated state, spermatozoa movement is of high amplitude, asymmetric flagellar movement, pronounced lateral head displacement and non-linear trajectory, allowing the sperm to penetrate the *cumulus oophorus* and zona pellucida surrounding the oocyte. Furthermore, hyperactive motility may enable the progressive movement through the oviduct by preventing stagnation, adding yet another benefit to the sperm function [62]. The biochemistry of hyperactivation is poorly understood, but it is known to involve a rise in cAMP activity and pH [58], increased generation of ROS, an initial influx of bicarbonate ions and an increase in intracellular Ca^{2+} concentrations [62].

Extracellular $O_2^{\bullet-}$ is considered nearly essential for hyperactivation in mammalian spermatozoa, as the presence of SOD, but not catalase, reduced the percentage of spermatozoa exhibiting hyperactivity in a variety of culture media [58]. *In vitro* experiments have also revealed that $O_2^{\bullet-}$ is a vital trigger of sperm motility hyperactivation [30]. At the same time, $NO^{\bullet}$ plays important roles in regulating hyperactivation in mammalian epididymis. H_2O_2 may interact with this process as well; however, its activity may be dependent upon $NO^{\bullet}$ regulation. This hypothesis was confirmed by *in vitro* experiments, according to which catalase vital against H_2O_2 toxicity prevents $NO^{\bullet}$-induced capacitation and hyperactivation [60].

4.4. Acrosome reaction

Acrosome reaction (AR) is related to the release of proteolytic enzymes, primarily acrosin and hyaluronidase, in order to degrade the zona pellucida of the oocyte. Once degraded, hyperactive motility propels the spermatozoa into the perivitelline space, at which point the spermatozoa may eventually fuse with the oocyte [63]. Compared to the slow, reversible process of capacitation, this is a permanent, fast-acting step associated with a respiratory burst (rapid extracellular $O_2^{\bullet-}$ production) increasing the tyrosine phosphorylation of specific proteins [57, 64]. $O_2^{\bullet-}$ produced *via* NADPH oxidase may dismutate into H_2O_2, and these two molecules may have a positive effect on the AR [6, 32, 64]. •NO has also been reported to increase the percentage of sperm undergoing the AR [37]. At the same time, results regarding the specific ROS are conflicting. The majority of studies note positive effects of H_2O_2 and negative effects of catalase, thus suggesting that H_2O_2 is the major species responsible for a proper AR [58, 64].

Moreover, ROS act as signal transducers in the AR. Elevated ROS production may occur upon interaction with the *cumulus oophorus*, thereby enhancing the signal for exocytosis initiated by either progesterone or the zona pellucida. *In vivo*, binding of the zona pellucida and a certain stimulus *via* progesterone on capacitated spermatozoa initiates this process and is associated with an influx of extracellular Ca^{2+} into the cytosol [6]. *In vitro* studies indicate that ROS can induce the Ca^{2+} influx and initiates the biochemical cascade associated with the AR [53, 64].

4.5. Sperm-oocyte fusion

A link exists between enhanced ROS levels and increased sperm-oocyte fusion. High rates of sperm-oocyte fusion are correlated with increased expression of phosphorylated tyrosine proteins [6], suggesting that sperm-oocyte fusion is related to the events of capacitation and AR. Both H_2O_2 and $O_2^{\bullet-}$ contribute to the increase in fertilization rates as revealed by the fact that the addition of catalase or SOD significantly decreased the fusogenicity, whereas the addition of H_2O_2 or $O_2^{\bullet-}$ significantly increased the fusogenicity [53, 64].

Ultimately, ROS are thought to increase membrane fluidity using two mechanisms: (1) de-esterification of membrane phospholipids and (2) activation of phospholipase A2 (PLA2) [65].

Once the zona pellucida and corona radiata are penetrated by the sperm cell, the oocyte prevents eventual polyspermy by turning the vitelline layer into a hard envelope. o,o-Dityrosine crosslinks catalyzed by ovoperoxidase lead to the formation of a single macromolecular structure acting as the envelope [66]. H_2O_2 serves as the substrate to ovoperoxidase to provide for the envelope formation. With our understanding of ROS and their spermicidal effect, H_2O_2 proves to be an effective spermicide agent against polyspermy [66, 67].

5. Oxidative stress (OS)

The term oxidative stress refers to a critical imbalance between ROS production and antioxidant defense mechanisms available to the biological system [15]. According to Sies [5], it is a disturbance in the prooxidant-antioxidant balance in favor of the former, leading to potential cellular damage.

Essentially, OS may result from:

1. Diminished antioxidants, e.g. mutations affecting antioxidant defense enzymes or toxic agents that deplete such mechanisms [5].
2. Increased ROS or RNS generation either by exposure to increased levels of toxins that act as reactive species themselves or are metabolized to induce further biological oxidation or

by excessive activation of 'natural' FR-generating systems (e.g. phagocytic oxidative outburst during chronic inflammatory diseases) [5, 15]. This mechanism is normally thought to be more relevant to mammalian diseases and is frequently the target of attempted therapeutic intervention.

OS can result in:

1. Adaptation: Usually by upregulation of antioxidant defense systems.
2. Cell and tissue injury: OS can cause damage to all molecular targets: DNA, proteins and lipids. Often it is not clear which is the first point of attack, since injury mechanisms may overlap [5].
3. Cell death: This process may occur by two mechanisms, necrosis or apoptosis. During necrotic cell death, the cell swells and ruptures, releasing its contents into surrounding areas and affecting adjacent cells. The intracellular content can include antioxidants such as catalase or glutathione (GSH) as well as prooxidants such as copper and iron. As such, necrosis may lead to further oxidative insults in the internal milieu [3–5, 15]. During apoptosis, the cell's own "suicide mechanism" gets activated. As such, apoptotic cells do not release their content into surrounding environment and apoptosis does not cause damage to the neighboring cells [5].

An intricate cellular architecture of spermatozoa renders them to be particularly sensitive to OS. Sperm plasma membranes contain large quantities of polyunsaturated fatty acids (PUFAs). On the other hand, their cytoplasm contains low concentrations of scavenging enzymes [68]. OS usually results in a decreased sperm motion and viability, accompanied by a rapid loss of ATP, axonemal damage, increased midpiece morphology defects, followed by alterations in the sperm capacitation and acrosome reaction [32]. Lipid peroxidation has been repeatedly postulated to be the key mechanism of ROS-induced sperm damage, possibly leading to male reproductive dysfunction [68].

5.1. Lipid peroxidation (LPO)

Sperm plasma membranes are largely composed of PUFAs, which are exceptionally susceptible to oxidative damage due to the presence of more than two carbon–carbon double bonds [68]. These fatty acids maintain the fluidity of membranes [69]. ROS attack PUFAs, leading to a cascade of chemical reactions called lipid peroxidation (LPO). As the LPO proceeds, more than 60% of PUFAs may be lost. LPO affects most prominent structural and functional characteristics of the membrane, including fluidity, ion gradients, receptor transduction, transport processes as well as enzymatic activities. As a result, properties that are crucial for a normal fertilization are impaired [68, 69].

LPO is a self-propagating process that may be divided into three phases: the initiation phase, the propagation phase and the termination phase. Before any of these processes takes place, $O_2^{\bullet-}$ is generated either intracellularly through the NADPH system or through leukocytes as an extracellular source. $O_2^{\bullet-}$ can be directly protonated to create the hydroperoxyl radical ($HO_2^{\bullet}$) or it can be converted into H_2O_2 *via* SOD. H_2O_2 may be subsequently converted into $OH^{\bullet}$ *via* the Fenton reaction involving ferrous iron. Generation of $OH^{\bullet}$ and $HO_2^{\bullet}$ mark the beginning of the initiation stage, as neither $O_2^{\bullet-}$ nor H_2O_2 is not energetically rich enough to initiate LPO directly [70]. During the initiation phase, one hydrogen is taken from unsaturated lipids to form lipid radicals. These radicals subsequently interact with oxygen to generate lipid $HO_2^{\bullet}$, which may be transformed into lipid peroxides through available antioxidants, stabilizing the sperm plasma membrane. Nevertheless, during the propagation stage, in the presence of a transition metal ion, lipid peroxides will be transformed into alkoxyl radical and $HO_2^{\bullet}$ through the Fenton and Haber-Weiss reaction, subsequently acting upon additional lipids until the damage is widespread and irreversible [68–70]. During the termination phase, two radicals react with each other to form a stable product and LPO finally ceases [70].

Numerous pathological effects of LPO on the sperm function are currently known. Overall, LPO causes DNA and protein damage through oxidation of lipid peroxyl or alkoxyl radicals. DNA fragmentation by LPO can occur *via* base modifications, strand breaks or crosslinks [71]. LPO generally results in loss of membrane fluidity and subsequently a decreased sperm motility and sperm-oocyte fusion [68–71].

Furthermore, during LPO, ROS initiate a cascade of events involving the xanthine and xanthine oxidase system and deplete the ATP production which may ultimately lead to sperm death [68].

5.2. DNA damage

The unique sperm chromatin packing alongside antioxidant molecules present in the seminal plasma provide notable protection to sperm DNA against oxidative damage. Nevertheless, spermatozoa lack any specific DNA repair mechanisms and hence depend on the oocyte for eventual DNA repair following fertilization. ROS-associated catalysis and apoptosis are considered to be the primary mechanisms that induce DNA fragmentation in spermatozoa [72].

DNA bases and phosphodiester backbones are believed to be most susceptible to ROS-associated peroxidative damage. At the same time, sperm mitochondrial DNA is more vulnerable to oxidative insults when compared to the nuclear genome [73]. Furthermore, because of the structure of the Y chromosome as well as its inability to repair double strand breaks, Y-bearing spermatozoa are more susceptible to DNA damage than X-carrying counterparts [74]. Y-bearing spermatogonia can be a target of mutations in the euchromatic Y region (Yq11), known as the azoospermia factor, resulting in infertility [75].

Various types of DNA abnormalities may occur in sperm that have been exposed to ROS artificially. These include base modifications, production of base-free sites, deletions, frame shifts, DNA crosslinks and chromosomal rearrangements. OS has also been associated with high frequencies of single- and double-strand DNA breaks. ROS can also cause gene mutations, such as point mutation and polymorphism, resulting in decreased semen quality. These changes may be observed especially during the prolonged meiotic prophase, when the spermatocytes are particularly sensitive to damage and widespread degeneration can occur [72–74]. Also, mutations in the mitochondrial DNA (mtDNA) may cause a defect of mitochondrial energy metabolism and therefore lower levels of mutant mtDNA may compromise sperm motility *in vivo* [76]. Other mechanisms such as denaturation and DNA base-pair oxidation may also be involved [74].

Increased DNA damage has become a serious issue during artificial reproduction techniques (ARTs), as it has been correlated with decreased fertilization rates *in vitro* and increased early embryo death. Unfortunately, no successful method to prevent or treat sperm DNA damage is currently available [77].

5.3. Protein oxidation

Proteins are a critical target for oxidation because of their abundance and high rate constants for interactions with diverse ROS. As such, protein damage is a major consequence of both intracellular and extracellular oxidative insults. ROS may attack both the side chains and backbone, and the extent of the insult depends on multiple factors. In some cases, the damage is limited to specific residues, whereas in case of other ROS, the damage is widespread and nonspecific [78].

Oxidative attacks on proteins generally result in site-specific amino acid modifications, fragmentation of the peptide chain, aggregation of cross-linked reaction products, altered electric charge and increased susceptibility or extreme tolerance to proteolysis [79].

The resulting products of protein oxidation include reactive hydroperoxides, which may be employed as biomarkers for protein oxidation *in vitro* and *in vivo*. As protein damage is usually non-repairable, oxidation may have deleterious consequences, including the loss (or sometimes gain) of enzymatic, structural or signaling function, fragmentation, unfolding, altered interactions with other proteins and modified turnovers. Generally, oxidized proteins are degraded by proteasomal and lysosomal pathways; however, in some cases, such altered material is poorly degraded and may accumulate within cells contributing to multiple mammalian pathologies [78, 79].

The amino acids in a peptide differ in their susceptibility to oxidative insults, while various ROS differ in their potential reactivity. Primary, secondary and tertiary protein structures alter the relative susceptibility of certain amino acids. Sulfur-containing amino acids and particularly thiol (–SH) groups are very susceptible to ROS-associated damage [79, 80].

According to Mammoto et al. [81], protein oxidation in spermatozoa leads to a blocked sperm-egg fusion, the capacity to penetrate the zona pellucida, as well as sperm-egg binding. Sinha et al. [80] showed that oligospermia is linked to a quantitative reduction in the SH-groups in spermatozoa. Thus, oxidation of the sperm SH-proteins may be a notable mechanism responsible for the suppressive effects of ROS on sperm functions.

5.4. Apoptosis

Usually, when cellular components undergo serious damage, apoptosis or programmed cell death is initiated. During spermatogenesis, abnormal spermatozoa are eliminated primarily through apoptosis. The exact mechanism of action is not fully understood yet; however, previous studies have speculated that ROS serve as an activator of the mitochondria to release the signaling cytochrome c [82, 83]. This molecule initiates a cascade of events involving caspases 3 and 9, eventually leading to sperm apoptosis. The Fas-protein may be also an integral component in the apoptotic pathway. When Fas-ligand or anti-Fas antibody binds to Fas, apoptosis is initiated [83]. An additional mechanism involves the inflammatory production of ROS, primarily hypochlorous acid (HOCl), which is a product of H_2O_2 and chloride ion. This molecule oxidizes a variety of cellular components, thus causing apoptosis [84]. Said et al. [85] emphasized that HOCl is associated with elevated levels of apoptotic markers in spermatozoa.

Numerous studies have focused to study apoptosis in spermatozoa. Various authors [35, 86] have reported increased ROS levels and apoptotic markers measured by fluorescence in samples of infertile subjects. In deer spermatozoa, it was demonstrated that H_2O_2 addition stimulates apoptosis, whereas $O_2^{\bullet -}$ and $OH^{\bullet}$ do not have this ability [86]. Meanwhile studies in primate, murine and boar spermatozoa indicated that $NO^{\bullet}$ was correlated with apoptosis possibly through caspase activation [87, 88].

On the other hand, in certain males, abortive apoptosis appears to fail in the clearance of spermatozoa that are marked for elimination by apoptosis. As such, the subsequent population of ejaculated spermatozoa may exhibit an array of anomalies consistent with characteristics typical for cells that are in the process of apoptosis. Apoptotic failures may lead to a decreased sperm count resulting in subfertility [82, 83].

5.5. Effects on sperm motility

Spermatozoa motility is an important prerequisite to secure their distribution in the female sexual system, followed by an effective passage through the cervical mucus and penetration into the egg [89]. Increased ROS levels have been repeatedly correlated with a decreased sperm motility [10–12, 90], although the exact mechanism involved is still not completely understood. One hypothesis suggests that H_2O_2 diffuses across the membranes into the cells and inhibits the activity of vital enzymes such as NADPH oxidase [6]. At the same time, a decreased G6PDH leads to a reduced availability of NADPH accompanied by a build-up of oxidized glutathione. Such changes may lead to a decline in the intracellular antioxidant levels and a subsequent peroxidation of membrane phospholipids [65].

Another hypothesis presents a series of interrelated events leading to a decreased phosphorylation of axonemal proteins, followed by sperm immobilization, both of which are linked to a reduced membrane fluidity crucial for sperm-oocyte fusion [10, 32]. When spermatozoa are incubated with selected ROS overnight, loss of motion characteristics observed is highly correlated with sperm LPO. Furthermore, the ability of antioxidants to revive sperm motility is evidence that LPO is a major cause for motility loss in spermatozoa [68, 69].

6. The role of antioxidants in male reproduction

Because ROS have both physiological and pathological functions, biological systems have developed defense systems to maintain ROS levels within a certain range. Whenever ROS levels become pathologically elevated, antioxidants scavenge them to minimize any potential oxidative damage [1].

Antioxidants are defined as molecules that dispose, scavenge and inhibit the formation of ROS or oppose their actions. According to Ďuračková [13], antioxidants can protect cells against OS *via* three mechanisms: prevention, interception and repair.

Antioxidants may be divided into two dominant categories:

- Enzymatic (e.g. superoxide dismutases, catalase and glutathione peroxidases).
- Non-enzymatic (e.g. vitamin C, vitamin E, vitamin A, carotenoids, albumin, glutathione, uric acid, pyruvate, etc.) [13].

Due to the size and small volume of cytoplasm, as well as the low concentrations of scavenging enzymes, spermatozoa have limited antioxidant defense possibilities. Mammalian spermatozoa predominantly contain enzymatic antioxidants, including SOD and glutathione peroxidases (GPx), which are mainly located in the midpiece. A few non-enzymatic antioxidants, such as vitamins C and E, transferrin and ceruloplasmin, are present in the plasma membrane of spermatozoa and act as preventive antioxidants [16].

Under normal circumstances, the seminal plasma is an important protectant of spermatozoa against any possible ROS formation and distribution. Seminal plasma contains both enzymatic antioxidants, as well as an array of non-enzymatic antioxidants (e.g. ascorbate, urate, vitamin E, pyruvate, glutathione, albumin, taurine and hypotaurine) [9].

Studies have shown that antioxidants protect spermatozoa from ROS generating abnormal spermatozoa, scavenge ROS produced by leukocytes, prevent DNA fragmentation, improve semen quality, reduce cryodamage to spermatozoa, block premature sperm maturation and generally stimulate sperm vitality [91, 92].

6.1. Superoxide dismutases (SOD)

Superoxide dismutases are metal-containing enzymes that catalyze the conversion of two superoxides into oxygen and hydrogen peroxide, which is less toxic than superoxide [1, 13]:

$$M^{(n+1)+} - SOD + O_2^{\bullet -} \rightarrow M^{n+} - SOD + O_2 \quad (1)$$

$$Mn^{+} - SOD + O_2^{\bullet -} + 2H^{+} \rightarrow M^{(n+1)+} - SOD + H_2O_2 \tag{2}$$

where M = Cu (n = 1); Mn (n = 2); Fe (n = 2); Ni (n = 2).

The enzymes are present in both intracellular and extracellular forms. The first intracellular form is the dimeric copper-zinc SOD, localized primarily in the cytosol and/or intermembrane space and containing copper and zinc (Cu/ZnSOD, SOD-1) in its active center. The second form is manganese SOD, which is found predominantly in the mitochondrial matrix and has manganese in its active center (MnSOD, SOD-2) [93].

The secretory tetrameric SOD (EC-SOD, SOD-3) may be detected in the extracellular space. The enzyme is associated with surface polysaccharides although it may also be found as a free molecule. Structurally, SOD-3 is similar to SOD-2; however, it has zinc and copper in its active center instead of manganese [1, 5, 15]. The cytosolic Cu/Zn-SOD is the dominant SOD isoenzyme found in the seminal plasma and spermatozoa [93].

SOD protects spermatozoa against spontaneous O_2 toxicity and lipid peroxidation [69]. The enzyme also prevents premature hyperactivation and capacitation induced by $O_2^{\bullet -}$ before ejaculating [10, 32].

Numerous studies have suggested a significant role for SOD in sperm motility both *in vivo* and *in vitro*. The addition of SOD to human and animal semen [94–96] has been shown to protect spermatozoa against the harmful effects of ROS and improve sperm motility and membrane integrity during liquid storage or cryopreservation. As such, it may be concluded that the SOD content in mature spermatozoa may be a good predictor of post-thaw motility recovery following sperm preservation.

6.2. Catalase (CAT)

Catalase catalyzes the decomposition of hydrogen peroxide to molecular oxygen and water, thereby completing the detoxifying reaction started by SOD. A characteristic feature of its structure is a heme system with centrally located iron [1, 13]:

$$H_2O_2 + Fe(III) - E \rightarrow H_2O + O = Fe(IV) - E(.+) \tag{3}$$

$$H_2O_2 + O = Fe(IV) - E(.+) \rightarrow H_2O + Fe(III) - E + O_2 \tag{4}$$

Fe()-E represents the iron center of the heme group attached to the enzyme.

CAT has been found in peroxisomes, mitochondria, endoplasmic reticulum and the cytosol in a variety of cells [93]. In semen, the enzyme was detected in human, bovine and rat spermatozoa, as well as seminal plasma, with the prostate as its source [97, 98].

Catalase activates sperm capacitation induced by nitric oxide [59, 60]. Furthermore, it plays an important role in decreasing lipid peroxidation and protecting spermatozoa during genitourinary inflammation [25].

Numerous studies have revealed a positive relationship between sperm motility and the presence of CAT in mammalian ejaculates. Also, positive correlations were observed between sperm morphology and protein expression of CAT in seminal plasma [98, 99]. Furthermore, CAT supplementation to fresh, processed and cryopreserved semen resulted in a higher sperm vitality, progressive motility and DNA integrity [100].

6.3. Glutathione peroxidase (GPx)

Glutathione peroxidases are a family of selenium-containing enzymes, which catalyze the reduction of H_2O_2 and organic peroxides, including phospholipid peroxides [93]. In their active site, the enzymes contain selenium in the form of selenocysteine.

The net reaction catalyzed by glutathione peroxidase may be represented as:

$$2GSH + H_2O_2 \rightarrow GS-SG + 2H_2O \qquad (5)$$

where GSH symbolizes reduced glutathione and GS-SG represents glutathione disulfide. The reaction is based on the oxidation of selenol of a selenocysteine residue by H_2O_2. This process leads to its derivation with selenic acid (RSeOH). This by-product is subsequently converted back to selenol through a two-step process that starts with a reaction comprising GSH to generate GS-SeR and water. A second GSH molecule then reduces the GS-SeR intermediate back to selenol, releasing GS-SG as a by-product [1, 5, 13]:

$$\begin{aligned} RSeH + H_2O_2 &\rightarrow RSeOH + H_2O \; RSeOH + GSH \\ &\rightarrow GS\text{-}SeR + H_2O \; GS\text{-}SeR + GSH \rightarrow GS\text{-}SG + RSeH \end{aligned} \qquad (6)$$

Glutathione reductase then reduces the oxidized glutathione to complete the cycle:

$$GS-SG + NADPH + H^+ \rightarrow 2\,GSH + NADP^+ \qquad (7)$$

The classic intracellular GPx1 is expressed in sperm nucleus, mitochondria and cytosol, as well as in the testes, prostate, seminal vesicles, vas deferens, epididymis, and has a significant relationship with sperm motility [101, 102].

More importantly, a direct relationship has been reported between male fertility and phospholipid hydroperoxide glutathione peroxidase (PHGPx; GPx4), a selenoprotein that is highly expressed in testicular tissue and has a prominent role in the formation of the mitochondrial capsule [51, 53, 54]. Glutathione peroxidases remove peroxyl ($ROO^\bullet$) radicals from various peroxides, including hydrogen peroxide [13].

6.4. Other enzymes

Other enzymes, such as glutathione reductase, ceruloplasmin or heme oxygenases, may also participate in the enzymatic control of oxygen radicals and their products. A short overview of minor antioxidant enzymes is provided in **Table 2**.

Glutathione reductase (GR)	• Location: Found in the epididymis, sertoli cells, vas deferens, seminal vesicles, epithelium and prostate gland [103, 104]. • Roles: Catalyzes reduction of oxidized glutathione. Maintains glutathione homeostasis. Altered in infertile men, and these alterations seem to be linked to sperm morphology [103–105].
Glutathione S-transferase (GST)	• Location: Most abundant in the seminiferous tubular fluid of mammalian testes, sperm acrosomes, human sperm and mouse spermatogenic cells [106–108]. • Roles: Detoxification enzymes, intracellular-binding proteins [106]. Involved in epididymal maturation, capacitation and sperm-oocyte interactions [107, 108].
Ceruloplasmin	• Location: Semen, probably of testicular origin [109]. • Roles: Cu-dependent ferroxidase, a fundamental bridge between Fe utilization and Cu status. Associated with the oxidation of ferrous ion into ferric [110]. Prevents non-enzymatic generation of superoxide and scavenges superoxide, hydroxyl and singlet oxygen [110, 111]. Has positive impact on sperm parameters and male fertility [112]. Serves as a marker of a proper seminiferous tubule function [109].
Transferrin	• Location: Seminal plasma [111, 113]. • Roles: Primary binding and transport protein for iron and regulates iron transport and storage [110]. Serves as a reliable index of seminiferous tubular function [111].
Heme oxygenase (HO)	• Location: Two forms of heme oxygenase, HO-1 and HO-2, were identified in human testis and seminal plasma [114, 115]. • Roles: HO is strongly induced by oxidant stress and protects against oxidative insults. Increases reduced glutathione levels, degrades heme and intervenes with the metabolism of biliverdin and bilirubin, which have potent antioxidant properties [116]. HO is highly expressed in fertile normozoospermic subjects with positive correlations to sperm concentration, motility and morphology. HO enzyme activity is related to spermatogenesis and sperm motility processes [114, 115].

Table 2. Overview of minor antioxidant enzymes.

6.5. Non-enzymatic antioxidants

Non-enzymatic antioxidants are also known as synthetic antioxidants or dietary supplements. The body's complex antioxidant system is affected by dietary intake of antioxidants, vitamins and minerals, such as vitamin C, vitamin E, zinc, selenium, taurine and glutathione.

6.5.1. Glutathione (GSH)

Glutathione is the most abundant thiol protein in mammalian cells [117]. Being an endogenous source, it is synthesized by the liver but it can also be derived from dietary sources such as fresh meat, fruits and vegetables. This molecule has three precursors: cysteine, glutamic acid and glycine. Its cysteine subunit provides and exposes -SH that directly scavenges free radicals. Once oxidized, GS-SG is then regenerated/reduced by glutathione reductase to complete the cycle [13].

High levels are found especially in the testis of rats [118] and the reproductive tract fluids and epididymal sperm of bulls [98]. GSH protects the cell membranes from lipid oxidation and prevents further formation of free radicals. Its deficit leads to instability of the sperm midpiece, which results in motility disorders [118]. Glutathione supplementation in infertile subjects has led to a significant improvement in sperm parameters and prevents oxidative damage to sperm DNA. A factor increasing the level of GSH is pantothenic acid, which by doing so also protects tissues against oxidative stress [117, 118].

6.5.2. *Vitamin C*

Vitamin C or ascorbic acid (AA) may be found in its reduced (ascorbate) as well as oxidized form (dehydroascorbic acid), both of which are easily interconvertible and biologically active. Vitamin C is found in citrus fruits, peppers, strawberries, tomatoes, broccoli, brussels sprouts and other leafy vegetables. AA is a water-soluble vitamin, and because of its hydrophilic nature, it has more effective scavenging properties at the plasma level than in the lipid bilayer [119].

Vitamin C has been used in the management of male infertility on empirical grounds, particularly in the presence of non-specific seminal infections [120]. Its presence in the seminal plasma of healthy males has been reported by various authors [121–123]. Chinoy et al. [124] stated that AA was essential for the structural and functional integrity of androgen-dependent reproductive organs. Low concentration of vitamin C showed significant degenerative changes in the testes, epididymis and vas deferens of scorbutic guinea pigs. On the other hand, excessive intake of vitamin C has been reported to cause reproductive failure in the men [125].

AA deficiency may lead to an increase in oxidative damage induced by ROS and a disturbed oxidative balance was observed in ejaculates of 25–45% of infertile men [123]. This was further corroborated by the association of decreased AA followed by an increase in the seminal plasma LPO as observed in a human trial [126, 127]. Moreover, it has been reported that AA supplementation leads to a significant reduction in the ROS concentration, sperm membrane LPO and DNA oxidation together with an increased sperm quality. The results of a recent animal experimental study indicate that vitamin C improves the activity of antioxidant enzymes and significantly reduces malondialdehyde (MDA) concentration in testicular structures [127].

6.5.3. *Vitamin E*

Vitamin E is a term that encompasses a group of potent, lipid-soluble tocol (tocopherol) and tocotrienol derivatives qualitatively exhibiting the biological activity of RRR-α-tocopherol. Structural analyses have revealed that molecules having vitamin E antioxidant activity include four tocopherols (α-, β-, γ- and δ-) and four tocotrienols (α-, β-, γ- and δ-) with α-tocopherol being the most abundant form in nature and mostly available in food, having the highest biological activity and reversing vitamin E deficiency symptoms. The molecular functions fulfilled specifically by α-tocopherol have yet to be fully described; however, the antioxidant feature is the flagship of the biological activity related to vitamin E [128].

Vitamin E is present within the seminal plasma and plasma membrane. It is a lipid soluble, chain-breaking antioxidant that able to terminate free radical chain reactions, particularly the peroxidation of PUFAs [129, 130].

Numerous reports emphasize on the role of α-tocopherol in the management of male infertility. A positive association was found between α-tocopherol in sperm plasma membranes and the percentage of motile, living and morphologically intact spermatozoa [129]. At the same time, α-tocopherol levels were decreased significantly in oligo- and azoospermic patients in comparison to normospermic controls [130].

A significant improvement in the *in vitro* ability of spermatozoa to bind the zona pellucida of unfertilized oocytes was found in men with high ROS production supplemented with vitamin E for 3 months [131]. Vitamin E supplementation may also play a role in reducing sperm DNA fragmentation and morphology defects [132].

6.5.4. Other non-enzymatic antioxidants

There are other substances which may contribute to the maintenance of oxidative homeostasis. The prime function of these compounds is not to combat the production or action of ROS; however, their presence may decrease the risk of OS development. Albumin, cysteine, taurine, zinc and selenium are the most known representatives. Furthermore, antioxidant substances isolated from natural resources, such as resveratrol, curcumin or lycopene, have recently emerged as suitable dietary supplements or therapeutics due to their chemical diversity, structural complexity, availability, lack of significant toxic effects and intrinsic biologic activity. A short overview of secondary non-enzymatic antioxidants is provided in **Table 3**.

N-acetyl-cysteine (NAC)	• A modified derivate of the sulfur-containing amino acid cysteine • Has the ability to reduce free radicals by acting with thiols and hydroxyl radicals. Plays a role as a precursor to glutathione [133] • Reduces seminal OS and sperm DNA damage [134]. When combined with selenium, NAC has a positive impact on sperm concentration and acrosome reaction [133, 134].
Carnitine	• A quaternary ammonium compound acting as a water-soluble antioxidant • Stimulates mitochondrial metabolism. Has the ability to shuttle long-chain lipids across the mitochondrial bilayer and start the process of ß-oxidation to create NADH and $FADH_2$ along with acetyl-CoA [135]. • Acts primarily in the epididymis. Prevents DNA damage and apoptosis during sperm maturation [136].
Taurine (2-aminoethanesulfonic acid)	• Found abundantly in the mammalian body, including testes and spermatozoa [137]. • Participates in bile salt formation, calcium binding and transport, osmoregulation and stabilization of biological membranes. A component of cellular antioxidant defenses [138]. • Taurine administration to semen prevents the loss of sperm motility and viability, promotion of the activity of reduced glutathione, GPx, SOD and CAT while concomitantly lowering LPO and morphological abnormalities of spermatozoa [137]
Zinc	• A trace element with high concentration in the seminal plasma [139]. • Serves as a cofactor to dihydrofolate reductase and methionine synthase needed for homocysteine recycling, membrane and DNA stabilization [140] • Acts as a cofactor for SOD and metallothioneins, assisting in scavenging superoxide and hydroxyl radicals [141].
Selenium	• A trace element positively correlated with increased levels of sperm concentration, motility and morphology [142]. • Cofactor of phospholipid hydroxyperoxide glutathione peroxidase, important for chromatin condensation and formation of the mitochondrial capsule [52–54]
Albumin	• A highly soluble protein containing 585 amino acids • A key element in the regulation of osmotic pressure and distribution of fluid between different compartments [143] and able to bind metals ions, fatty acids, drugs and hormones. • Stimulates spermatozoa motility, eliminates free radicals and protects membrane integrity from heat shock during semen cryopreservation [144, 145]

Bilirubin	• End product of heme metabolism via heme oxygenase-1, biliverdin and biliverdin reductase [146] • May protect vitamin A and linoleic acid from oxidative destruction due to an extended system of conjugated double bonds and a reactive hydrogen atom [147]
Uric acid	• Final enzymatic product of the degradation of purine nucleosides and free bases • Despite being a major antioxidant in the plasma, both correlates with and predicts OS development. It may function either as an antioxidant (primarily in plasma) or pro-oxidant (primarily within the cell) [148]. • A powerful scavenger of singlet oxygen, peroxyl and hydroxyl radicals in the hydrophilic environment, but loses an ability to scavenge lipophilic radicals and cannot break the radical chain propagation within lipid membranes [149]
Resveratrol (3,5,4′-Trihydroxystilbene)	• A polyphenol that belongs to the stilbene family and is found in grapes, berries, pistachios, plums, peanuts and wines [150]. • A free radical scavenger and a potent antioxidant, promotes the activities of a variety of antioxidant enzymes and increases the antioxidant capacity [150] • Copper and iron chelator preventing the Fenton reaction [151] • Stimulates and protects spermatocytes and spermatozoa against LPO, reduces apoptosis of germinal cells [152] and protects against environmental toxins [153] • Enhances spermatogenesis by stimulating the hypothalamic-pituitary-gonadal axis without adverse effects, triggers penile erection and enhances blood testosterone levels, testicular sperm count and epididymal sperm motility [151, 152]
Lycopene (ψ,ψ-Carotene)	• One of over 600 carotenoids found in nature, present in tomatoes, watermelons and pink grapefruits [154]. • A highly unsaturated straight chain hydrocarbon with a total of 13 double bonds, 11 of which are conjugated making the molecule to be twice as potent singlet oxygen quencher as ß-carotene and 10 times more active in comparison to α-tocopherol [154]. • LYC administration leads to a significant improvement of semen parameters (sperm concentration, motility and morphology) in patients with idiopathic infertility, antibody-mediated infertility as well as with different sperm abnormalities [155, 156] • In vitro LYC supplementation has led to an increased post-thaw spermatozoa survival and DNA stability [157], together with an improved sperm morphology and membrane integrity [158].

Table 3. Overview of minor non-enzymatic antioxidants.

7. Strategies to reduce oxidative stress in male reproduction

Antioxidant supplementation has proven to be effective against male reproductive dysfunction *in vivo*. Recent reports have acclaimed significant attention due to the quality of their study design and demonstrated compelling evidence regarding the efficacy of antioxidants towards improving semen parameters. On the other hand, numerous clinical trials studying the effects of dietary antioxidants on semen parameters are still uncontrolled, focus on rather on healthy individuals or have indirect end-points of success. The dose and duration of antioxidant administration also need to be thoroughly examined and standardized. **Table 4** presents the most effective doses for the treatment of male subfertility based on currently available studies that explored the impact of antioxidant supplementation on sperm parameters.

Vitamin C	• 13 infertile patients received 1000 mg of vitamin C twice daily for a maximum of 2 months. Vitamin C supplementation improved sperm count, motility and morphology [159] • 115 men with clinical varicocele and abnormal semen analyses were recruited. After surgery, the subjects received 250 mg vitamin C for 2 months. Vitamin C supplementation following surgery resulted in a better motility and morphology. Prior to surgery, vitamin C was not effective on the sperm count, but it improved sperm motility and morphology [160]
Vitamin E	• 110 asthenozoospermic patients received 300 mg of vitamin E daily over a period of 26 weeks. At the end of the experiment, sperm motility increased, while LPO decreased in the studied population [161]
Vitamin C and vitamin E	• 1000 mg vitamin C and 800 mg vitamin E were administered to 31 subjects diagnosed with asthenozoospermia and normal or only moderately reduced sperm concentration for a period of 56 days. The treatment did not affect sperm concentration, motility and morphology [162] • 64 men with unexplained infertility and an elevated percentage of DNA-fragmented spermatozoa received 1 g vitamin C and 1 g vitamin E daily for 2 months. No differences in basic sperm parameters were found following antioxidant treatment; however, the percentage of DNA-fragmented spermatozoa was markedly reduced [163].
Vitamins A, C, E, N-acetyl-cysteine and zinc	• 20 post-varicocelectomy oligospermic patients were subjected to a daily administration of 0.06 IU/kg of vitamin A, 3 mg/kg of vitamin C, 0.2 mg/kg of vitamin E, 10 mg/kg of NAC and 0.01 mg/kg of zinc over a period of 13 weeks. Sperm count increased by 20-fold, and of the 20 subjects, 6 of the originally infertile men had sperm counts greater than 20million/mL post-treatment [164]
Glutathione	• 600 mg of GSH per day given to 11 men suffering from dyspermia associated with unilateral varicocele or germ-free genital tract inflammation over 2 months lead to an improvement in sperm kinetics and higher sperm concentration [165].
Carnitine	• 3 g/day of L-carnitine was administered to 100 asthenozoospermic men. After 4 months of treatment, a significant improvement was observed in sperm concentration, motility and morphology [166]. • 2 g/day of carnitine administered for 6 months led to a significant improvement in sperm concentration and motility in 100 patients with oligoasthenoteratozoospermia [167], while the following year an increased sperm count and motility were found in 56 infertile men after a combined daily treatment with 2 g carnitine and 1 g acetyl-L-carnitine supplemented for 6 months [168] • No improvements in semen quality was detected in 26 men diagnosed with asthenozoospermia who underwent 6 months of daily treatment with 2 g L-carnitine and 1 g L-acetyl-carnitine [169]
Selenium	• No positive effects were found in 33 subfertile men following 3 months of treatment with 200 μg/day of selenium [170]
Selenium and Vitamins	• 9 oligoasthenoteratozoospermic men were supplemented for a period of 6 months with selenium and vitamin E, leading to improvements in sperm motility, morphology and viability, although the concentration did not change significantly [171] • 46 oligoasthenoteratozoospermic and 16 subfertile patients received selenium alone or in combination with vitamins A, C and E at daily doses of 100 μg, 1 mg, 10 mg and 15 mg, respectively. No improvement was observed in sperm concentration after 3 months, although the motility was increased in the treated subjects [172] • 28 infertile men were supplemented daily by vitamin E (400 mg) and selenium (225 μg) during 3 months. Following treatment, a significant decrease of LPO was observed together with an improvement of sperm motility [173]
N-acetyl-cysteine	• No improvements in sperm parameters were observed after 3 months of 600 mg/day administration of NAC to 27 infertile men [174]. • Supplementation of 600 mg/day of NAC to 60 patients diagnosed with idiopathic infertility seemed to improve sperm motility, volume, viscosity and seminal oxidative status [175].

Zinc sulfate ($ZnSO_4$)	• Administration of 250 mg of $ZnSO_4$ twice daily for 3 months to 50 asthenozoospermic patients resulted in a higher sperm count and membrane integrity. $ZnSO_4$ also played an immunological role as T-helper cytokines and interleukin-4 levels increased in the experimental group and TNF-α and antisperm antibodies decreased [176]
Coenzyme Q10	• Supplementation of 60 mg/day of coenzyme Q10 for 103 days led to an increase in the fertilization rate but had no effect on motility, morphology or concentration in 17 patients with low fertilization rates due to male factor infertility [177] • 60 patients with idiopathic asthenozoospermia who received 200 mg/day of coenzyme Q10 demonstrated significant improvement in motility after 6 months of treatment [178]

Table 4. Most pronounced studies on the effects of oral antioxidant supplementation on male infertility.

ROS-induced damage may have significant clinical implications in the context of ARTs. Numerous reports have indicated that significantly increased ROS levels may occur in response to repeated cycles of centrifugation involved in conventional sperm preparation techniques used for ARTs [179]. Spermatozoa selected for ART often face OS and a high risk for DNA damage. When intrauterine insemination or *in vitro* fertilization (IVF) is used, such damage does not represent a cause of concern as damage to the sperm membrane lipids ensures that fertilization will not occur. However, in case of intracytoplasmic sperm injection is used, this natural selection barrier may be overlooked and sperm with DNA damage may be directly injected into the ovum [77].

Selection of an effective sperm preparation technique is important to minimize ROS overgeneration and eventual oxidative insults to the male gamete. The density gradient technique is able to separate leukocytes and immature or damaged spermatozoa from normal spermatozoa, which may be subsequently used in ARTs [77, 179, 180].

Assisted reproduction techniques may benefit from *in vitro* supplementation of antioxidants [180]. Various antioxidants such as vitamin E, vitamin C, cysteine, taurine and hypotaurine present in the culture medium have been shown to improve the developmental ability of the embryos by counteracting the effects of ROS [93, 180].

In cases of IVF, incubation times of more than 16–20 hours have been correlated with increased oxidative damage. Shortening the insemination timeframes (up to 1–2 hours or less) may reduce ROS overgeneration in culture media and possibly improve fertilization, embryogenesis and pregnancy rates [77, 179].

8. Methods for detecting reactive oxygen species

Because high levels of ROS have been associated with a decreased male infertility, measuring ROS levels in semen is an important part of the initial evaluation as well as follow-up of men with reproductive dysfunction [10–12]. Chemiluminescence and flow cytometry are currently the most common techniques in clinical andrology to assess and study seminal OS.

Chemiluminescence measures light emitted following administration of specific reagents to a semen sample. Two major probes currently used to assess ROS generation by spermatozoa are luminol (5-amino-2,3-dihydro-1,4-phthalazinedione) and lucigenin (10,10′-dimethyl-9,9′-biacridinium dinitrate). Lucigenin is membrane-impermeable and responsive to ROS, particularly $O_2^{\bullet-}$, in the extracellular space. Inversely, luminol is relatively membrane-permeable and reacts with a variety of ROS, including $O_2^{\bullet-}$, H_2O_2 and $OH^{\bullet}$ intracellularly as well as extracellularly. Chemiluminescent assays are sensitive, convenient for diagnostic purposes and have relatively well-established normal ranges [11, 12]. Nevertheless, significant set up costs have to be taken into consideration, and the data generated by chemiluminescence must be interpreted carefully because a variety of factors can affect the signals obtained [181].

A possible solution to the disadvantages associated with the chemiluminescence approach can be found in a variety of redox-sensitive fluorescence probes that can be loaded into spermatozoa and subsequently monitored by flow cytometry [182]. Two probes can be used. Dihydroethidium or hydroethidine is a non-fluorescent probe that is oxidized by the superoxide to become ethidium bromide, which will stain the mitochondrial and nuclear DNA [183, 184]. The other fluorescent probe is 2,7-dichlorofluorescein diacetate, a stable non-fluorescent cell-permeable probe that de-esterifies in the presence of intracellular H_2O_2 to form 2,7-dichlorofluorescein [183]. Other ROS such as peroxynitrite, HOCl, and $OH^{\bullet}$ can also oxidize this probe [184]. Flow cytometry has a higher specificity, accuracy, sensitivity and reproducibility than fluorescent microscopy or chemiluminescence. A large number of cells can easily be analyzed, leading to high specificity and sensitivity [185]. One major disadvantage is that sophisticated and expensive hardware is needed. Also, the results do not quantify the target ROS but simply indicate the percentage of cells exhibiting a high level of activity [182].

Other methods to assess the oxidative balance in semen include indirect measurements such as the total antioxidant assay. This protocol is based on the ability of all antioxidants present in the sample to cease the oxidation of 2,20-azino-di-3-ethylbenzthiazoline sulfonate (ABTS) to $ABTS^{+}$ by metmyoglobin. Hence, the antioxidants suppress oxidative processes to a degree that is proportional to their final concentration, which may be detected at 750 nm [186]. Another option is to assess the activity of antioxidant enzymes (SOD, CAT, GPx) or the redox potential defined by the ratio of oxidized and reduced glutathione using commercially available assay kits. A popular option is the measurement of oxidative end-products, including protein carbonyls [187], lipid hydroperoxides [188], MDA [98] and oxidative DNA adduct 8-hydroxy 2-deoxyguanosine [189].

Despite a remarkable progress in the evolution and design of new techniques to evaluate seminal OS, more straight-forward and accessible assays with well-defined and clinically significant physiological ranges reflecting normal sperm functions have yet to be introduced in order for oxidative stress to become a standard sub- or infertility marker in andrology laboratories.

9. Conclusions

Oxygen toxicity is an inherent double-edged sword to aerobic life. Increased oxidative insults to sperm lipids, proteins and DNA are associated with alterations of signal transduction mechanisms crucial for fertility. The origin of ROS generation and the etiologies of increased ROS in men with low sperm quality are becoming increasingly clear, offering multiple management and/or treatment options. Recent evidence suggests that spermatozoa possess an inherent ability to generate ROS essential for the fertilization process. A variety of defense mechanisms against ROS overproduction encompassing antioxidant enzymes, vitamins and other biologically active molecules are involved in biological systems. A balance of the benefits and risks from free radical production seems to be crucial for the sperm survival and function. As male infertility continues to play an increasing role in contributing to the inability to conceive in couples of reproductive age, it is pivotal for andrologists to fully comprehend the importance of thoroughly evaluating seminal oxidative profiles in order to provide a better care for male patients with reproductive dysfunction. Although the therapeutic use of antioxidants appears attractive, clinicians need to be aware of exaggerated claims of antioxidant benefits by various commercial supplements for fertility purposes until proper multicenter trials have been completed. However, initial data emphasizing on the potential of antioxidant supplementation in improving semen quality and conception rates are indeed encouraging.

Acknowledgements

This study was supported by the Slovak Research and Development Agency grants APVV-15-0543 and APVV-15-0544.

List of abbreviations

AA	Ascorbic acid
ABTS	2,20-azino-di-3-ethylbenzthiazoline sulfonate
AR	Acrosome reaction
ARTs	Artificial reproduction techniques
ATP	Adenosine triphosphate
Ca^{2+}	Calcium
cAMP	Cyclic adenosine monophosphate
CAT	Catalase
Fe^{2+}	Ferrous ion
Fe^{3+}	Ferric ion
FR	Free radical
G6PD	Glucose-6-phosphate dehydrogenase

GPx	Glutathione peroxidases
GSH	Glutathione
GS-SG	Glutathione disulfide
H^+	Hydrogen
H_2O_2	Hydrogen peroxide
HCO_3^-	Bicarbonate
$HO_2^\bullet$	Hydroperoxyl radical
HOCl	Hypochlorous acid
ICSI	Intracytoplasmic sperm injection
IVF	*In vitro* fertilization
LPO	Lipid peroxidation
MDA	Malondialdehyde
mtDNA	Mitochondrial DNA
NADPH	ß-nicotinamide adenine dinucleotide phosphate
$NO^\bullet$	Nitric oxide
O_2	Oxygen
$O_2^{\bullet-}$	Superoxide
$OH^\bullet$	Hydroxyl radical
$ONOO^-$	Peroxynitrite
OS	Oxidative stress
PHGPx	Phospholipid hydroperoxide glutathione peroxidase
PLA2	Phospholipase A2
PMN	Polymorphonuclear
PUFAs	Polyunsaturated fatty acids
RNS	Reactive nitrogen species
$ROO^\bullet$	Peroxyl radical
ROS	Reactive oxygen species
-SH	Thiol
SOD	Superoxide dismutase
WHO	World Health Organization

Author details

Eva Tvrdá*, Peter Massanyi and Norbert Lukáč

*Address all correspondence to: evina.tvrda@gmail.com

Department of Animal Physiology, Faculty of Biotechnology and Food Sciences, Slovak University of Agriculture in Nitra, Slovakia

References

[1] Sies H. Strategies of antioxidant defense. European Journal of Biochemistry. 1993;**215**: 213-219

[2] Boveris A, Chance B. The mitochondrial generation of hydrogen peroxide. General properties and effect of hyperbaric oxygen. Biochemical Journal. 1973;**134**:707-716

[3] Chance B, Sies H, Boveris H. Hydroperoxide metabolism in mammalian organs. Physiological Reviews. 1979;**59**:527-605

[4] Makker K, Agarwal A, Sharma R. Oxidative stress & male infertility. Indian Journal of Medical Research. 2009;**129**:357-367

[5] Sies H. Oxidative stress: Oxidants and antioxidants. Experimental Physiology. 1997;**82**: 291-295

[6] Aitken RJ. Molecular mechanisms regulating human sperm function. Molecular Human Reproduction. 1997;**3**:169-173

[7] Chen H, Zhao HX, Huang XF, Chen GW, Yang ZX, Sun WJ, Tao MH, Yuan Y, Wu JQ, Sun F, Dai Q, Shi HJ. Does high load of oxidants in human semen contribute to male factor infertility? Antioxidants & Redox Signaling. 2012;**16**:754-759. DOI: 10.1089/ars.2011

[8] Aitken RJ, De Iuliis GN, Finnie JM, Hedges A, McLachlan RI. Analysis of the relationships between oxidative stress, DNA damage and sperm vitality in a patient population: Development of diagnostic criteria. Human Reproduction 2010;**25**:2415-2426. DOI: 10.1093/humrep/deq214

[9] Aitken RJ, Roman SD. Antioxidant systems and oxidative stress in the testes. Oxidative Medicine and Cellular Longevinity. 2008;**1**:15-24

[10] Zini A, de Lamirande E, Gagnon C. Reactive oxygen species in the semen of infertile patients: Levels of superoxide dismutase- and catalase-like activities in seminal plasma and spermatozoa. International Journal of Andrology. 1993;**16**:183-188

[11] Agarwal A, Mulgund A, Sharma R, Sabanegh E. Mechanisms of oligozoospermia: An oxidative stress perspective. Systems Biology in Reproductive Medicine. 2014a;**60**:206-126. DOI: 10.3109/19396368.2014.918675

[12] Agarwal A, Tvrda E, Sharma R. Relationship amongst teratozoospermia, seminal oxidative stress and male infertility. Reproductive Biology and Endocrinology. 2014b;**12**:45. DOI: 10.1186/1477-7827-12-45

[13] Ďuračková Z. Free radicals and antioxidants for non-experts. In: Laher I, editor. Systems Biology of Free Radicals and Antioxidants. 1st ed. Berlin Heidelberg: Springer Verlag; 2014. p. 3-38. DOI: 10.1007/978-3-642-30018-9_2

[14] Hermes-Lima M. Oxygen in biology and biochemistry: Role of free radicals. In: Storey KB, editor. Functional Metabolism: Regulation and Adaptation. Hoboken, New Jersey, USA: John Wiley & Sons, 2004, pp. 319-368. ISBN: 0-471-410909-X

[15] Halliwell B. Free radicals and other reactive species in disease. Encyclopedia of Life Sciences. 2005;**1**:1-9

[16] Agarwal A, Prabakaran SA. Mechanism, measurement, and prevention of oxidative stress in male reproductive physiology. Indian Journal of Experimental Biology. 2005;**43**:963-974

[17] Whittington K, Ford WC. Relative contribution of leukocytes and of spermatozoa to reactive oxygen species production in human sperm suspensions. International Journal of Andrology. 1999;**22**:229-235

[18] Wolff H. The biologic significance of white blood cells in semen. Fertility and Sterility. 1995;**63**:1143-1157

[19] Ochsendorf FR. Infections in the male genital tract and reactive oxygen species. Human Reproduction Update. 1999;**5**:399-420

[20] Shekarriz M, Sharma RK, Thomas Jr AJ, Agarwal A. Positive myeloperoxidase staining (Endtz test) as an indicator of excessive reactive oxygen species formation in semen. Journal of Assisted Reproduction and Genetics. 1995;**12**:70-74

[21] Cooper TG, Noonan E, von Eckardstein S, Auger J, Baker HW, Behre HM, Haugen TB, Kruger T, Wang C, Mbizvo MT, Vogelsong KM. World Health Organization reference values for human semen characteristics. Human Reproduction Update. 2010;**16**:231-245. DOI: 10.1093/humupd/dmp048

[22] Henkel R, Kierspel E, Stalf T, Mehnert C, Menkveld R, Tinneberg HR, Schill WB, Kruger TF. Effect of reactive oxygen species produced by spermato – zoa and leukocytes on sperm functions in non-leukocytospermic patients. Fertility and Sterility. 2005;**83**:635-642

[23] Wolff H, Politch JA, Martinez A, Haimovici F, Hill JA, Anderson DJ. Leukocytospermia is associated with poor semen quality. Fertility and Sterility. 1990;**53**:528-536

[24] Sharma RK, Pasqualotto AE, Nelson DR, Thomas Jr AJ, Agarwal A. Relationship between seminal white blood cell counts and oxidative stress in men treated at an infertility clinic. Journal of Andrology. 2001;**22**:575-283

[25] Plante M, de Lamirande E, Gagnon C. Reactive oxygen species released by activated neutrophils, but not by deficient spermatozoa, are sufficient to affect normal sperm motility. Fertility and Sterility. 1994;**62**:387-393

[26] Gatti JL, Castella S, Dacheux F, Ecroyd H, Métayer S, Thimon V, Dacheux JL. Post-testicular sperm environment and fertility. Animal Reproduction Science. 2004;**82-83**:321-339

[27] Aitken J, Krausz C, Buckingham D. Relationships between biochemical markers for residual sperm cytoplasm, reactive oxygen species generation, and the presence of leukocytes and precursor germ cells in human sperm suspensions. Molecular Reproduction and Development. 1994;**39**:268-279

[28] Gil-Guzman E, Ollero M, Lopez MC, Sharma RK, Alvarez JG, Thomas AJ Jr, Agarwal A. Differential production of reactive oxygen species by subsets of human spermatozoa at different stages of maturation. Human Reproduction. 2001;**16**:1922-1930

[29] Cho ChL, Esteves SC, Agarwal A. Novel insights into the pathophysiology of varicocele and its association with reactive oxygen species and sperm DNA fragmentation. Asian Journal of Andrology. 2016;**18**:186-193. DOI: 10.4103/1008-682X.170441

[30] Du Plessis SS, Agarwal A, Halabi J, Tvrda E. Contemporary evidence on the physiological role of reactive oxygen species in human sperm function. Journal of Assisted Reproduction and Genetics. 2015;**32**:509-520. DOI: 10.1007/s10815-014-0425-7

[31] Shiraishi K, Matsuyama H, Takihara H. Pathophysiology of varicocele in male infertility in the era of assisted reproductive technology. International Journal of Urology. 2012;**19**:538-550. DOI: 10.1111/j.1442-2042.2012.02982.x

[32] de Lamirande E, Jiang H, Zini A, Kodama H, Gagnon C. Reactive oxygen species and sperm physiology. Reviews of Reproduction. 1997;**2**:48-54

[33] Koppers AJ, De Iuliis GN, Finnie JM. Significance of mitochondrial reactive oxygen species in the generation of oxidative stress in spermatozoa. Journal of Clinical Endocrinology & Metabolism. 2008;**93**:3199-3207. DOI: 10.1210/jc.2007-2616

[34] Armstrong JS, Bivalacqua TJ, Chamulitrat W, Sikka S, Hellstrom WJ. A comparison of the NADPH oxidase in human sperm and white blood cells. International Journal of Andrology. 2002;**25**:223-229

[35] Richer S, Ford W. A critical investigation of NADPH oxidase activity in human spermatozoa. Molecular Human Reproduction. 2001;**7**:237-244

[36] Said TM, Agarwal A, Sharma RK, Mascha E, Sikka SC, Thomas AJ Jr. Human sperm superoxide anion generation and correlation with semen quality in patients with male infertility. Fertility and Sterility. 2004;**82**:871-877

[37] Herrero MB, Gagnon C. Nitric oxide: A novel mediator of sperm function. Journal of Andrology. 2001;**22**:349-356

[38] Marques-Pinto A, Carvalho D. Human infertility: Are endocrine disruptors to blame? Endocrine Connections. 2013;**2**:R15-R29

[39] Wirth JJ, Mijal RS. Adverse effects of low level heavy metal exposure on male reproductive function. Systems Biology in Reproductive Medicine. 2010;**56**:147-167. DOI: 10.3109/19396360903582216

[40] La Vignera S, Condorelli RA, Vicari E, D'Agata R, Calogero AE. Effects of the exposure to mobile phones on male reproduction: A review of the literature. Journal of Andrology. 2012;**33**:350-356. DOI: 10.2164/jandrol.111.014373

[41] Taha EA, Ez-Aldin AM, Sayed SK, Ghandour NM, Mostafa T. Effect of smoking on sperm vitality, DNA integrity, seminal oxidative stress, zinc in fertile men. Urology. 2012;**80**:822-825. DOI: 10.1016/j.urology.2012.07.002

[42] Saleh RA, Agarwal A, Sharma RK, Nelson DR, Thomas AJ Jr. Effect of cigarette smoking on levels of seminal oxidative stress in infertile men: A prospective study. Fertillity and Sterility. 2002;**78**:491-499

[43] Gholinezhad CM, Colagar AH. Seminal plasma lipid peroxidation, total antioxidant capacity, and cigarette smoking in asthenoteratospermic men. Journal of Men's Health. 2011;**8**:43-49. DOI: 10.1016/j.jomh.2010.09.230

[44] Jensen TK, Swan S, Jørgensen N, Toppari J, Redmon B, Punab M, Drobnis EZ, Haugen TB, Zilaitiene B, Sparks AE, Irvine DS, Wang C, Jouannet P, Brazil C, Paasch U, Salzbrunn A, Skakkebæk NE, Andersson AM. Alcohol and male reproductive health: A cross-sectional study of 8344 healthy men from Europe and the USA. Human Reproduction. 2014;**29**:1801-1809. DOI: 10.1093/humrep/deu118

[45] Jang MH, Shin MC, Shin HS, Kim KH, Park HJ, Kim EH, Kim CJ. Alcohol induces apoptosis in TM3 mouse Leydig cells via bax-dependent caspase-3 activation. European Journal of Pharmacology. 2002;**449**:39-45

[46] Jensen TK, Heitmann BL, Jensen MB, Halldorsson TI, Andersson AM, Skakkebaek NE, Joensen UN, Lauritsen MP, Christiansen P, Dalgard C, Lassen TH, Jorgensen N. High dietary intake of saturated fat is associated with reduced semen quality among 701 young Danish men from the general population. American Journal of Clinical Nutrition. 2013;**97**:411-418. DOI: 10.3945/ajcn.112.042432

[47] Afeiche MC, Bridges ND, Williams PL, Gaskins AJ, Tanrikut C, Petrozza JC, Hauser R, Chavarro JE. Dairy intake and semen quality among men attending a fertility clinic. Fertility and Sterility. 2014;**101**:1280-1287. DOI: 10.1016/j.fertnstert.2014.02.003

[48] Qin DD, Yuan W, Zhou WJ, Cui YQ, JQ W, Gao ES. Do reproductive hormones explain the association between body mass index and semen quality? Asian Journal of Andrology. 2017;**9**:827-834

[49] Dadkhah H, Kazemi A, Nasr-Isfahani MH, Ehsanpour S. The relationship between the amount of saturated fat intake and semen quality in men. Iranian Journal of Nursing and Midwifery Research. 2017;**22**:46-50. DOI: 10.4103/1735-9066.202067

[50] Hadjkacem Loukil L, Hadjkacem H, Bahloul A, Ayadi H. Relation between male obesity and male infertility in a Tunisian population. Andrologia. 2014;**47**:282-285. DOI: 10.1111/and.12257

[51] Ford WC. Regulation of sperm function by reactive oxygen species. Human Reproduction Update. 2004;**10**:87-399

[52] Erenpreiss J, Spano M, Erenpreisa J, Bungum M, Giwercman A. Sperm chromatin structure and male fertility: Biological and clinical aspects. Asian Journal of Andrology. 2006;**8**:11-29

[53] Aitken RJ, Ryan AL, Baker MA, McLaughlin EA. Redox activity associated with the maturation and capacitation of mammalian spermatozoa. Free Radical Biology and Medicine. 2004;**36**:994-1010

[54] Amaral A, Lourenço B, Marques M, Ramalho-Santos J. Mitochondria functionality and sperm quality. Reproduction. 2013;**146**:R163-R174. DOI: 10.1530/REP-13-0178

[55] Zini A, San Gabriel M, Baazeem A. Antioxidants and sperm DNA damage: A clinical perspective. Journal of Assisted Reproduction and Genetics. 2009;**26**:427-432. DOI: 10.1007/s10815-009-9343-5

[56] Menezo Y. 2007. Antioxidants to reduce sperm DNA fragmentation: An unexpected adverse effect. Reproductive Biomedicine Online. 2007;**14**:418-421

[57] de Lamirande E, Leclerc P, Gagnon C. Capacitation as a regulatory event that primes spermatozoa for the acrosome reaction and fertilization. Molecular Human Reproduction. 1997;**3**:175-194

[58] de Lamirande E, Gagnon C. Human sperm hyperactivation and capacitation as parts of an oxidative process. Free Radicals in Biology and Medicine. 1993;**14**:157-166

[59] Rivlin J, Mendel J, Rubinstein S, Etkovitz N, Breitbart H. Role of hydrogen peroxide in sperm capacitation and acrosome reaction. Biology of Reproduction. 2004;**70**:518-522

[60] Zini A, de Lamirande E, Gagnon C. Low levels of nitric oxide promote human sperm capacitation in vitro. Journal of Andrology. 1995;**16**:424-431

[61] Aitken RJ. The capacitation-apoptosis highway: Oxysterols and mammalian sperm function. Biology of Reproduction. 2011;**85**:9-12. DOI: 10.1095/biolreprod.111.092528

[62] Suarez SS. Control of hyperactivation in sperm. Human Reproduction Update. 2008;**14**:647-657. DOI: 10.1093/humupd/dmn029

[63] Baldi E, Luconi M, Bonaccorsi L, Muratori M, Forti G. Intracellular events and signaling pathways involved in sperm acquisition of fertilizing capacity and acrosome reaction. Frontiers in Bioscience. 2000;**5**:110-123

[64] de Lamirande E, Tsai C, Harakat A, Gagnon C. Involvement of reactive oxygen species in human sperm acrosome reaction induced by A23187, lysophosphatidylcholine, and biological fluid ultrafiltrates. Journal of Andrology. 1998;**19**:585-594

[65] Griveau JF, Le Lannou DL. Reactive oxygen species and human spermatozoa: Physiology and pathology. International Journal of Andrology. 1997;**20**:61-69

[66] Min L. The biology and dynamics of mammalian cortical granules. Reproductive Biology and Endocrinology. 2011;**9**:149. DOI: 10.1186/1477-7827-9-149

[67] Gadella BM. Interaction of sperm with the zona pellucida during fertilization. Society for Reproduction and Fertility. 2010;**67**:267-287

[68] Aitken RJ, Clarkson JS, Fishel S. Generation of reactive oxygen species, lipid peroxidation and human sperm function. Biology of Reproduction. 1989;**40**:183-197

[69] Alvarez JG, Touchstone JC, Blasco L, Storey BT. Spontaneous lipid peroxidation and production of hydrogen peroxide and superoxide in human spermatozoa. Superoxide dismutase as major enzyme protectant against oxygen toxicity. Journal of Andrology. 1987;**8**:338-348

[70] Ayala A, Muñoz MF, Argüelles S. Lipid peroxidation: Production, metabolism, and signaling mechanisms of malondialdehyde and 4-hydroxy-2-nonenal. Oxidative Medicine and Cellular Longevity. 2014;**2014**:1-31. DOI: 10.1155/2014/360438

[71] Aitken RJ, Wingate JK, De Iuliis GN, Kopper AJ, McLaughlin EA. Cis-unsaturated fatty acids stimulate reactive oxygen species generation and lipid peroxidation in human spermatozoa. In Journal of Clinical Endocrinology & Metabolism. 2006;**91**, 14154-14163. DOI: 10.1210/jc.2006-1309

[72] Agarwal A, Said TM. Oxidative stress, DNA damage and apoptosis in male infertility: A clinical approach. BJU International. 2005;**95**:503-507. DOI: 10.1111/j.1464-410X.2005.05328.x

[73] Wright C, Milne S, Leeson H. Sperm DNA damage caused by oxidative stress: Modifiable clinical, lifestyle and nutritional factors in male infertility. Reproductive Biomedicine Online. 2014;**28**:684-703. DOI: 10.1016/j.rbmo.2014.02.004

[74] Hosen B, Islam R, Begum F, Kabir Y, Howlader ZH. Oxidative stress induced sperm DNA damage, a possible reason for male infertility. Iranian Journal of Reproductive Medicine. 2015;**13**:525-532

[75] Shirakawa T, Fujisawa M, Kanzaki M, Okada H, Arakawa S, Kamidono S. Y chromosome (Yq11) microdeletions in idiopathic azoospermia. International Journal of Urology. 1997;**4**:198-201

[76] Kumar DP, Sangeetha N. Mitochondrial DNA mutations and male infertility. Indian Journal of Human Genetics. 2009;**15**:93-97. DOI: 10.4103/0971-6866.60183

[77] Bach PV, Schlegel PN, Sperm DNA. Damage and its role in IVF and ICSI. Basic and Clinical Andrology. 2016;**26**:15. DOI: 10.1186/s12610-016-0043-6

[78] Davies MJ. Oxidative damage to proteins. In: Chatgilialoglu C, Studer A, editors. Encyclopedia of Radicals in Chemistry, Biology and Materials. 1st ed. New York, USA: Wiley; 2012. p. 93-109. 2324 p. DOI: 10.1002/9781119953678.rad045

[79] Berlett BS, Stadtman ER. Protein oxidation in aging, disease, and oxidative stress. The Journal of Biological Chemistry. 1997;**272**:20313-20316. DOI: 10.1074/jbc.272.33.20313

[80] Sinha S, Pradeep KG, Laloraya M, Warikoo D. Over-expression of superoxide dismutase and lack of surface-thiols in spermatozoa: Inherent defects in oligospermia. Biochemical and Biophysical Research Communications. 1991;**174**:510-517

[81] Mammoto A, Masumoto N, Tahara M, Ikebuchi Y, Ohmichi M, Tasaka K, Miyake A. Reactive oxygen species block sperm-egg fusion via oxidation of sperm sulfhydryl proteins in mice. Biology of Reproduction. 1996;**55**:1063-1068

[82] Shaha C, Tripathi R, Mishra DP. Male germ cell apoptosis: Regulation and biology. Philosophical Transactions of the Royal Society of London. 2010;**365**:1501-1515. DOI: 10.1098/rstb.2009.0124

[83] Shukla KK, Mahdi AA, Rajender S. Apoptosis, spermatogenesis and male infertility. Frontiers in Bioscience. 2012;**4**:746-754

[84] Vissers MC, Pullar JM, Hampton MB. Hypochlorous acid causes caspase activation and apoptosis or growth arrest in human endothelial cells. Biochemical Journal. 1999;**344**:443-449

[85] Said TM, Paasch U, Glander HJ, Agarwal A. Role of caspases in male infertility. Human Reproduction Update. 2004;**10**:39-51

[86] Martínez-Pastor F, Aisen E, Fernández-Santos MR, Esteso MC, Maroto-Morales A, García-Alvarez O, Garde JJ. Reactive oxygen species generators affect quality parameters and apoptosis markers differently in red deer spermatozoa. Reproduction. 2009;**137**:225-235. DOI: 10.1530/REP-08-0357

[87] Moran JM, Madejón L, Ortega Ferrusola C, Peña FJ. Nitric oxide induces caspase activity in boar spermatozoa. Theriogenology. 2008;**70**:91-96. DOI: 10.1016/j.theriogenology.2008.02.010

[88] Johnson C, Jia Y, Wang C, Lue Y, Swerdloff RS, Zhang X, Hu Z, Li Y, Sinha Hikim AP. Role of caspase 2 in apoptotic signaling in primate and murine germ cells. Biology of Reproduction. 2008;**79**:806-814. DOI: 10.1095/biolreprod.108.068833

[89] Elia J, Imbrogno N, Delfino M, Mazzilli R, Rossi T, Mazzilli F. The importance of the sperm motility classes-future directions. The Open Andrology Journal. 2010;**2**:42-43

[90] Armstrong JS, Rajasekaran M, Chamulitrat W, Gatti P, Hellstrom WJ, Sikka SC. Characterization of reactive oxygen species induced effects on human spermatozoa movement and energy metabolism. Free Radical Biology & Medicine. 1999;**26**:869-880

[91] Twigg J, Irvine DS, Houston P, Fulton N, Michael L, Aitken RJ. Iatrogenic DNA damage induced in human spermatozoa during sperm preparation: Protective significance of seminal plasma. Molecular Human Reproduction. 1998;**4**:439-445

[92] Zareba P, Colaci DS, Afeiche M, Gaskins AJ, Jørgensen N, Mendiola J, Swan SH, Chavarro JE. Semen quality in relation to antioxidant intake in a healthy male population. Fertility and Sterility. 2013;**100**:1572-1579. DOI: 10.1016/j.fertnstert.2013.08.032

[93] Walczak-Jedrzejowska R, Wolski JK, Slowikowska-Hilczer J. The role of oxidative stress and antioxidants in male fertility. Central European Journal of Urology. 2013;**66**:60-67. DOI: 10.5173/ceju.2013.01.art19

[94] Asadpour R, Jafari R, Tayefi-Nasrabadi H. The effect of antioxidant supplementation in semen extenders on semen quality and lipid peroxidation of chilled bull spermatozoa. Iranian Journal of Veterinary Research. 2012;**13**:246-249

[95] Perumal P. Effect of superoxide dismutase on semen parameters and antioxidant enzyme activities of liquid stored (5°C) mithun (Bos Frontalis) semen. Journal of Animals. 2014;**2014**:1-9. DOI: 10.1155/2014/821954

[96] Buffone MG, Calamera JC, Brugo-Olmedo S, De Vincentiis S, Calamera MM, Storey BT, Doncel GF, Alvarez JG. Superoxide dismutase content in sperm correlates with motility recovery after thawing of cryopreserved human spermatozoa. Fertility and Sterility. 2012;**97**:293-298. DOI: 10.1016/j.fertnstert.2011.11.012

[97] Jeulin C, Soufir JC, Weber P, Laval-Martin D, Calvayrac R. Catalase activity in human spermatozoa and seminal plasma. Gamete Research. 1989;**24**:185-196

[98] Tvrdá E, Kňažická Z, Lukáčová J, Schneidgenová M, Goc Z, Greń A, Szabó C, Massányi P, Lukáč N. The impact of lead and cadmium on selected motility, prooxidant and antioxidant parameters of bovine seminal plasma and spermatozoa. Journal of Environmental Science and Health Part A. 2013;**48**:1292-1300. DOI: 10.1080/10934529.2013.777243

[99] Macanovic B, Vucetic M, Jankovic A, Stancic A, Buzadzic B, Garalejic E, Korac A, Korac B, Otasevic V. Correlation between sperm parameters and protein expression of antioxidative defense enzymes in seminal plasma: A pilot study. Disease Markers. 2015;**2015**:1-5. DOI: 10.1155/2015/436236

[100] Moubasher AE, El Din AME, Ali ME, El-Sherif WT, Gaber HD. Catalase improves motility, vitality and DNA integrity of cryopreserved human spermatozoa. Andrologia. 2013;**45**:135-139. DOI: 10.1111/j.1439-0272.2012.01310.x

[101] Imai H, Nakagawa Y. Biological significance of phospholipid hydroperoxide glutathione peroxidase (PHGPx, GPx4) in mammalian cells. Free Radical Biology and Medicine. 2003;**34**:145-169

[102] Jelezarsky L, Vaisberg C, Chaushev T, Sapundjiev E. Localization and characterization of glutathione peroxidase (GPx) in boar accessory sex glands, seminal plasma, and spermatozoa and activity of GPx in boar semen. Theriogenology. 2008;**69**:139-145

[103] Fujii J, Ito JI, Zhang X, Kurahashi T. Unveiling the roles of the glutathione redox system in vivo by analyzing genetically modified mice. Journal of Clinical Biochemistry and Nutrition. 2011;**49**:70-78. DOI: 10.3164/jcbn.10-138SR

[104] Garrido N, Meseguer M, Alvarez J, Simón C, Pellicer A, Remohí J. Relationship among standard semen parameters, glutathione peroxidase/glutathione reductase activity, and mRNA expression and reduced glutathione content in ejaculated spermatozoa from fertile and infertile men. Fertility and Sterility. 2004;**82**:1059-1066

[105] Kaneko T, Iuchi Y, Kobayashi T, Fujii T, Saito H, Kurachi H, Fujii J. The expression of glutathione reductase in the male reproductive system of rats supports the enzymatic basis of glutathione function in spermatogenesis. European Journal of Biochemistry. 2002;**269**:1570-1578

[106] Gopalakrishnan B, Aravinda S, Pawshe CH, Totey SM, Nagpal S, Salunke DM, Shaha C. Studies on glutathione S-transferases important for sperm function: Evidence of catalytic activity-independent functions. Biochemical Journal. 1998;**329**:231-241

[107] Kumar R, Singh VK, Atreja SK. Glutathione-S-transferase: Role in buffalo (*Bubalus bubalis*) sperm capacitation and cryopreservation. Theriogenology. 2014;**81**:587-598. DOI: 10.1016/j.theriogenology.2013.11.012

[108] Hemachand T. Functional role of sperm surface glutathione S-transferases and extracellular glutathione in the haploid spermatozoa under oxidative stress. FEBS Letters. 2003;**538**:14-18

[109] Orlando C, Caldini AL, Barni T, Wood WG, Strasburger CJ, Natali A, Maver A, Forti G, Serio M. Ceruloplasmin and transferrin in human seminal plasma: Are they an index of seminiferous tubular function? Fertility and Sterility. 1985;**43**:290-294

[110] Roeser HP, Lee GR, Nacht S, Cartwright GE. The role of ceruloplasmin in iron metabolism. Journal of Clinical Investigation. 1970;**49**:2408-2417

[111] Galdston M, Feldman JG, Levytska V, Magnůsson B. Antioxidant activity of serum ceruloplasmin and transferrin available iron-binding capacity in smokers and nonsmokers. American Review of Respiratory Disease. 1987;**135**:783-787

[112] Akalın PP, Bülbül B, Çoyan K, Başpınar N, Kırbaş M, Bucak MN, Güngör S, Öztürk C. Relationship of blood and seminal plasma ceruloplasmin, copper, iron and cadmium concentrations with sperm quality in merino rams. Small Ruminant Research. 2015;**133**:135-139. DOI: 10.1016/j.smallrumres.2015.08.019

[113] Wojtczak M, Dietrich GJ, Irnazarow I, Jurecka P, Słowińska M, Ciereszko A. Polymorphism of transferrin of carp seminal plasma: Relationship to blood transferrin and sperm motility characteristics. Comparative Biochemistry and Physiology – Part B. 2007;**148**:426-431

[114] Abdel Aziz MT, Mostafa T, Roshdy N, Hosni H, Rashed L, Sabry D, Abdel Nasser T, Abdel Azim O, Abdel Gawad O. Heme oxygenase enzyme activity in human seminal plasma of fertile and infertile males. Andrologia. 2008;**40**:292-297. DOI: 10.1111/j.1439-0272.2008.00856.x

[115] Abdel Aziz MT, Mostafa T, Atta H, Kamal O, Kamel M, Hosni H, Rashed L, Sabry D, Waheed F. Heme oxygenase enzyme activity in seminal plasma of oligoasthenoteratozoospermic males with varicocele. Andrologia. 2010;**42**:236-241. DOI: 10.1111/j.1439-0272.2009.00983.x

[116] Turkseven S, Kruger A, Mingone CJ, Kaminski P, Inaba M, Rodella LF, Ikehara S, Wolin MS, Abraham NG. Antioxidant mechanism of heme oxygenase-1 involves an increase in superoxide dismutase and catalase in experimental diabetes. American Journal of Physiology – Heart and Circulatory Physiology. 2005;**289**:H701-H707

[117] Irvine DS. Glutathione as a treatment for male infertility. Reviews of Reproduction. 196;**1**:6-12

[118] Meseguer M, Martínez-Conejero JA, Muriel L, Pellicer A, Remohí J, Garrido N. The human sperm glutathione system: A key role in male fertility and successful cryopreservation. Drug Metabolism Letters. 2007;**1**:121-126

[119] Chambial S, Dwivedi S, Shukla KK, John PJ, Sharma P. Vitamin C in disease prevention and cure: An overview. Indian Journal of Clinical Biochemistry. 2013;**28**:314-328. DOI: 10.1007/s12291-013-0375-3

[120] Mathur V, Murdia A, Hakim AA, Suhalka ML, Shaktawat GS, Kothari LK. Male infertility and the present status of its management by drugs. Journal of Postgraduate Medicine. 1979;**25**:90-96

[121] Colagar AH, Marzony ET. Ascorbic acid in human seminal plasma: Determination and its relationship to sperm quality. Journal of Clinical Biochemistry and Nutrition. 2009;**45**:144-149. DOI: 10.3164/jcbn.08-251

[122] Das P, Choudhari AR, Dhawan A, Singh R. Role of ascorbic acid in human seminal plasma against the oxidative damage to the sperms. Indian Journal of Clinical Biochemistry. 2009;**24**:312-315. DOI: 10.1007/s12291-009-0058-2

[123] Song GJ, Norkus EP, Lewis V. Relationship between seminal ascorbic acid and sperm DNA integrity in infertile men. International Journal of Andrology. 2006;**29**:569-575

[124] Chinoy MR, Sharma JD, Sanjeevan AG, Chinoy NJ. Structural changes in male reproductive organs and spermatozoa of scorbutic guinea pigs. Proceedings of the National Academy of Sciences, India. 1983:**B49**628-B49635

[125] Paul PK, Datta-Gupta PN. Beneficial or harmful effects of a large dose of vitamin C on the reproductive organs of the male rat depending upon the level of food intake. Indian Journal of Experimental Biology. 1978;**16**:18-21

[126] Akmal M, Qadri JQ, Al-Waili NS, Thangal S, Haq A, Saloom KY. Improvement in human semen quality after oral supplementation of vitamin C. Journal of Medicinal Food. 2006;**9**:440-442

[127] Jelodar G, Nazifi S, Akbari A. The prophylactic effect of vitamin C on induced oxidative stress in rat testis following exposure to 900 MHz radio frequency wave generated by a BTS antenna model. Electromagnetic Biology and Medicine. 2013;**32**:4094-4016. DOI: 10.3109/ 15368378.2012.735208

[128] Chow CK, Chow-Johnson HS. Antioxidant function and health implications of vitamin E. The Open Nutrition Journal. 2013;**7**:1-6

[129] Bolle P, Evandri MG, Saso L. The controversial efficacy of vitamin E for human male infertility. Contraception. 2002;**65**:313-315

[130] Moilanen J, Hovatta O, Lindroth L. Vitamin E levels in seminal plasma can be elevated by oral administration of vitamin E in infertile men. International Journal of Andrology. 1993;**16**:165-166

[131] Kessopoulou E, Powers HJ, Sharma KK, Pearson MJ, Russell JM, Cooke ID, Barratt CLA. Double-blind randomized placebo cross-over controlled trial using the antioxidant vitamin E to treat reactive oxygen species associated male infertility. Fertility and Sterility. 1995;**64**:825-831

[132] Suleiman SA, Ali ME, Zaki ZM, El-Malik EM, Nasr MA. Lipid peroxidation and human sperm motility: Protective role of vitamin E. Journal of Andrology. 1996;**17**:530-537

[133] Ciftci H, Verit A, Savas M, Yeni E, Erel O. Effects of N-acetylcysteine on semen parameters and oxidative/antioxidant status. Urology. 2009;**74**:73-76. DOI: 10.1016/j.urology.2009.02.034

[134] Safarinejad MR, Safarinejad S. Efficacy of selenium and/or N-acetyl-cysteine for improving semen parameters in infertile men: A double-blind, placebo controlled, randomized study. Journal of Urology. 2009;**181**:741-751. DOI: 10.1016/j.juro.2008.10.015

[135] Ahmed SD, Karira KA, Jagdesh AS. Role of L-carnitine in male infertility. Journal of the Pakistan Medical Association. 2011;**61**:732-736

[136] Aliabadi E, Mehranjani MS, Borzoei Z, Talaei-Khozani T, Mirkhani H, Tabesh H. Effects of L-carnitine and L-acetyl-carnitine on testicular sperm motility and chromatin quality. Iranian Journal of Reproductive Medicine. 2012;**10**:77-82

[137] Holmes RP, Goodman HO, Shihabi ZK, Jarow JP. The taurine and hypotaurine content of human semen. Journal of Andrology. 1992;**13**:289-292

[138] Bidri M, Choay P. Taurine: A particular aminoacid with multiple functions. Annales Pharmaceutiques Francaises. 2003;**61**:385-391

[139] Zhao J, Dong X, Hu X, Long Z, Wang L, Liu Q, Sun B, Wang Q, Wu Q, Lia L. Zinc levels in seminal plasma and their correlation with male infertility: A systematic review and meta-analysis. Scientific Reports. 2016;**6**:22386. DOI: 10.1038/srep22386

[140] Santiago Y, Chan E, Liu PQ, Orlando S, Zhang L, Urnov FD, Holmes MC, Guschin D, Waite A, Miller JC, Rebar EJ, Gregory PD, Klug A, Collingwood TN. Targeted gene knockout in mammalian cells by using engineered zinc-finger nucleases. Proceedings of the National Academy of Sciences of USA. 2008;**105**:5809-5814. DOI: 10.1073/pnas.0800940105

[141] Powell SR. The antioxidant properties of zinc. Journal of Nutrition. 2000;**130**:1447S-1454S

[142] Boitani C, Puglisi R. Selenium, a key element in spermatogenesis and male fertility. Advances in Experimental Medicine and Biology. 2008;**636**:65-73. DOI: 10.1007/978-0-387-09597-4_4

[143] Bourdon E, Blache D. The importance of proteins in defense against oxidation. Antioxidants & Redox Signaling. 2001;**3**:293-311

[144] Elzanaty S, Erenpreiss J, Becker C. Seminal plasma albumin: Origin and relation to the male reproductive parameters. Andrologia. 2007;**39**:60-65

[145] Uysal O, Bucak MN. Effects of oxidized glutathione, bovine serum albumin, cysteine and lycopene on the quality of frozen-thawed ram semen. Acta Veterinaria Brunensis. 2007;**76**:383-390. DOI: 10.2754/avb200776030383

[146] Sedlak TW, Snyder SH. Bilirubin benefits: Cellular protection by a biliverdin reductase antioxidant cycle. Pediatrics. 2004;**113**:1776-1782

[147] Neuzil J, Stocker R. Free and albumin-bound bilirubin are efficient co-antioxidants for alpha-tocopherol, inhibiting plasma and low density lipoprotein lipid peroxidation. Journal of Biological Chemistry. 1994;**269**:16712-16719

[148] Sautin YY, Johnson RJ. Uric acid: The oxidant-antioxidant paradox. Nucleosides, Nucleotides & Nucleic Acids. 2008;**6**:608-619. DOI: 10.1080/15257770802138558

[149] Muraoka S, Miura T. Inhibition by uric acid of free radicals that damage biological molecules. Pharmacology & Toxicology. 2003;**93**:284-289

[150] de la Lastra CA, Villegas I. Resveratrol as an antioxidant and pro-oxidant agent: Mechanisms and clinical implications. Biochemical Society Transactions. 2007;**35**:1156-1160

[151] Baur JA, Sinclair DA. Therapeutic potential of resveratrol: The in vivo evidence. Nature Reviews Drug Discovery. 2010;**6**:493-506

[152] Shin S, Jeon JH, Park D, Jang MJ, Choi JH, Choi BH, Joo SS, Nahm SS, Kim JC, Kim YB. Trans-resveratrol relaxes the corpus cavernosum ex vivo and enhances testosterone levels and sperm quality in vivo. Archives of Pharmacal Research. 2008;**31**:83-87

[153] Tvrdá E, Kováčik A, Tušimová E, Massányi P, Lukáč N. Resveratrol offers protection to oxidative stress induced by ferrous ascorbate in bovine spermatozoa. Journal of Environmental Science and Health Part A. 2015;**50**:1440-1451. DOI: 10.1080/10934529.2015.1071153

[154] Agarwal S, Rao AV. Tomato lycopene and its role in human health and chronic diseases. Canadian Medical Association Journal. 2000;**163**:739-744

[155] Filipcikova R, Oborna I, Brezinova J, Novotny J, Wojewodka G, De Sanctis JB, Radova L, Hajduch M, Radzioch D. Lycopene improves the distorted ratio between AA/DHA in the seminal plasma of infertile males and increases the likelihood of successful pregnancy. Biomedical Papers of the Medical Faculty of the University Palacký, Olomouc, Czech Republic. 2013;**157**:1-6. DOI: 10.5507/bp.2013.007

[156] Gupta NP, Kumar R. Lycopene therapy in idiopathic male infertility – A preliminary report. International Urology and Nephrology. 2002;**34**:369-372

[157] Zini A, San Gabriel M, Libman J. Lycopene supplementation in vitro can protect human sperm deoxyribonucleic acid from oxidative damage. Fertility and Sterility. 2010;**94**:1033-1036. DOI: 10.1016/j.fertnstert.2009.04.004

[158] Tvrdá E, Kováčik A, Tušimová E, Paál D, Mackovich A, Alimov J, Lukáč N. Antioxidant efficiency of lycopene on oxidative stress-induced damage in bovine spermatozoa. Journal of Animal Science and Biotechnology. 2016;**7**:50. DOI: 10.1186/s40104-016-0113-9

[159] Akmal M, Qadri JQ, Al-Waili NS, Thangal S, Haq A, Saloom KY. Improvement in human semen quality after oral supplementation of vitamin C. Journal of Medicinal Food. 2006;**9**:440-442

[160] Cyrus A, Kabir A, Goodarzi D, Moghimi M. The effect of adjuvant vitamin C after varicocele surgery on sperm quality and quantity in infertile men: A double blind placebo controlled clinical trial. International Brazilian Journal of Urology. 2015;**41**:230-238. DOI: 10.1590/S1677-5538.IBJU.2015.02.07

[161] Suleiman SA, Ali ME, Zaki ZM, El-Malik EM, Nasr MA. Lipid peroxidation and human sperm motility: Protective role of vitamin E. Journal of Andrology. 1996;**17**:530-537

[162] Rolf C, Cooper TG, Yeung CH, Nieschlag E. Antioxidant treatment of patients with asthenozoospermia or moderate oligoasthenozoospermia with high-dose vitamin C and vitamin E: A randomized, placebo-controlled, double-blind study. Human Reproduction. 1999;**14**:1028-1033

[163] Greco E, Iacobelli M, Rienzi L, Ubaldi F, Ferrero S, Tesarik J. Reduction of the incidence of sperm DNA fragmentation by oral antioxidant treatment. Journal of Andrology. 2005;**26**:349-353

[164] Paradiso Galatioto G, Gravina GL, Angelozzi G, Sacchetti A, Innominato PF, Pace G, Ranieri G, Vicentini C. May antioxidant therapy improve sperm parameters of men with persistent oligospermia after retrograde embolization for varicocele? World Journal of Urology. 2008;**26**:97-102

[165] Lenzi A, Culasso F, Gandini L, Lombardo F, Dondero F. Placebo-controlled, double-blind, cross-over trial of glutathione therapy in male infertility. Human Reproduction. 1993;**8**: 1657-1662

[166] Costa M, Canale D, Filicori M, D'lddio S, Lenzi A. L-carnitine in idiopathic asthenozoospermia: A multicenter study. Italian study group on Carnitine and male infertility. Andrologia. 1994;**26**:155-159

[167] Lenzi A, Lombardo F, Sgrò P, Salacone P, Caponecchia L, Dondero F, Gandini L. Use of carnitine therapy in selected cases of male factor infertility: A double-blind crossover trial. Fertility and Sterility. 2003;**79**:292-300

[168] Lenzi A, Sgrò P, Salacone P, Paoli D, Gilio B, Lombardo F, Santulli M, Agarwal A, Gandini L. A placebo-controlled double-blind randomized trial of the use of combined l-carnitine and l-acetyl-carnitine treatment in men with asthenozoospermia. Fertility and Sterility. 2004;**81**:1578-1584

[169] Sigman M, Glass S, Campagnone J, Pryor JL. Carnitine for the treatment of idiopathic asthenospermia: A randomized, double-blind, placebo-controlled trial. Fertility and Sterility. 2006;**85**:1409-1414

[170] Iwanier K, Zachara BA. Selenium supplementation enhances the element concentration in blood and seminal fluid but does not change the spermatozoal quality characteristics in subfertile men. Journal of Andrology. 1995;**16**:441-447

[171] Vézina D, Mauffette F, Roberts KD, Bleau G, Selenium-vitamin E. Supplementation in infertile men. Effects on semen parameters and micronutrient levels and distribution. Biological Trace Element Research. 1996;**53**:65-83

[172] Scott R, MacPherson A, Yates RW, Hussain B, Dixon J. The effect of oral selenium supplementation on human sperm motility. British Journal of Urology. 1998;**82**:76-80

[173] Keskes-Ammar L, Feki-Chakroun N, Rebai T, Sahnoun Z, Ghozzi H, Hammami S, Zghal K, Fki H, Damak J, Bahloul A. Sperm oxidative stress and the effect of an oral vitamin E and selenium supplement on semen quality in infertile men. Archives of Andrology. 2003;**49**:83-94

[174] Comhaire FH, Christophe AB, Zalata AA, Dhooge WS, Mahmoud AM, Depuydt CE. The effects of combined conventional treatment, oral antioxidants and essential fatty acids on sperm biology in subfertile men. Prostaglandins, Leukotrienes & Essential Fatty Acids. 2000;**63**:159-165

[175] Ciftci H, Verit A, Savas M, Yeni E, Erel O. Effects of N-acetylcysteine on semen parameters and oxidative/antioxidant status. Urology. 2009;**74**:73-76. DOI: 10.1016/j.urology.2009.02.034

[176] Omu AE, Al-Azemi MK, Kehinde EO, Anim JT, Oriowo MA, Mathew TC. Indications of the mechanisms involved in improved sperm parameters by zinc therapy. Medical Principles and Practice. 2008;**17**:108-116. DOI: 10.1159/000112963

[177] Lewin A, Lavon H. The effect of coenzyme Q10 on sperm motility and function. Molecular Aspects of Medicine. 1997;**18**:S213-S219

[178] Balercia G, Buldreghini E, Vignini A, Tiano L, Paggi F, Amoroso S, Ricciardo-Lamonica G, Boscaro M, Lenzi A, Littarru G. Coenzyme Q10 treatment in infertile men with idiopathic asthenozoospermia: A placebo-controlled, double-blind randomized trial. Fertility and Sterility. 2009;**91**:1785-1792. DOI: 10.1016/j.fertnstert.2008.02.119

[179] Agarwal A, Said TM, Bedaiwy MA, Banerjee J, Alvarez JG. Oxidative stress in an assisted reproductive techniques setting. Fertility and Sterility. 2006;**86**:503-512

[180] Sikka SC. Role of oxidative stress and antioxidants in andrology and assisted reproductive technology. Journal of Andrology. 2004;**25**:5-18

[181] Kobayashi H, Gil-Guzman E, Mahran AM. Quality control of reactive oxygen species measurement by luminol-dependent chemiluminescence assay. Journal of Andrology. 2001;**22**:568-574

[182] Aitken RJ, De Iuliis GN, Baker MA. Direct methods for the detection of reactive oxygen species in human semen samples. In: Agarwal A, Aitken RJ, Alvarez JG, editors. Studies on Men's Health and Fertility, Oxidative Stress in Applied Basic Research and Clinical

Practice. 1st ed. New York: Springer Science+Business Media, LLC; 2012. p. 275-299. DOI: 10.1007/978-1-61779-776-7_14

[183] Rothe G, Valet G. Flow cytometric analysis of respiratory burst activity in phagocytes with hydroethidine and 2′, 7′-dichlorofluorescein. Journal of Leukocyte Biology. 1990;**47**: 440-448

[184] De Iuliis GN, Wingate JK, Koppers AJ, McLaughlin EA, Aitken RJ. Definitive evidence for the nonmitochondrial production of superoxide anion by human spermatozoa. Journal of Clinical Endocrinology and Metabolism. 2006;**91**:1968-1975

[185] Myhre O, Andersen JM, Aarnes H, Fonnum F. Evaluation of the probes 2′,7′-dichlorofluorescein diacetate, luminol, and lucigenin as indicators of reactive species formation. Biochemical Pharmacology. 2003;**65**:1575-1582

[186] Mancini A, Milardi D, Bianchi A. Increased total antioxidant capacity in seminal plasma of varicocele patients: A multivariate analysis. Archives of Andrology. 2007;**53**:37-42

[187] Stadtman ER, Oliver CN. Metal-catalyzed oxidation of proteins. Physiological consequences. Journal of Biological Chemistry. 1991;**266**:2005-2008

[188] Jiang ZY, Hunt JV, Wolf SP. Detection of lipid hydroperoxides using fox method. Analytical Biochemistry. 1992;**202**:384-389

[189] Takagi Y, Nikaido T, Toki T, Kita N, Kanai M, Ashida T, Ohira S, Konishi I. Levels of oxidative stress and redox-related molecules in the placenta in preeclampsia and fetal growth restriction. Virchows Archiv. 2004;**444**:49-55

Permissions

All chapters in this book were first published in SFP, by InTech Open; hereby published with permission under the Creative Commons Attribution License or equivalent. Every chapter published in this book has been scrutinized by our experts. Their significance has been extensively debated. The topics covered herein carry significant findings which will fuel the growth of the discipline. They may even be implemented as practical applications or may be referred to as a beginning point for another development.

The contributors of this book come from diverse backgrounds, making this book a truly international effort. This book will bring forth new frontiers with its revolutionizing research information and detailed analysis of the nascent developments around the world.

We would like to thank all the contributing authors for lending their expertise to make the book truly unique. They have played a crucial role in the development of this book. Without their invaluable contributions this book wouldn't have been possible. They have made vital efforts to compile up to date information on the varied aspects of this subject to make this book a valuable addition to the collection of many professionals and students.

This book was conceptualized with the vision of imparting up-to-date information and advanced data in this field. To ensure the same, a matchless editorial board was set up. Every individual on the board went through rigorous rounds of assessment to prove their worth. After which they invested a large part of their time researching and compiling the most relevant data for our readers.

The editorial board has been involved in producing this book since its inception. They have spent rigorous hours researching and exploring the diverse topics which have resulted in the successful publishing of this book. They have passed on their knowledge of decades through this book. To expedite this challenging task, the publisher supported the team at every step. A small team of assistant editors was also appointed to further simplify the editing procedure and attain best results for the readers.

Apart from the editorial board, the designing team has also invested a significant amount of their time in understanding the subject and creating the most relevant covers. They scrutinized every image to scout for the most suitable representation of the subject and create an appropriate cover for the book.

The publishing team has been an ardent support to the editorial, designing and production team. Their endless efforts to recruit the best for this project, has resulted in the accomplishment of this book. They are a veteran in the field of academics and their pool of knowledge is as vast as their experience in printing. Their expertise and guidance has proved useful at every step. Their uncompromising quality standards have made this book an exceptional effort. Their encouragement from time to time has been an inspiration for everyone.

The publisher and the editorial board hope that this book will prove to be a valuable piece of knowledge for researchers, students, practitioners and scholars across the globe.

List of Contributors

Kristina Lasiene
Department of Histology and Embryology, Academy of Medicine, Lithuanian University of Health Sciences, Kaunas, Lithuania

Lozano Hernández Jesús Ricardo
Cátedra de Fisiopatología, Facultad de Farmacia y Bioanálisis, Universidad de Los Andes, Mérida, Venezuela

Qiuqin Tang
State Key Laboratory of Reproductive Medicine, Department of Obstetrics, Nanjing

Maternity and Child Health Care Hospital Affiliated to Nanjing Medical University, Nanjing, China

Wei Wu, Jing Zhang and Rong Fan
State Key Laboratory of Reproductive Medicine, Institute of Toxicology, School of Public

Mu Liu
School of Basic Medical Sciences, Nanjing Medical University, Nanjing, China

Rosanna Chianese
Department of Experimental Medicine sec. "F. Bottazzi", University of Campania "L. Vanvitelli", Italy

Rosaria Meccariello
Department of Movement Sciences and Wellbeing, University of Naples "Parthenope", Naples, Italy

Qiuqin Tang, and Mu Liu
State Key Laboratory of Reproductive Medicine, Department of Obstetrics, Nanjing
Maternity and Child Health Care Hospital Affiliated to Nanjing Medical University, Nanjing, China

Wei Wu, Jing Zhang and Rong Fan
State Key Laboratory of Reproductive Medicine, Institute of Toxicology, School of Public Health, Nanjing Medical University, Nanjing, China

Mu Liu
School of Basic Medical Sciences, Nanjing Medical University, Nanjing, China

Rosanna Chianese
Department of Experimental Medicine sec. "F. Bottazzi", University of Campania "L. Vanvitelli", Italy

Rosaria Meccariello
Department of Movement Sciences and Wellbeing, University of Naples "Parthenope", Naples, Italy

Yona Barak
Dr Yona Barak Laboratories Ltd., Rosh Ha'Ayin, Israel

Adrian Ellenbogen
Rappaport School of Medicine, Technion-Israel Institute of Technology, Haifa, Israel
IVF Unit, Hillel Yaffe Medical Center, Hadera, Israel
Meuheded Female Health Center, Bnai-Brack, Israel

Mari Carmen Uribe and Sergio Gracia-Fernández
Department of Compared Biology, Sciences Faculty, Laboratory of Biology of Reproduction, Universidad Nacional Autónoma de México, Mexico City, Mexico

Annalisa De Angelis and Anna Chiara De Luca
Institute of Protein Biochemistry - National Research Council, Naples, Italy

Maria Antonietta Ferrara and Giuseppe Coppola
Institute for Microelectronics and Microsystems - National Research Council, Naples, Italy

DMAB Dissanayake
Department of Obstetrics and Gynaecology, Faculty of Medicine Ragama, University of Kelaniya, Sri Lanka

Elizaveta E. Bragina
Department of Electron Microscopy, AN Belozersky Institute of Physico-Chemical
Biology, MV Lomonosov Moscow State University, Moscow, Russia

Elena N. Bocharova
Moscow Scientific and Practical Center of Dermatology, Moscow, Russia

Luigi Montano
Andrology Unit of the "San Francesco d'Assisi" Hospital, ASL Salerno, Oliveto Citra, Salerno, Italy

Paolo Bergamo
National Research Council (CNR), Institute of Food Sciences, Avellino, Italy

Maria Grazia Andreassi
National Research Council (CNR), Institute of Clinical Physiology, Pisa, Italy

Stefan Lorenzetti
Department of Food Safety, Nutrition and Veterinary Public Health, Istituto Superiore di Sanità (ISS), Rome, Italy

Eva Tvrdá, Peter Massanyi and Norbert Lukáč
Department of Animal Physiology, Faculty of Biotechnology and Food Sciences, Slovak University of Agriculture in Nitra, Slovakia

Index